NEUROSURGICAL SYNDROMES OF THE BRAIN

Neurosurgical Syndromes of the Brain

By

CHARLES W. NEEDHAM, M.D.

Assistant Professor of Neurosurgery
UCLA School of Medicine and
Harbor General Hospital
Los Angeles, California

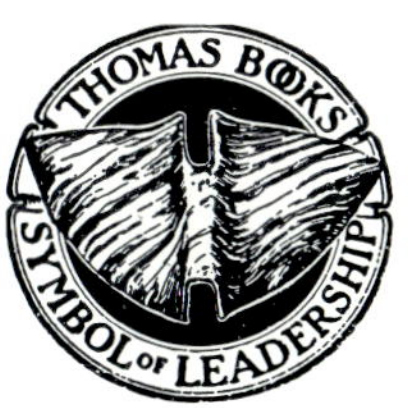

CHARLES C THOMAS · PUBLISHER
Springfield · Illinois · U.S.A.

Published and Distributed Throughout the World by

CHARLES C THOMAS • PUBLISHER
BANNERSTONE HOUSE
301-327 East Lawrence Avenue, Springfield, Illinois, U.S.A.

ISBN 0-398-02369-7

Library of Congress Catalog Card Number: 76-187668

With THOMAS BOOKS *careful attention is given to all details of manufacturing and design. It is the Publisher's desire to present books that are satisfactory as to their physical qualities and artistic possibilities and appropriate for their particular use.* THOMAS BOOKS *will be true to those laws of quality that assure a good name and good will.*

Printed in the United States of America
N-1

This book is dedicated to my dear wife Connie, my son Andrew, and my daughters Susan, Jennifer and Sarah.

". . . upon the principles of cerebral localization is founded that which may be called 'regional diagnosis' of encephalic diseases, that ideal toward the realization of which . . . should be directed all the efforts of clinical teaching."

J.M. Charcot
Lectures on Localization in Diseases of the Brain
(Delivered at the Faculté de Médecine, Paris, 1875)

ACKNOWLEDGMENTS

I WISH TO EXPRESS my deep appreciation to those men responsible for my neurosurgical training. I would like to thank Theodore Rasmussen, the Director of the Montreal Neurological Institute. I owe a great debt to my Chiefs of Service, Gilles Bertrand and Joseph Stratford. I also received instruction from William Feindel, Phanor Perot, Henry Garretson, Charles Branch and Robert Ford. I want to especially thank my good friend Frank LeBlanc. I have great respect for the wisdom of the senior neurosurgeons Wilder Penfield and Arthur Elvidge and for the senior neurologist Francis McNaughton. I owe my understanding of neuroradiology to Donald McRae and Roméo Ethier.

I would like to thank my secretaries, Mrs. Nancy Sanders and Mrs. Sheryl Turner, for their many hours devoted to the typing of this manuscript. I appreciate the photographic assistance of Mr. Tom Lotto. The drawings are my own.

I acknowledge my debt to the literature. The mass of the printed word has become enormous. I have attempted to be concise in the presentation of this method of diagnosis. I have tried to be selective in the inclusion of references.

It has been my great privilege to be able to care for patients afflicted with surgical lesions of the nervous system. Much is learned at the bedside.

CHARLES WILLIAM NEEDHAM

CONTENTS

NEUROSURGICAL SYNDROMES OF THE BRAIN

CHAPTER 1

INTRODUCTION

THE SUCCESSFUL SURGICAL TREATMENT of neurological disease depends upon early diagnosis and precise localization of pathology. The neurosurgeon has become increasingly dependent upon the methods of neuroradiology. As Leeds and Taveras (1969) note, "carotid angiography in the diagnosis of intracranial space occupying lesions. . .has become the most important neuroradiologic procedure." It demands emphasis, however, that the neurological surgeon is first and foremost a neurologist with special skills. Clinical neurological diagnosis remains primary, and early accurate localization is the first objective of the surgical neurologist.

High degrees of integration often allow the normal, undisturbed functions of the brain to escape the confines of localization. The "experiments of disease" however, constitute disintegration, with segregation of localizable symptom-sign clusters of disturbed function. These are the syndromes. Localization of a lesion is very different from localization of function. The primary neurosurgical concern is the pragmatic value of clinical signs in arriving at early and accurate diagnosis. The neurosurgical syndromes are made even more characteristic by their separate angiographic and pneumographic deformities. In terms of the temporal development of symptoms, the spatial distribution of signs, and the characteristics of the contrast study, each neurosurgical syndrome may be defined by its individual "development-deficit-deformity."

Flavor is added to the syndromes by the fact that the presenting signs may include the following:

1. Focal or localizing signs.
2. Nonlocalizing signs.
3. Satellite signs.
4. False-localizing signs.
5. Combined signs.
6. Sign-silence.

Thus a patient with an aneurysm may describe premonitory headache but present no neurological deficit ("sign-silence"). Alternatively, focal oculomotor paralysis may result from pressure of the aneurysm sac upon the third cranial nerve ("localizing sign"). Rupture of the aneurysm with subarachnoid bleeding leads to stiff neck and retinal hemorrhage ("nonlocalizing signs"). Blood clot in the vicinity of the leaking aneurysm may lead to paralyses of neighboring cranial nerves ("satellite signs"). The intracranial hemorrhage may produce arterial spasm with distal infarction, intracerebral hematoma with transtentorial herniation, or impaired cerebrospinal fluid (CSF) circulation with hydrocephalus. Any such result may cause focal signs at a distance from the primary lesion ("false-localizing signs").

Adding still further interest is the irritative or destructive effect of a given lesion, resulting in

1. Positive-released signs.
2. Positive ictal signs.
3. Negative-paretic signs.
4. Negative-postictal signs.

Spasticity occurs as a positive sign of release from a normally inhibiting control. Positive neurologic discharge also occurs during the aura and ictus of epileptic seizures, which may be of sharp localizing value. Paralysis in its broadest sense is the negative neurologic disturbance. It may occur in isolation or as a postictal event (Todd's paralysis). It is difficult to place a positive or negative label upon disturbances of the mental sphere occurring with focal pathology. However, modern methods of neuropsychology have demonstrated high degrees of localizing significance in certain disturbances of the "higher cortical functions."

Positive or negative, focal or nonfocal, satellite or falsely localizing signs may occur with or without elevated CSF pressure. Clinical hydrocephalus similarly may occur with or without increased pressure. Elevated intracranial pressure may be associated with "sign-silence," or may accentuate, compound or mask signs already present. The array of signs may similarly be clouded by impairment of sensorium from stupor to deeply comatose states.

Localization in neurological surgery requires syndrome analysis. The need for early diagnosis demands rapid recognition of the neurosurgical syndromes from the hundreds of neurological and neuromedical disorders. Thus both uremia and brain tumor may produce headache, vomiting, papilledema, seizures and paralysis. Cerebrovascular thrombosis with infarction may be closely simulated by tumor, hematoma or abscess. Brain abscess without fever or cellular response can occur. Intracerebral or chronic subdural hematomas may present as clear spinal fluid stroke syndromes. Brain neoplasm may initially reveal its presence by infarction or hemorrhage. Prompt neurosurgical consultation should be considered whenever regional diagnosis is possible. The clinical suspicion of elevated intracranial pressure, even in the absence of focal signs, requires urgent neurosurgical attention.

Fully half of all intracranial tumors in the adult involve the massive frontal lobes of the brain. The frontal lobes are frequent points of impact in automotive trauma. The frontal region is a common site of brain abscess. Epileptic seizures are a frequent manifestation of the frontal mass lesion. Yet the rostral majority of the frontal lobe is relatively "silent" clinically. The symptoms and signs of intracranial hypertension are often long delayed when the responsible mass is frontal in location. In the interest of early diagnosis of surgically treatable frontal lesions, heavy emphasis is placed upon frontal signs and frontal satellite regions. Chapter 2 deals with the "frontobasal syndromes" and includes lesions involving the orbital cortex, olfactory tracts, optic nerves, the bony floor of the anterior fossa, the fronto-ethmoidal and anterior sphenoidal sinuses, the cranio-orbital junction and the orbit. Chapter 3 is concerned with the "frontopolar syndromes," including the prefrontal lobes anterior to the coronal suture, the frontal sinus, the anterior third of the sagittal sinus and falx. Chapter 4 considers the "frontodorsal syndromes" and neurosurgical lesions involving the oculomotor, premotor, supplementary and rolandic motor regions, the central third of the sagittal sinus and falx, and the cranial vertex. Chapter 5 is an analysis of the "frontolateral syndromes" and the importance of Broca's area, the frontal operculum, the precentral face region and lesions adjacent to the pterion of the skull.

The mass lesion with which the neurosurgeon has to deal often does not respect the anatomist's division of the cerebrum into lobes. Certain tumors are frontoparietal or frontotemporal. Nonetheless, there is a definite clinical and surgical usefulness in the lobar concept as it has been traditionally employed. Chapter 6 deals with the "parietal syndromes" and lesions involving the postcentral sensory region, superior parietal lobule and supramarginal gyrus. The caudal portion of the central third of the sagittal sinus is considered in conjunction with the parietal lobe. Anatomical divisions between the parietal, posterior temporal and occipital lobe are largely artificial. Chapter 7, concerning the "caudal cerebral syndromes," is designed to reveal the signs of lesions which involve this confluent posterior parieto-temporo-occipital region. Focal lesions involving Wernicke's area, the angular gyrus and the occipital pole are discussed. Craniodural regional landmarks include the posterior third of the sagittal sinus and falx, straight sinus, transverse sinus, tentorial base and caudal cranial vault. Chapter 8 is concerned with the "temporal syndromes" and considers the temporal pole, uncus and amygdala, temporal lobe and hippocampus, middle fossa and tentorial edge. Neurosurgical syndromes involving the optic radiation are examined in both Chapters 7 and 8.

The "central cerebral syndromes" constitute the subject matter of Chapter 9 and include striatal, capsular and thalamic signs. Neurosurgical mass lesions typically involve these deep structures in combination: the "thalamic tumor" is rarely confined to the thalamus. The deep "capsular" intracerebral hematoma invariably extends beyond the internal capsule. Chapter 10 is a discussion of the "perichiasmatic syndromes" and includes lesions compressing the basal optic pathway and hypothalamus. Pituitary tumors, suprasellar and parasellar tumors and aneurysms are presented. Chapter 11, on the "posterior fossa syndromes" consists of an analysis of neurosurgical lesions involving the cerebellum, brain stem, cerebellopontine angle, cranial nerves, clivus and foramen magnum. Chapter 12 deals with the "syndromes of intracranial hypertension" and considers the clinical details of the symptoms and signs of elevated intracranial pressure. The varieties of hydrocephalus, cerebral edema and intracranial hemorrhage which transcend a strictly regional analysis are included in this final chapter.

The text is a system of regional diagnosis of the cephalic syndromes amenable to modern neurosurgical therapy. Each syndrome is analyzed in outline form to facilitate rapid recognition. The essential neuroanatomy is included, along with blood supply and infarction syndromes. Regional structure and satellite syndromes are emphasized. Relevant neurophysiology is presented in capsule form. Characteristic features in development, varieties of neurological deficit, and deformities in angiography and pneumography are itemized. Significant plain x-ray findings are included. Ancillary procedures are noted only if they make highly characteristic diagnostic contributions.

The development of syndromes varies from an onset which is most sudden to that which is most insidious. The "brain tumor suspect" usually has had progressively worsening symptoms or signs during several weeks or months preceding neurosurgical evaluation. More acute presentations are associated with intraneoplastic hemorrhage or acute ventricular obstruction. More chronic presentations may result from the slowly growing meningiomas. Brain tumor syndromes can be closely simulated by the brain abscess and chronic subdural hematoma. The traumatic and vascular syndromes account for many cases of sudden development. The time scale and sequence of events are as important to accurate diagnosis as the type and distribution of neurological deficits. Each syndrome presents a temporospatial array of symptoms and signs. In subsequent chapters, syndrome development is listed according to rapidity of evolution. The order of listing is a flexible one and indicates general trends of development rather than rigid time scales.

The system of regional diagnosis is most valuable when a high degree of clinical and radiological correspondence is detected. The "development-deficit-deformity" technique is used in terms of symptoms, signs and angiographic or pneumographic study of the individual case. A diagram (Fig. 1)

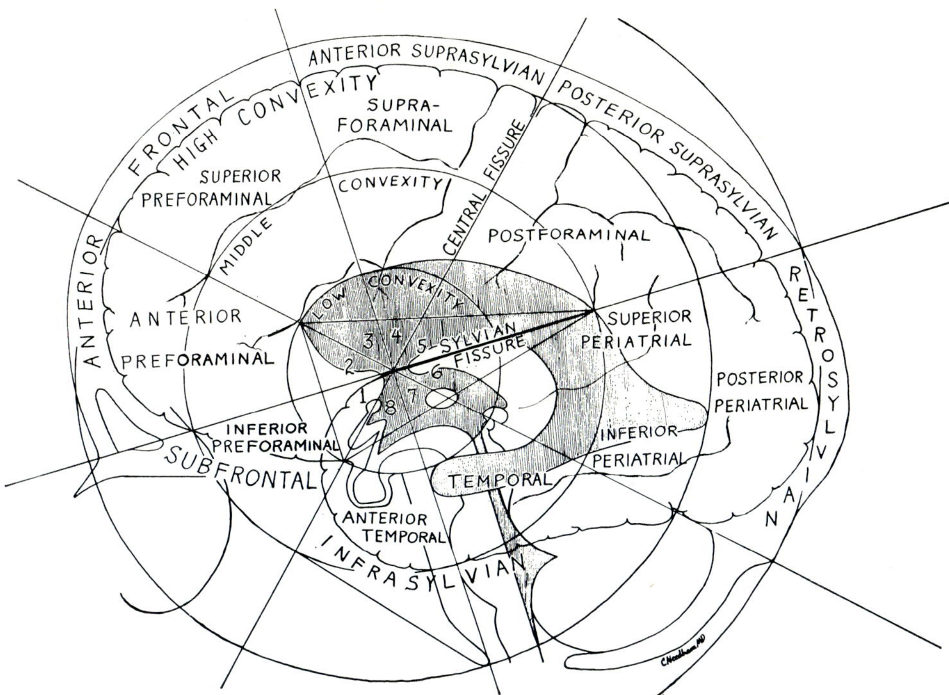

Figure 1. A guide to cerebral correlation. The diagram employs the foramen of Monro as the center of intersecting lines and concentric circles. Note the angiographic and pneumographic identification of sectors (numbers adjacent to the foramen of Monro) and ventricular structure. The convexities, fissures and sylvian triangle are also indicated (see text).

is employed as a conceptual guide in the correlation of neurological signs with contrast study deformities. The diagram is designed to be a practical clinical tool rather than a quantitative measure. Variability in the human brain and in its surgical pathology is an important limiting factor in the use of this diagnostic template. However, as a correlative guide the diagram has practical value for the neurosurgeon. The center of Figure 1 is the foramen of Monro. This interventricular foramen is critical because of a number of factors.

1. It marks the point of union of the anterior horn and body of the lateral ventricle.
2. It is the junction of the lateral and third ventricles.
3. It indicates the anterior pole of the thalamus.
4. It is located at the center of the angiographic "sylvian triangle." This triangle is composed of middle cerebral arteries upon the buried cortex of the insula of Reil (Fig. 2).

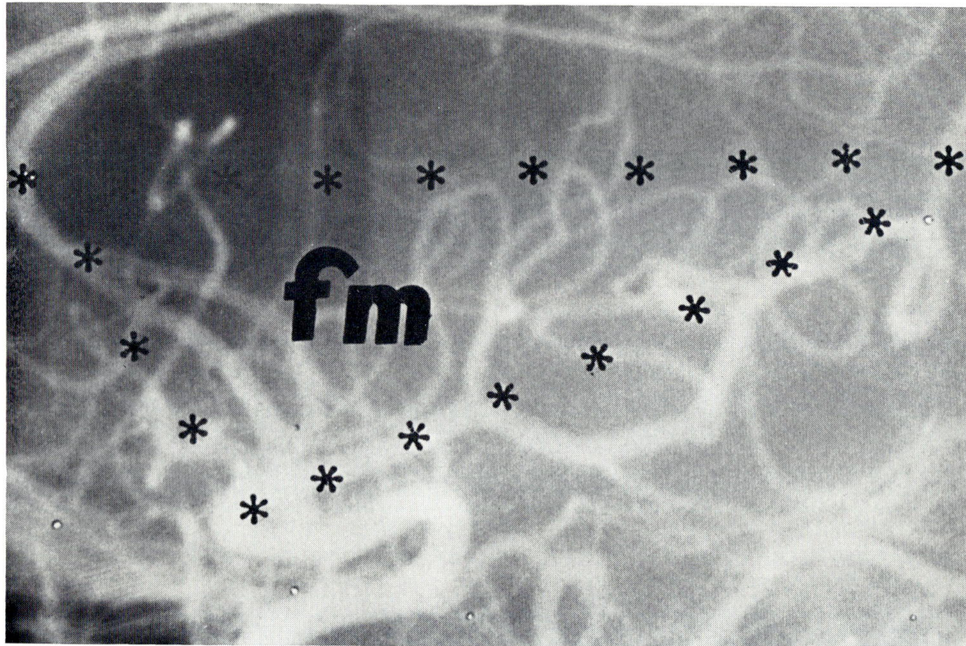

Figure 2. The sylvian triangle and foramen of Monro. A lateral view of a combined air-angiogram indicates the position of the foramen of Monro deep to the center of the angiographic sylvian triangle. Air fills the anterior horns to a point just to the foramen. Middle cerebral arteries on the insula of Reil form the sylvian triangle.

5. It is indicated on the venous phase of the angiogram by the point of union of the thalamostriate vein (floor of the lateral ventricle) with the internal cerebral vein (roof of the third ventricle) to form the "venous angle."

6. Four equidistant lines (premotor, rolandic, sylvian and posterior fossa lines) have been constructed to intersect at the foramen of Monro.

7. Four concentric circles (internal, middle, external and extreme circles) have been constructed with the foramen of Monro as their common center.

The four lines delineate eight sectors (see numbers adjacent to foramen of Monro in Fig. 1) which are designated according to angiographic or pneumographic study:

Angiogram	*Sector*	*Pneumogram*
Subfrontal	1	Inferior preforaminal
Anterior frontal	2,3	Anterior and superior preforaminal
Anterior suprasylvian	4	Supraforaminal
Posterior suprasylvian	5	Postforaminal
Retrosylvian	6	Periatrial
Infrasylvian	7,8	Temporal and anterior temporal

Another diagram indicates that the four intersecting lines have additional value in terms of the ventricular system (Fig. 3). The "premotor line" indicates the plane dividing the anterior horn from the body of the lateral ventricle. The "rolandic line" is projected through the anterior wall of the third ventricle (lamina terminalis). The "sylvian line" marks the plane of division between the body and atrium of the lateral ventricle. The "posterior fossa line" lies on a plane separating the temporal horn from the atrium.

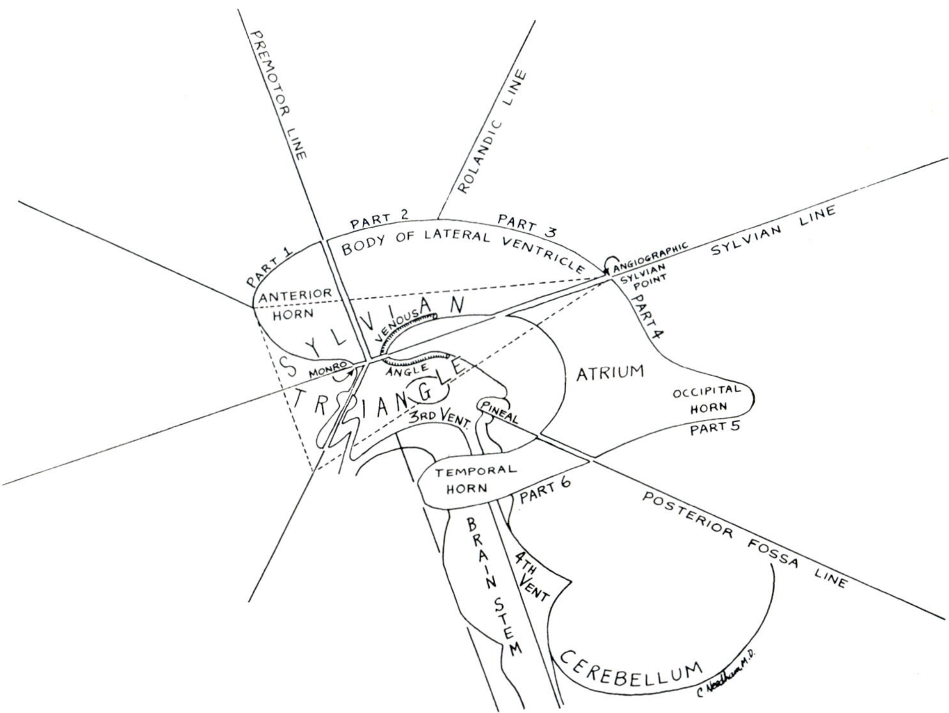

Figure 3. The venous angle and foramen of Monro. The venous angle consists of the thalamostriate vein crossing the floor of the lateral ventricle (between caudate head and thalamus) and the internal cerebral vein in the roof of the third ventricle. The angle is formed at the foramen of Monro. The sylvian triangle is projected upon the foramen and venous angle for air and angiographic arterial and venous phase correlation. The lines (see Fig. 1) defining the cerebral sectors are identified.

The approximate normal position of the foramen of Monro can be estimated from a plain lateral skull x-ray with calcified pineal. Major cerebral landmarks can, in turn, be derived. At the anterior apex of the third ventricle, the foramen of each side converges toward the midline. Since the foramen and ventricles are not visible on plain x-ray, the derivation employs the midline tuberculum sella and calcified pineal. A "tuberculum-pineal line" forms the hypotenuse of a right-angled triangle. Legs of equal length ascend at angles of 45° from tuberculum and pineal to join at an angle of 90° at the foramen of Monro. It should be emphasized again that normal craniocerebral variation, and especially the distortion brought about by tumor, will modify this derivation to varying degree. The construction of an idealized model is nonetheless of value for correlative purposes. The "internal circle" (Fig. 1) can then be delineated, using the foramen of Monro as the center point and the foramen-pineal distance as a radius. A line passing through the foramen of Monro, parallel to the tuberculum-pineal line, indicates the plane of the sylvian fissure. Inspection of Figure 1 reveals how the sylvian triangle, and thereby the insula overlying the basal ganglia, can be placed into perspective. While the thalamus just begins at the level of the foramen of Monro, half of the corpus striatum lies rostral, and half caudal, to the foraminal level. The foramen of Monro is thus a key correlative point whose position can be derived from the plain x-ray, the arteriogram, venogram and pneumogram. The cerebral convexity divisions are apparent in both lateral (Fig. 1) and anteroposterior (AP) views (Fig. 4). Three of these lie above the sylvian fissure:

1. High convexity (and parasagittal).
2. Middle convexity.
3. Low convexity.
4. Temporal convexity.

The correlation of cerebral landmarks in both plain and contrast studies, especially when combined with the use of stereoscopic views, will soon create a three-dimensional mental image of the brain. This is a valuable asset to the neurosurgeon and includes a stereo-portrait of major deep cerebral structures and their relationship to the ventricular system. Study of the cerebral hemisphere (Fig. 5), the cerebral midline (Fig. 6), and normal brain sections (Figs. 7-13) in which only major landmarks are labelled will reinforce this image. The recognition of characteristic landmark distortions produced by the intracranial mass, brain edema, herniation and hydrocephalus is a critical part of diagnostic neurosurgery. The repeated effort to correlate clinical, radiological and other ancillary signs with operative findings in each individual case develops diagnostic acumen. It is hoped that this volume will contribute to that cause.

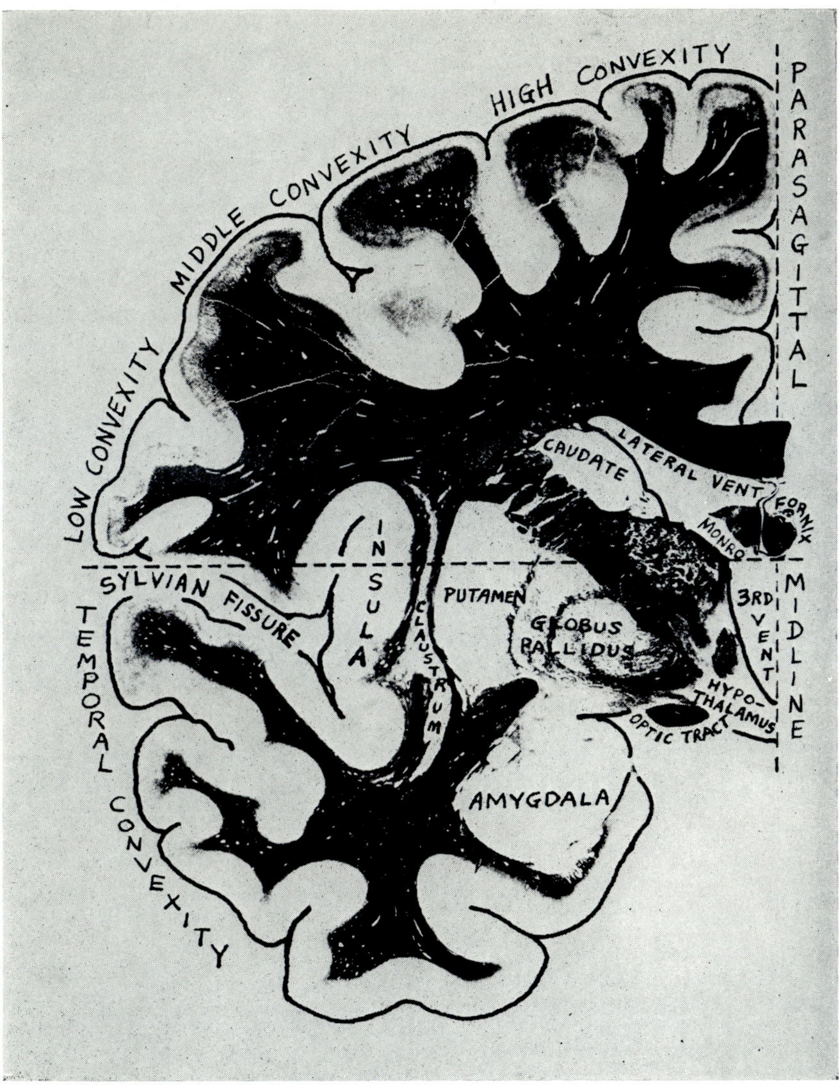

Figure 4. The cerebral convexities in coronal view. The parasagittal – high, middle, low and temporal convexities are indicated. Note the position of the basal ganglia between the insula (i.e. sylvian triangle) and the third ventricle (i.e. venous angle – foramen of Monro). The thalamus begins just behind the coronal level of the foramen of Monro and extends caudally. In contrast, the corpus stratum is bisected by the coronal-foraminal plane shown. The rostral half of the basal ganglia, including the caudate head, lies ahead of the foraminal level, while the caudal half of the lenticular nucleus and the entire thalamus lie behind.

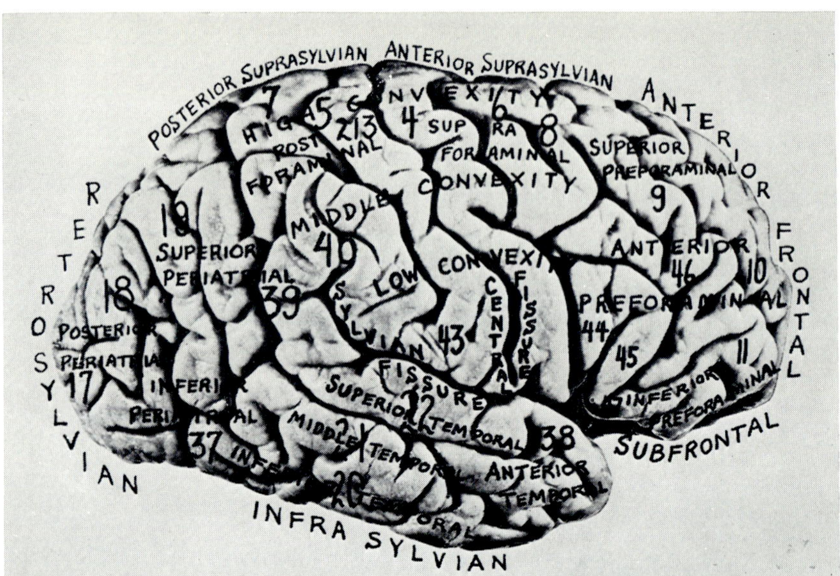

Figure 5. The cerebral hemisphere. A lateral view of the cerebral hemisphere to correlate angiographic and pneumographic regions. The cortical areas are numbered according to Brodmann.

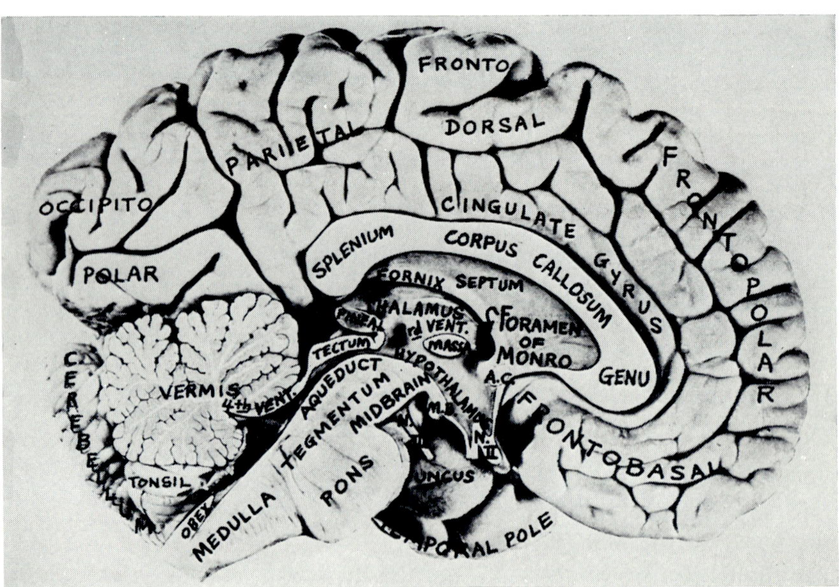

Figure 6. The midline of the brain. This medial view depicts the relation of the cerebral midline to the brain stem and cerebellum. Note the position of the foramen of Monro at the anterior apex of the third ventricle; at this point, the foramen on each side approaches the midline. The position of the thalamus behind the foramen and the hypothalamus below the foramen are indicated. The optic chiasm immediately behind and below the frontobasal region, and the oculomotor nerve medial to the temporal uncus, are important relationships. The septum pellucidum prevents a view of the lateral ventricle, but the third ventricle, aqueduct and fourth ventricle are well seen.

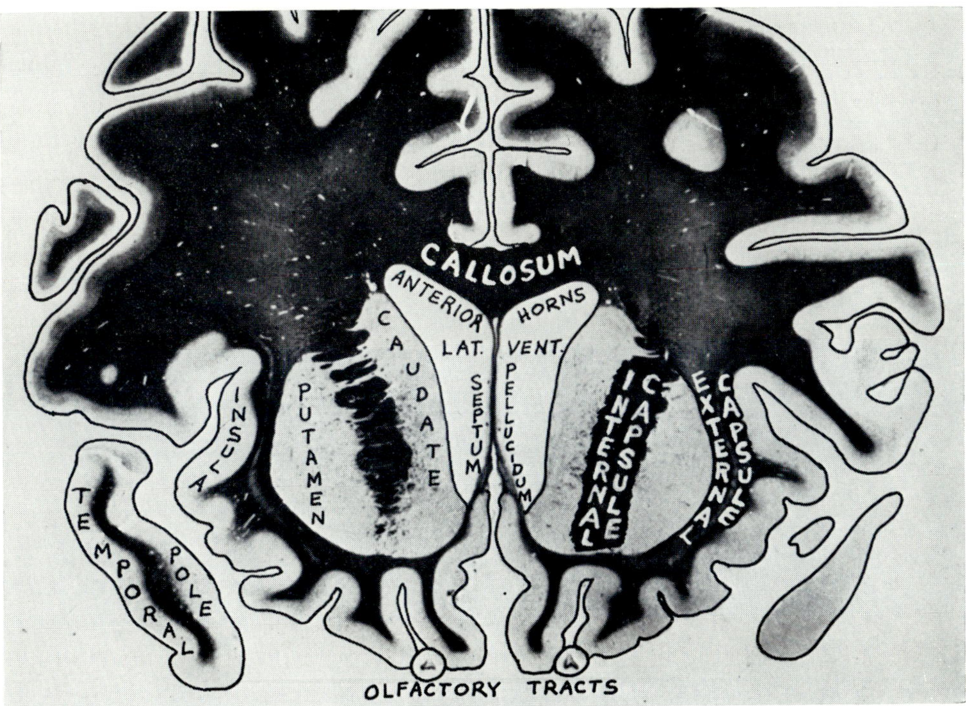

Figure 7. Coronal section of the cerebral hemispheres through the rostral caudate-putamen. This is a first sample coronal section through the rostral basal ganglia. This is the level of the anterior horns and temporal tips. A considerable portion of frontal lobe, the frontal pole (i.e. prefrontal region), lies rostral to this section. The structures shown are telencephalic. The caudate-putamen is a continuous structure pierced by the internal capsule. The caudate heads, corpus callosum and septum constitute the boundaries of the anterior horns. Note the relation of the olfactory tracts to the frontal base.

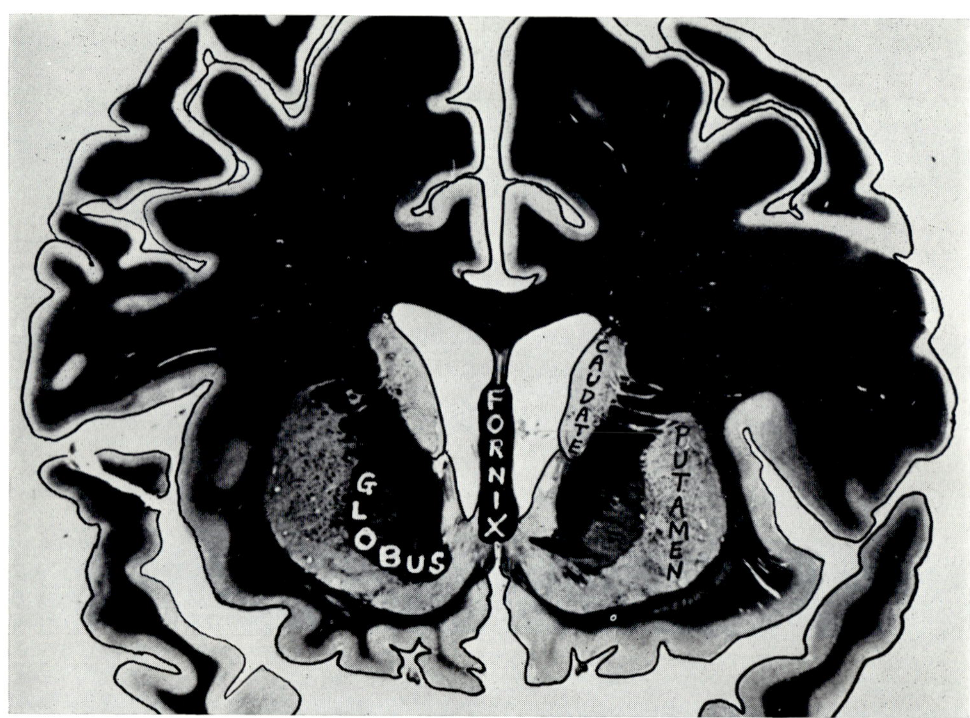

Figure 8. Coronal section of the cerebral hemispheres through the rostral globus pallidus. The globus pallidus appears just medial to the putamen. Both structures constitute the lenticular nucleus. The section lies just rostral to the level of the foramen of Monro.

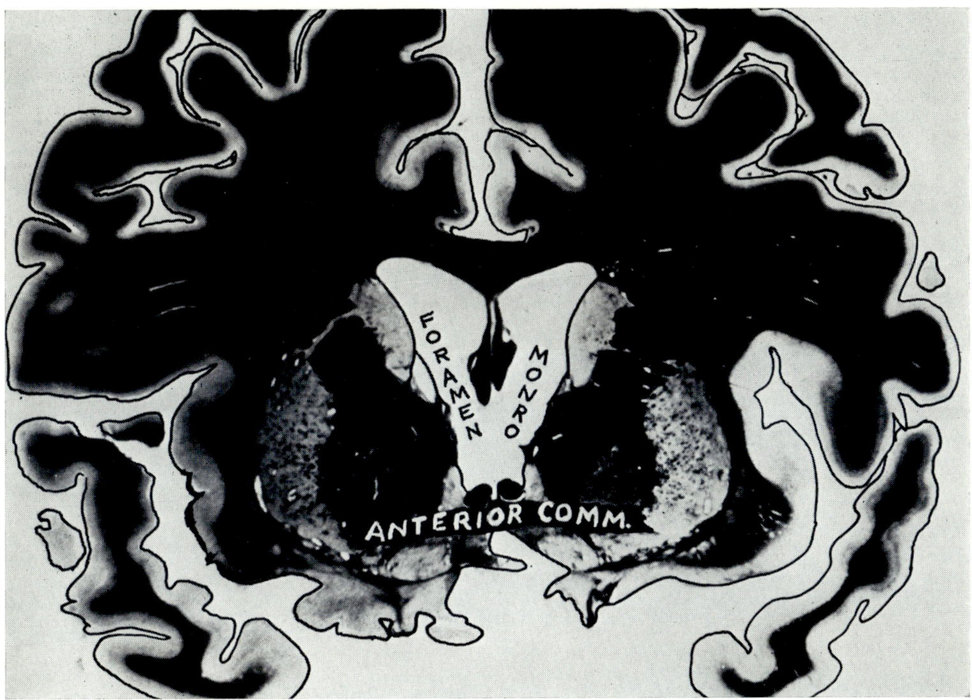

Figure 9. Coronal section of the cerebral hemispheres through the foramen of Monro. The anterior commissure lies closely adjacent to the foramen of Monro. The foramen on each side joins the lateral ventricle to the anterior apex of the third ventricle. The diencephalon begins just caudal to this level.

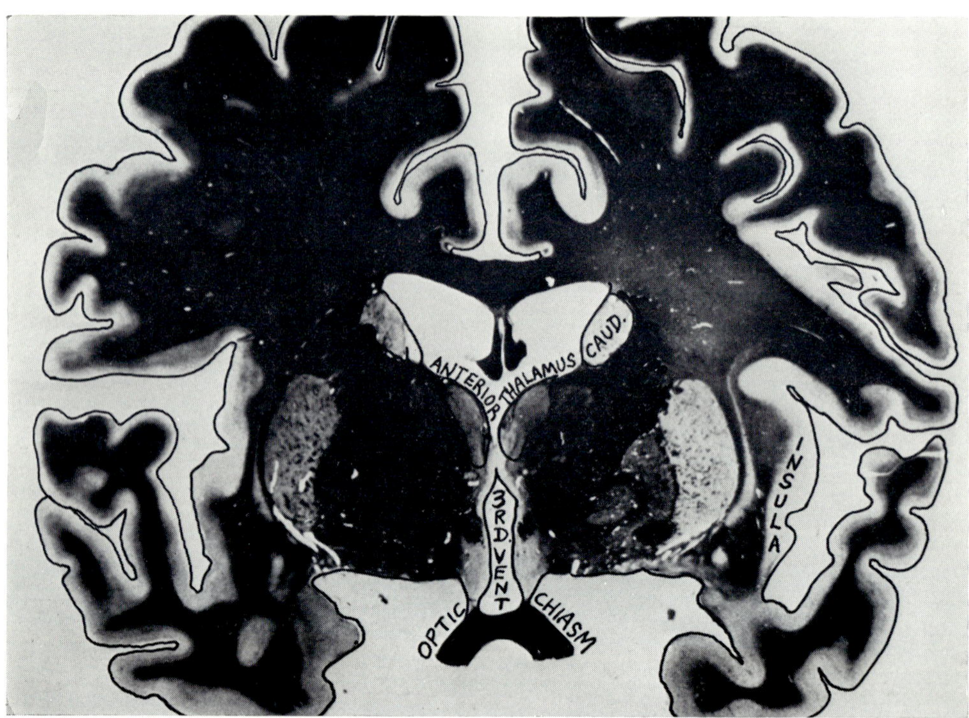

Figure 10. Coronal section of the cerebral hemispheres through the anterior thalamus. This section shows the anterior tubercle of the dorsal thalamus and the suprachiasmatic hypothalamus. The optic chiasm forms the floor of the anterior third ventricle. The lateral wall of the body (i.e. postforaminal) of the lateral ventricle is formed by the body of the caudate and the thalamus.

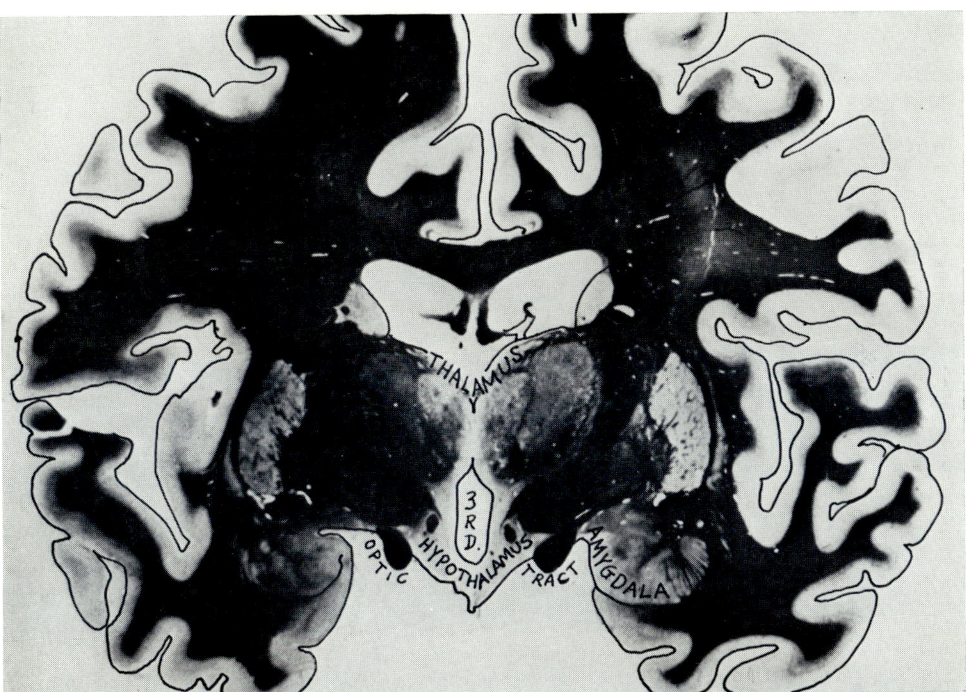

Figure 11. Coronal section of the cerebral hemispheres through the amygdala. The amygdala is shown lying medial in the temporal pole. The temporal horn of the lateral ventricle is not yet apparent. The amygdala is just lateral to the hypothalamus and optic tract, and just beneath the caudal half of the lenticular nucleus. The massa intermedia connects the thalamus on each side. The thalamic and hypothalamic boundaries of the third ventricle are evident.

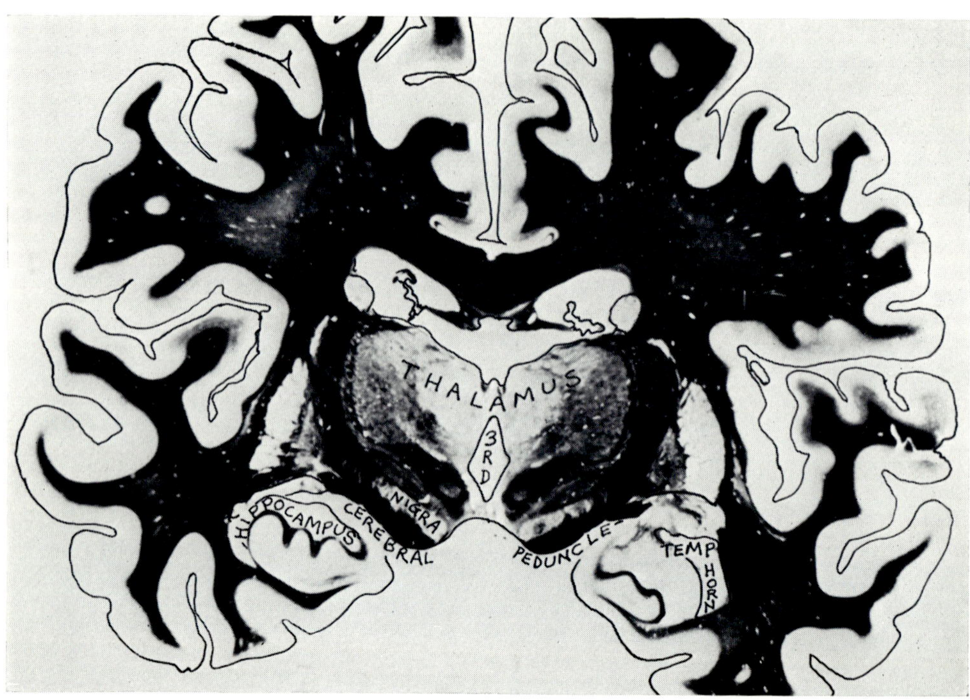

Figure 12. Coronal section of the cerebral hemispheres through the cerebral peduncle. The cerebral peduncles connect the cerebrum with the brain stem. At this level, the dorsal thalamus is quite prominent compared to the relatively smaller caudal pole of the lenticular nucleus. The hippocampus and temporal horn of the lateral ventricle have replaced the amygdala. Note the close relationship of the hippocampal gyrus (i.e. medial temporal surface) to the cerebral peduncle (i.e. and the pyramidal tract within the basis pedunculi). The substantia nigra, and red nucleus above it, extend across the brain stem-cerebral junction.

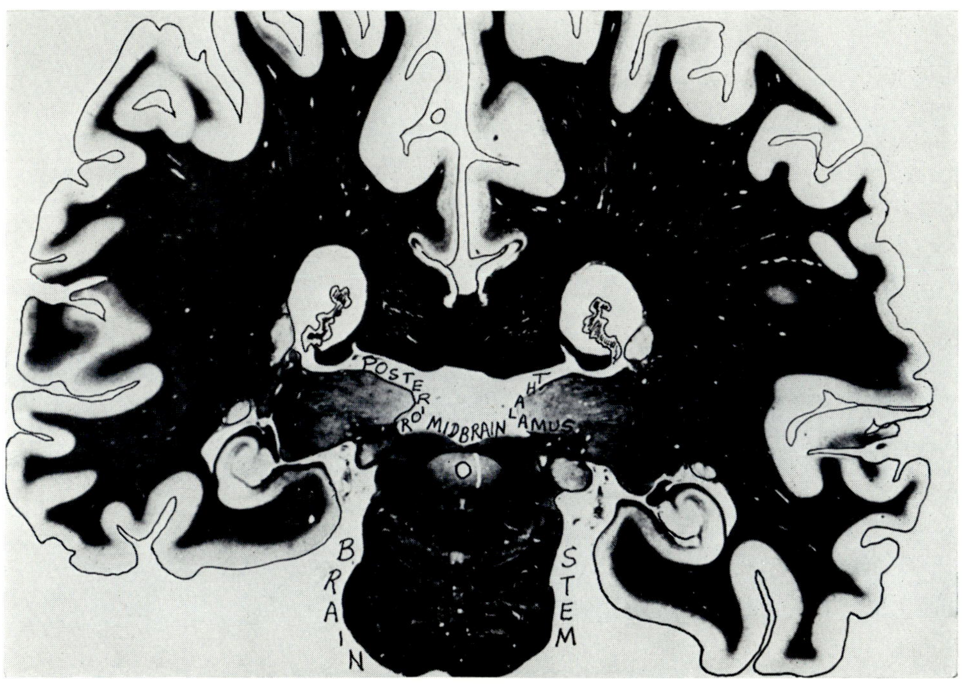

Figure 13. Coronal section of the cerebral hemispheres with attached brain stem. The posterior pole of the thalamus is evident, but the lenticular nucleus is not. The third ventricle is no longer evident, but the aqueduct is noted in the mesencephalon. The basis pontis is attached to the midbrain, since the section is coronal to the cerebrum, and the brain stem is cut in the same cerebral plane. Standard brain stem transverse sections are not cut in this cerebral coronal plane. The body and temporal horns of the lateral ventricle have not yet united (i.e. the atrium lies at a still more caudal level).

CHAPTER 2

FRONTOBASAL SYNDROMES

Anatomical and Physiological Correlates

Sector: 1; orbitofrontal region adjacent to the floor of the anterior fossa (Fig. 14)

Angiogram: Subfrontal

Pneumogram: Inferior Preforaminal

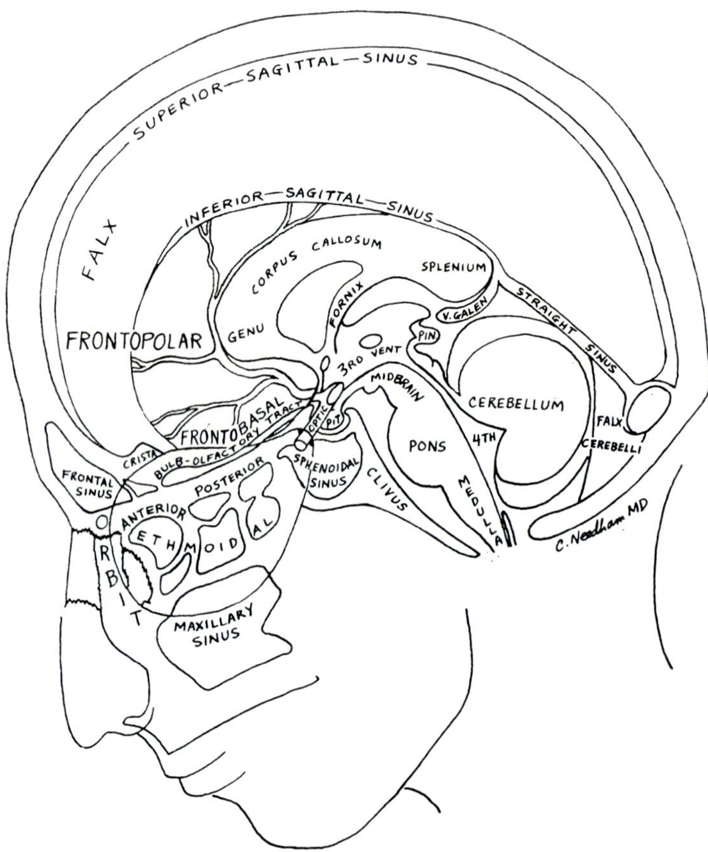

Figure 14. Frontobasal regional anatomy. The frontobasal region and its relation to the paranasal sinuses, orbit and sella are depicted. The positions of the first and second cranial nerves are noted. The anterior falx is relatively narrow. The mesial course of the anterior cerebral artery is indicated.

Neuroanatomy of the Frontobasal Region

A. Afferents
   1. Dorsomedial nucleus of dorsal thalamus—inferior thalamic peduncle.
   2. Reticular formation of midbrain and pons.
   3. Posterior hypothalamus.
   4. Temporal pole-uncinate fasciculus.

B. Efferents
   1. Dorsomedial nucleus of dorsal thalamus—orbitothalamic tract.
   2. Hypothalamus and tegmentum—medial forebrain bundle.
   3. Putamen and caudate, ipsilateral.
   4. Temporal pole—uncinate fasciculus.

Blood Supply of Frontobasal Region

A. Arterial
   1. Anterior cerebral.
      a. Ganglionic branches to anterior perforated substance.
      b. Recurrent artery of Heubner (medial striate artery)—to orbital cortex and anterior perforated substance; to caudate head, anterior limb of internal capsule, and putamen.
      c. Cortical branches—to orbital cortex.
   2. Middle cerebral.
      a. Ganglionic branches—to caudate head, genu and posterior limb of internal capsule, putamen and globus pallidus.
      b. Artery of Charcot (lateral striate artery of hypertension)—to lateral border of lenticular nucleus.
      c. Cortical orbitofrontal branches—to orbital surface of basal frontal region and lateral surface of frontal pole.

B. Venous
   1. Basal vein of Rosenthal—formed by union of deep basal veins (anterior cerebral vein, deep middle cerebral vein and lenticulostriate veins) at the anterior perforated substance; joins the great vein of Galen.
   2. Deep basal veins—also drain into cavernous sinus, sphenoparietal sinus and sylvian veins.

Infarction Syndromes of Arterial Occlusion in the Frontobasal Region

The infarct typically extends beyond or may be totally beyond the confines of this region, producing distant signs.

A. Occlusion of main trunk of anterior cerebral artery (proximal to Heubner's artery)
   1. Contralateral hemiplegia.
   2. Contralateral cortical sensory deficit in the leg.

3. Frontal ataxia.
4. Incontinence, grasp reflex, mental confusion.
5. Occlusion of left main trunk—aphasia, right hemiplegia and left apraxia.

B. Heubner's artery alone
1. Contralateral paralysis of face, tongue and shoulder.
2. Frontal ataxia.
3. Rigidity.

C. Occlusion of the anterior cerebral artery distal to the anterior communicating artery
1. Contralateral leg paralysis.
2. Contralateral cortical sensory deficit in the leg.
3. Incontinence.
4. Grasp reflex, mental confusion, expressive dysphasia—if proximal and left-sided; not present in distal callosomarginal occlusion (paracentral lobule infarction) .

D. Bilateral proximal anterior cerebral occlusion
1. Coma, akinetic mutism, catotonia.
2. Paraplegia.
3. Hypertonus of upper extremities.
4. Pseudobulbar palsy.

E. Proximal middle cerebral occlusion
1. Contralateral hemiplegia.
2. Contralateral hemisensory deficit.
3. Contralateral homonymous hemianopia.
4. Global aphasia—major hemisphere.
5. Coma—acute occlusion of main trunk.

F. Occlusion of orbitofrontal artery alone
1. Expressive dysphasia, major hemisphere.
2. Contralateral facial weakness.

Neurophysiology of the Frontobasal Region

A. Stimulation
1. Autonomic—respiratory arrest, hyper- or hypotension, increased gastric motility.
2. Sleep production—basal forebrain suppressor system.

B. Ablation
1. Hyperactive motor behavior—orbital lesion.
2. Bradykinetic motor state—subpallidal lesion.
3. Decreased gastric motility.
4. Sham rage.

NEUROSURGICAL SYNDROMES OF THE FRONTOBASAL REGION

Development

A. Traumatic—craniocerebral injury commonly produces an acute contre-coup subfrontal contusion against the orbital plate with associated temporopolar contusion. Fracture of the anterior fossa may result in coup subfrontal contusion, laceration or hematoma.

B. Aneurysm rupture, anterior communicating (Fig. 15) —sudden visual

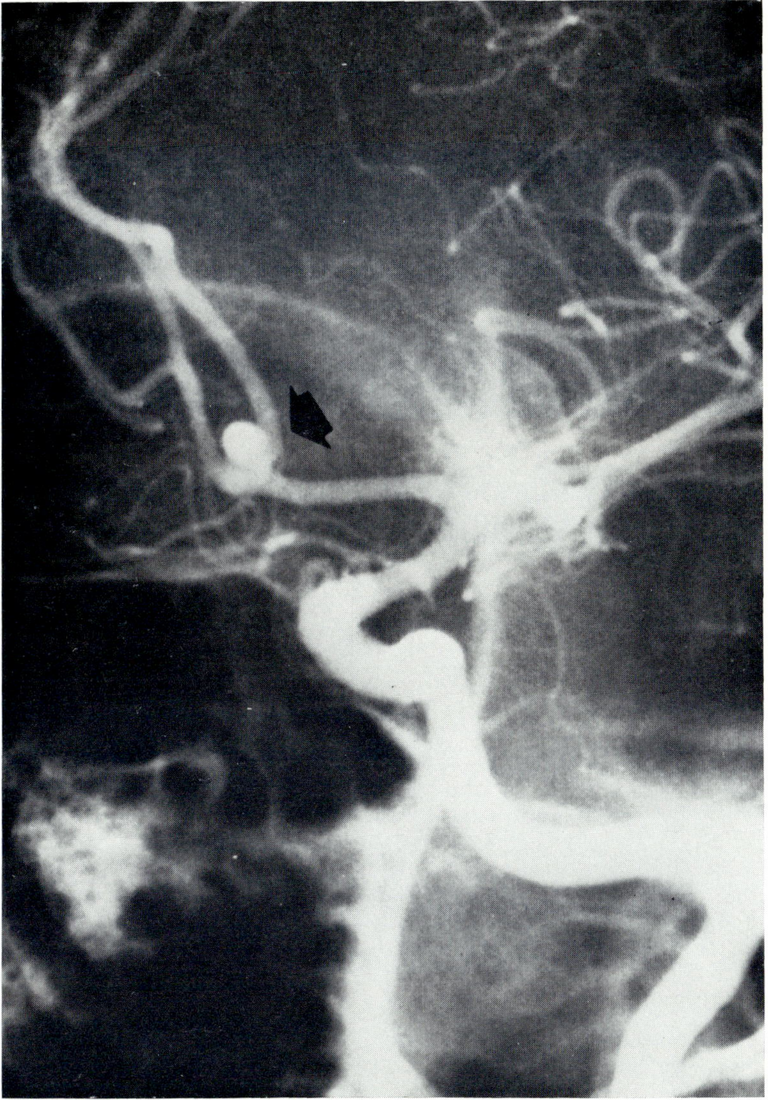

Figure 15. Anterior communicating aneurysm. An oblique film shows this midline aneurysm. The aneurysm lies between the optic chiasm and the posterior part of the frontobasal region, at its juncture with the anterior hypothalamus.

disturbances or loss of consciousness with a paucity of localizing signs, and stiff neck are characteristic.

C. Pituitary apoplexy—hemorrhage into the sella and subfrontal region producing an acute diplopia, visual loss, hypotension and hypopituitarism may occur from a chromophobe adenoma.

D. Brain abscess—the abscess may present clinically with relative rapidity during an acute cerebritis or ventricular rupture. Frontal, ethmoidal or sphenoidal sinus infection may be responsible. Osteomyelitis, epidural or subdural empyema or meningitis may be associated. A "silent" frontobasal abscess with subacute or chronic development is not uncommon.

E. Intracerebral glioma—a frontobasal glioma (Fig. 16) usually presents a history dating back weeks or months. Generalized seizures may precede detection of the tumor by months or even years. The most common cerebral glioma in the adult is the glioblastoma multiforme (astrocytoma, grade 3 or 4). Glioblastomas show a particular predilection for the adult frontal lobe. The glioblastoma and the oligodendroglioma may occasionally present suddenly as a result of intraneoplastic hemorrhage. Lower grade astrocytomas (grade 1 or 2) occur in the cerebral hemispheres of both adults and children. Cerebral ependymoma is more common in childhood, but also occurs in adults. Any of these gliomas may

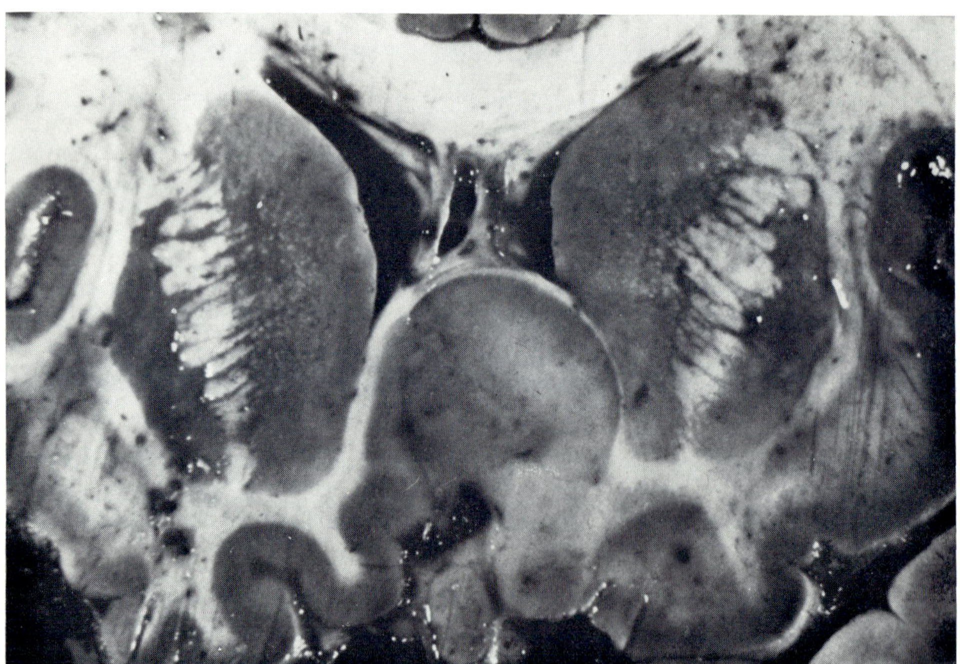

Figure 16. Frontobasal glioma. This frontobasal glioma extends into the septum. The floor of the anterior horn is elevated. A cavum septi pellucidi is also present.

produce a frontobasal syndrome. A bilateral frontobasal-septal syndrome with marked mental disturbance can occur.

F. Basal meningioma—this slowly growing extracerebral tumor produces a gradually progressive frontobasal syndrome. They are less common than the parasagittal or convexity meningiomas. They arise from the dura in the region of the olfactory groove (Fig. 17) or tuberculum sella (Fig. 18). They are uncommon in childhood. The usual patient is an

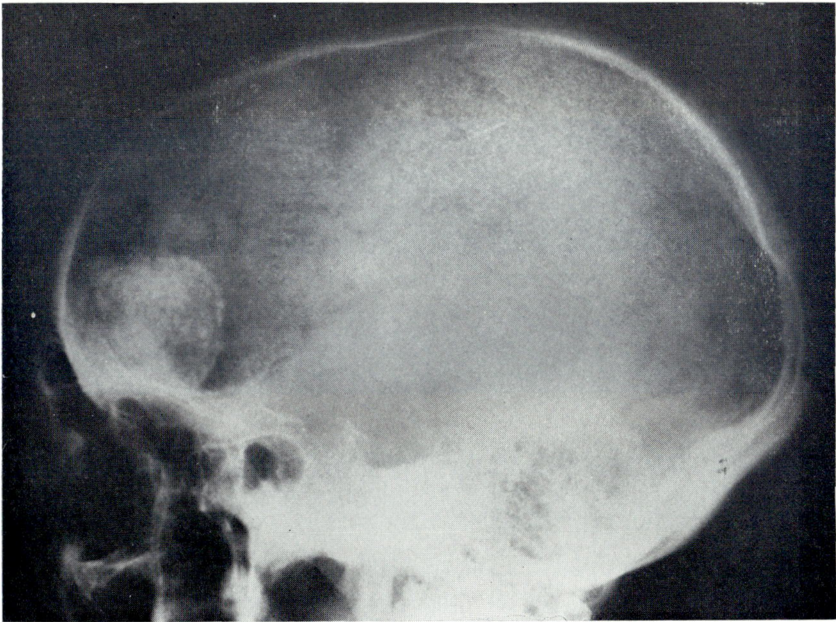

Figure 17. Olfactory meningioma. Tumor calcification arising from the floor of the anterior fossa with adjacent hyperostosis is present.

adult woman of middle age. Tuberculum and inner sphenoid ("clinoidal") meningiomas have a shorter course due to proximity to the optic nerve. The frontal base may be secondarily involved by "infra-alar herniation." An anterior falx meningioma may, for example, gradually dislocate the frontal base over the sphenoid ridge and into the middle fossa.

Deficits of Frontobasal Syndromes

"Sign-silence" is common, especially with lesions of intermediate or gradual onset; neurological and psychological deficits which may occur however, include the following:

A. Behavioral signs

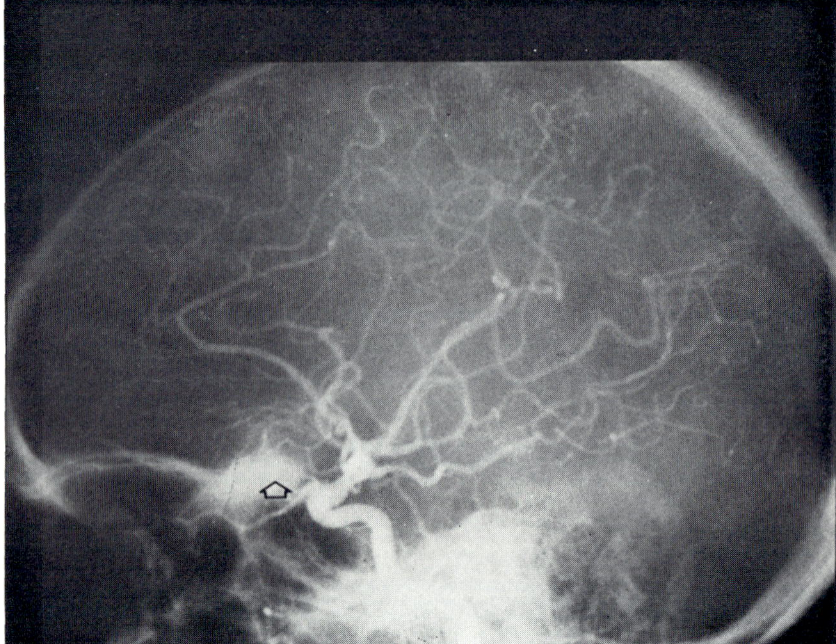

Figure 18. Tuberculum meningioma. Tumor vessels, elevation of the proximal anterior cerebral artery, and hyperostosis in the region of the tuberculum sella indicate the presence of this posterior frontobasal meningioma.

1. Loss of inhibition.
2. Impulsive laughter or crying.
3. Moria ("witzelsucht")—pointless silly joking associated with euphoria.
4. Rage attacks.
5. Impaired recent memory.

B. Ictal signs
   1. Epilepsy—seizures may be the earliest sign of a frontal tumor.
   2. Grand mal—this is the form of generalized convulsion beginning with an initial loss of consciousness. There is no lateralizing ictal sign. It is non adversive. It was termed a "highest level seizure" by Jackson. Such seizures occur with frontobasal, deep cerebral, midline and brain stem irritative foci. The frontobasal tumor, especially when eccentric, may produce generalized convulsions with prominent lateralizing signs. The term "grand mal," however, should be reserved for the unconscious, nonadversive, nonlateralized generalized attack. Any of the following cerebral seizures may terminate in generalized convulsion; note should be made of their localizing value.
      a. Unconscious, nonadversive-frontobasal and deep cerebral midline.

b. Unconscious, adversive-frontopolar.
c. Conscious, adversive or jacksonian focal motor (arm, leg) —frontodorsal.
d. Jacksonian focal motor (face) —frontolateral or temporal.
e. Jacksonian focal sensory—parietal.
f. Visual seizures—caudal cerebral (parieto-temporo-occipital).
g. Psychomotor seizures—hallucinatory attacks with déjà vu, parosmia and automatism are almost always of temporal lobe type. Occasionally, similar attacks are seen in irritative frontobasal or cingulate lesions.

C. Motor signs
1. Hyperkinetic, restless motor activity—this is often seen in an acute orbital cortex contusion or with rupture of an anterior communicating aneurysm. It must be differentiated from restlessness due to intracranial hypertension, meningeal irritation or transtentorial herniation.
2. Bradykinetic motor activity—this usually indicates involvement of deep subcortical white matter or extension to the basal ganglia.
3. Akinetic mutism—a speechless state without significant spontaneous movements of the extremities associated with an alert oculomotor system can occur with deep intracerebral frontobasal lesions. Involvement is usually mesial (cingulate gyrus) or bilateral.
4. Catatonia—a plastic state with maintained abnormal postures of the extremities indicates deep subcortical extension.
5. Expressive aphasia or dysphasia indicates convexity, opercular or subcortical extension, major hemisphere.
6. Facial weakness, contralateral—extension to either convexity.
7. Pseudobulbar syndrome—extension to frontal operculum, bilaterally.

D. Hypothalamic—autonomic signs
1. Hyperphagia, hypermotility.
2. Polydipsia, polyuria.
3. Hyperthermia, vasodilatation, diaphoresis.

E. Cranial nerve signs
1. Anosmia, unilateral—meningioma of the olfactory groove or middle sphenoid ridge.
2. Anosmia, bilateral—meningioma of the olfactory groove or severe hydrocephalus.
3. Anosmia of traumatic or nasal origin—may be unilateral or bilateral.
4. Optic atrophy—unilateral loss of visual acuity with central or paracentral scotoma and pallor of the optic disc.
5. Foster Kennedy syndrome—this includes ipsilateral optic atrophy and

contralateral papilledema. The olfactory meningioma or frontal glioma can produce this unusual combination.

6. Papilledema—may be absent despite the presence of elevated pressure due to a frontal mass. Many large frontal tumors are of course associated with bilateral papilledema at the time of clinical presentation.

F. Trauma signs

1. Naso-oral hemorrhage—often due to fracture of the floor of the anterior and/or middle fossa. CSF rhinorrhea may be obscured by the hemorrhage. "Target sign" is a central red blood-tinged area surrounded by a pink CSF ring, the specimen being collected upon white gauze.
2. CSF rhinorrhea—usually due to a fracture of the anterior fossa in the cribriform region. Less often due to a fracture in the middle fossa extending into the sphenoid sinus. The sphenoid sinus may have a large lateral wing extending into the middle fossa. CSF rhinorrhea may result from fracture of the pituitary fossa and even with posterior fossa fractures in the petrous bone (middle ear—eustachian tube—nasopharynx) with "paradoxical rhinorrhea." Rhinorrhea may only be noted when the patient leans forward in the sitting position with the head flexed.
3. Bilateral "panda-bear sign"—ecchymosis and swelling of both upper and lower lids of both eyes, especially if delayed in appearance, indicates a transverse fracture of the lesser wings of the sphenoid.
4. Infraorbital ecchymosis—with swelling of the lower lid out of proportion to the upper lid, discoloration indicates a fracture of the orbital floor or walls.
5. Supraorbital ecchymosis—with swelling of the upper lid much in excess of lower lid, discoloration indicates a fracture of the orbital roof.
6. Periorbital subcutaneous emphysema—indicates a fronto-ethmoidal sinus fracture and is usually associated with ecchymosis. Sinus fracture may be present without palpable emphysema.
7. Maxillofacial and nasal root fractures—these are commonly associated with subfrontal contusion. Malar fracture may be indicated by a palpable irregularity in the inferior orbital margin. This sign is only present early, before marked regional swelling prevents its detection.
8. Direct (soft-tissue) ocular injury—this commonly produces swelling and ecchymosis ("black-eye") of both upper and lower lids with subconjunctival hemorrhage. Corneal abrasion, a dilated pupil and intraocular hemorrhage may occur. When ecchymosis of the lids appears on a delayed basis, a fracture of the anterior fossa and orbit, rather than direct ocular injury, should be suspected.

9. Traumatic anosmia—unilateral or bilateral.
10. Traumatic blindness—may be secondary to the following:
    a. Hemorrhage into the optic nerve sheath with eventual optic atrophy; a basal skull fracture with a fracture of the anterior clinoid is often associated.
    b. Contrecoup contusion of the optic nerve in the optic foramen with optic atrophy.
    c. Intracranial hemorrhage with papilledema and secondary optic atrophy.
    d. Retrobulbar hemorrhage—unilateral exophthalmos.
    e. Retinal detachment, intraocular hemorrhage, trauma to lens or cornea.

G. Satellite syndromes—the syndromes of the cranio-orbital junction are conveniently considered with those of the frontal base. The intracranial fossae which bound the orbit include the anterior fossa, the middle fossa and the pituitary fossa (sella). The "orbital apex," containing the neurovascular stem of the eye, is located at the point of convergence of these three cranial fossae (Figs. 14 and 19).
   1. Orbital apex syndrome—the neurovascular structures passing through both the optic foramen and the superior orbital fissure are involved.
      a. Optic foramen syndrome.
         (1) Optic nerve and ophthalmic artery.
         (2) Central visual loss, optic atrophy, blindness.
         (3) Anterior clinoid—superior to optic foramen; clinoid (inner sphenoid) meningioma.
         (4) Sphenoid sinus—medial to optic foramen; mucocele, nasopharyngeal neoplasm.
         (5) Superior orbital fissure—inferolateral to optic foramen (see below).
         (6) Hyperostosis of optic foramen—foraminal meningioma.
         (7) Enlargement of optic foramen—glioma of optic nerve, neurofibroma.
      b. Superior orbital fissure syndrome.
         (1) Contents.
            (a) Cranial nerves—oculomotor, trochlear, first division of trigeminal, abducens.
            (b) Sympathetic nerves—filaments from cavernous plexus.
            (c) Arteries—orbital branch of middle meningeal artery, recurrent branch of lacrimal artery.
            (d) Ophthalmic veins.

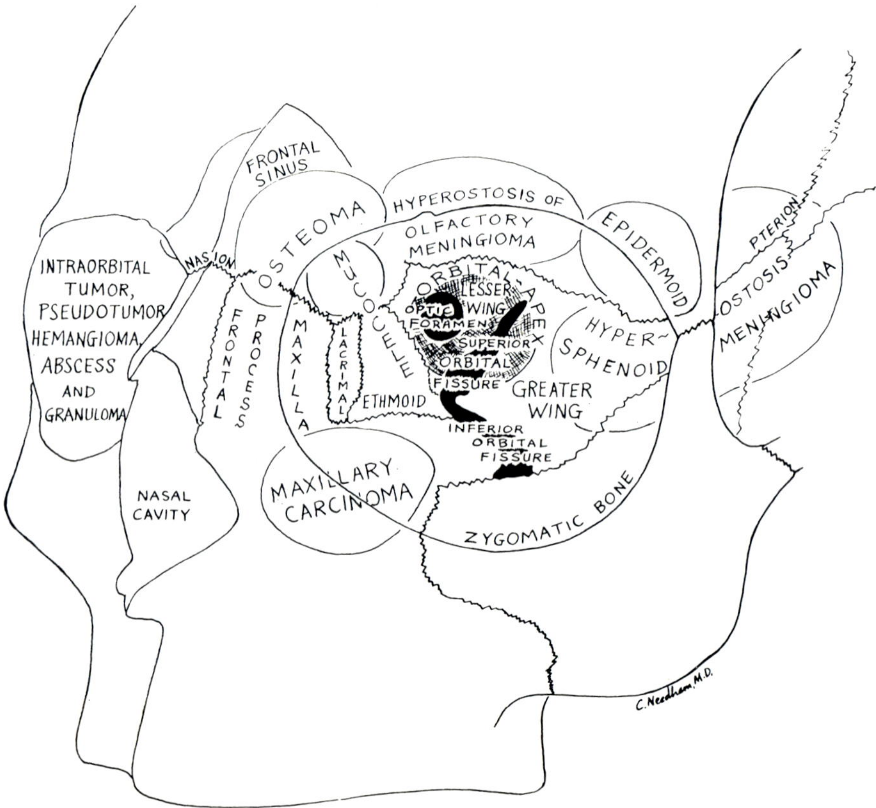

Figure 19. Intraorbital-extraorbital masses. The characteristic locations of mass lesions which involve the orbit and adjacent structure are shown. The "orbital apex," including the neurovascular stem of the eye, lies at the juncture of the anterior, middle and pituitary fossae of the skull (see Fig. 14). The optic foramen and superior orbital fissure are depicted within the shaded orbital apex.

(2) Signs.
 (a) Internal and external ophthalmoplegia—fixed, staring nonreactive eye with a dilated pupil.
 (b) First division trigeminal hypesthesia, pain; corneal anesthesia, keratitis.
 (c) Exophthalmos—engorged ophthalmic veins.

(3) Obstruction of superior orbital fissure—may be associated with pathological widening of the fissure due to erosion of sphenoid.
 (a) Infraclinoid aneurysm (Fig. 20).
 (b) Meningioma.
 (c) Pituitary adenoma.
 (d) Chordoma.

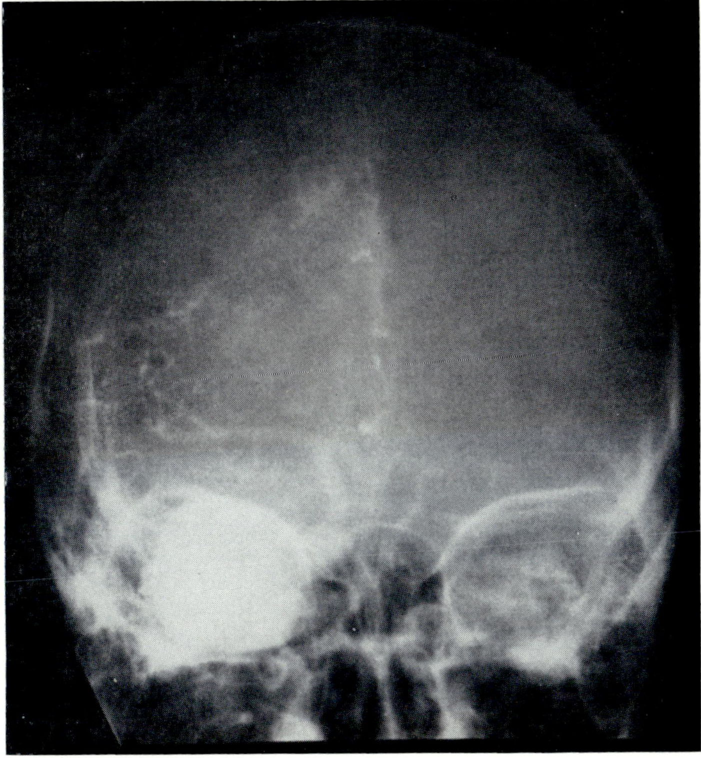

Figure 20. Giant infraclinoid aneurysm at the orbital apex. The aneurysm compressed the optic, oculomotor, trochlear, abducens and trigeminal (ophthalmic division) nerves in addition to obstructing the venous drainage of the orbit.

(e) Mucocele of sphenoid sinus.
(f) Intraorbital tumor.

2. Infraclinoid syndrome—anterior cavernous sinus syndrome.
   a. Equivalent to orbital apex syndrome.
   b. Erosion of anterior clinoid by internal carotid aneurysm in anterior part of cavernous sinus.
3. Petrosphenoidal crossway syndrome.
   a. Cranial nerves two through six.
   b. Resembles orbital apex syndrome but pain is in the distribution of the second trigeminal division.
   c. Extension of a pharyngeal neoplasm through the foramen lacerum into the cranial cavity is the most common source.
4. Unilateral exophthalmos syndrome.
   a. Traumatic exophthalmos.
      (1) Fracture of orbital roof with retrobulbar hematoma—early exophthalmos (fracture of orbital floor—enophthalmos).

(2) Carotid-cavernous fistula—delayed exophthalmos (Fig. 21); pulsating exophthalmos with bruit; pulsation and proptosis

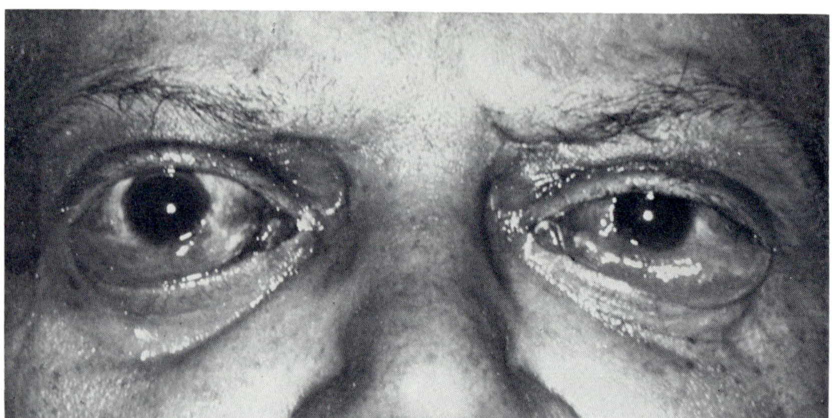

Figure 21. Exophthalmos and carotid-cavernous fistula. Bilateral exophthalmos with periocular swelling occurred after a traumatic carotid-cavernous fistula.

may be minimal or extreme; bruit diminished by carotid compression; exophthalmos may be bilateral with unilateral fistula (patent circular sinus) ; it may even be contralateral to fistula; bilateral fistulae are rare.

b. Vascular exophthalmos.
   (1) "Spontaneous" carotid-cavernous fistula—rupture of arteriosclerotic intracavernous carotid.
   (2) Anterior cavernous sinus syndrome—large intracavernous nonfistulous carotid aneurysm with orbital apex venous block.
   (3) Hemangioma of the orbit (Fig. 22)—compressibility of orbital content; satellite hemangioma of conjunctiva or skin may be associated; proptosis which changes with posture or straining.

c. Inflammatory exophthalmos.
   (1) Panophthalmitis.
   (2) Orbital cellulitis and orbital abscess.
   (3) Pseudotumor of the orbit.
   (4) Cavernous sinus thrombosis.

d. Exophthalmos and meningioma.
   (1) Orbital roof—hyperostosis of olfactory groove meningioma; proptosis with ipsilateral anosmia.
   (2) Orbital lateral wall—hyperostosis of greater wing of sphenoid; pterion meningioma "en plaque" occurring almost exclusively in women; bony mass in the temporal region may occur years before exophthalmos is noted.

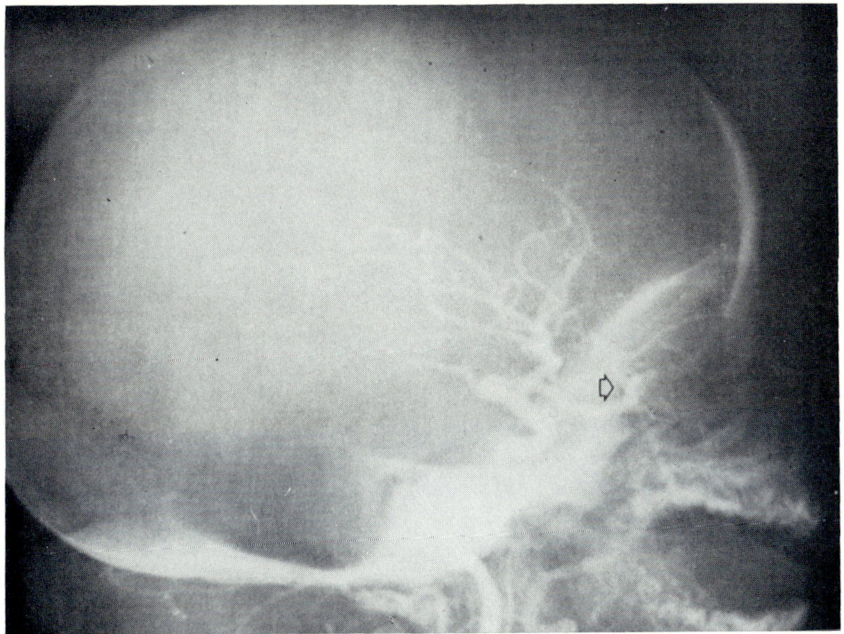

Figure 22. Hemangioma of the orbit. An enlarged ophthalmic artery and increased retro-ocular vascularity are evident.

(3) Orbital apex—venous block or intraorbital extension of inner ridge (clinoidal) sphenoid meningioma.

(4) Intraorbital—optic sheath meningioma (sheath of Schwalbe).

e. Exophthalmos, bony overgrowth, and tumors of the orbital walls.

(1) Hyperostosis of meningioma—begins in inner table.

(2) Benign osteoma—begins in outer table, usually with involvement of paranasal sinuses (Fig. 23).

(3) Fibrous dysplasia—pseudo-osteoma, asymmetrical thickening of orbit, facio-orbit or entire cranial base; both dense and lucent bone lesions.

(4) Albright's syndrome—polyostotic fibrous dysplasia, multiple skeletal lesions, café-au-lait spots, sexual precocity in females.

(5) Leontiasis ossea—craniofacial hyperostosis with foraminal obstruction, proptosis and sinus block.

(6) Osteochondroma—may be isolated or part of skeletal lesions of Ollier's syndrome.

(7) Osteoclastoma—giant cell tumor; more common in the mandible or maxillary antrum.

(8) Hemangioma of bone.

f. Exophthalmos and bony defect.

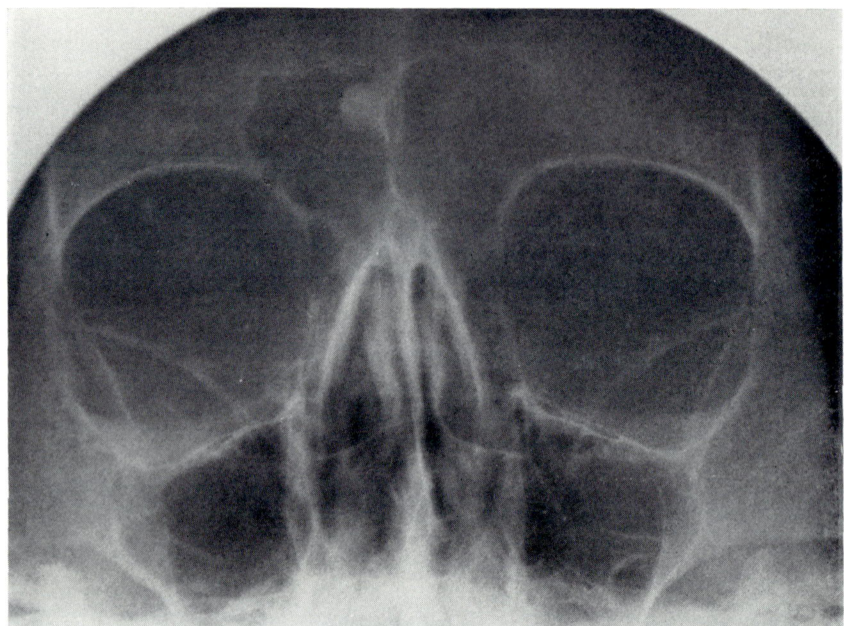

Figure 23. Osteoma. This small osteoma exhibits a characteristic location: the frontal sinus.

(1) Orbital encephalocele.
(2) Congenital defect of sphenoid wing—isolated or with von Recklinghausen's disease (neurofibromatosis).
(3) Sphenoid defect with neurofibroma (intraorbital) or dumbbell neurofibroma (intraorbital-intracranial).

g. Exophthalmos and intraorbital tumor.
(1) Neuroblastoma of infancy and early childhood—initial signs are usually due to metastases. Bone pain, fever, diarrhea, abdominal mass and proptosis commonly occur. Craniocerebral metastases also may be noted. Primary neuroblastoma of the adrenal is most common.
(2) Retinoblastoma—in infancy and childhood. This malignant tumor produces a "white pupil," blindness and enlargement of the globe. It is sometimes bilateral and may spread intracranially or distantly.
(3) Retinal anlage tumor—rare infantile tumor of the maxilla, orbit or skull which does not metastasize but may locally erode bone.
(4) Optic nerve glioma of childhood—visual loss precedes proptosis; enlargement of optic foramen; signs of von Reckling-

hausen's neurofibromatosis with café au lait spots may be present; may have intracranial extension to chiasm, optic tract and hypothalamus.

(5) Sarcoma of optic sheath—spread to opposite orbit and distant metastases.

(6) Malignant melanoma of choroid—distant metastases may result including intracranial spread especially to the meninges. Primary melanoma of the brain is rare. Cerebral melanoma usually is metastatic from an occult or obvious primary.

(7) Histiocytosis X—diabetes insipidis, multiple cranial and skeletal defects, orocutaneous and pulmonary lesions in childhood (Hand-Schüller-Christian syndrome) ; eosinophilic granuloma —older children and adults.

(8) Orbital epidermoid—dorsolateral.

(9) Orbital mucocele—dorsomedial.

Deformities (Angiographic and Pneumographic) of the Frontobasal Syndromes

A. Angiographic deformities

1. Extracerebral subfrontal mass (e.g. meningioma) .

a. Elevation (lateral view) .

(1) Anterior cerebral artery, proximal segment.

(2) Frontopolar artery.

(3) Pericallosal artery, at genu of corpus callosum.

(4) Above arteries appear taut.

(5) Pericallosal genu forms an acute angle due to basal arterial elevation.

(6) Middle cerebral orbitofrontal artery—only with lateral subfrontal mass.

(7) Septal vein.

b. Depression (lateral view) .

(1) Carotid siphon.

(2) Ophthalmic artery, proximal segment.

c. Posterior displacement (lateral view) .

(1) Carotid bifurcation.

(2) Anterior communicating artery.

(3) Internal cerebral vein, anterior segment; may produce narrow venous angle due to "humping" of internal cerebral vein.

d. Midline shift—anterior cerebral artery (AP view) .

(1) No shift—small or midline subfrontal mass.

(2) No shift, but anterior cerebral reaches midline as taut arch—extracerebral midline mass.

(3) Round shift—any frontal mass.

(4) Angular shift—only a subfrontal and extracerebral mass.

e. Angiographic meningioma signs.

(1) Arterial "sunburst sign"—multiple radially oriented small arteries of supply from the "hilus" of the meningioma produce this effect.

(2) Homogeneous "tumor cloud" with a peripheral zone of increased density.

(3) Longer persistence of the tumor cloud into the late angiographic phase than in gliomas.

(4) Extreme vascularity, tortuosity and enlargement of the vessels of supply.

(5) Extracerebral blood supply from meningeal and scalp branches of the external carotid artery.

(a) Middle meningeal artery—from the maxillary branch of the external carotid; it may enlarge the foramen spinosum; the frontal branches of the middle meningeal are unusually prominent.

(b) Accessory meningeal artery—enters through the foramen ovale as a branch of the middle meningeal or maxillary artery.

(c) Meningeal branches from the superficial temporal artery of the scalp.

(6) Meningeal branches not ordinarily seen which arise from the internal carotid system.

(a) Meningeal branch from the carotid siphon.

(b) Anterior meningeal branch—enters through the ethmoid foramen of the cribriform plate of the anterior fossa; a branch of the anterior ethmoidal artery, in turn a branch of the ophthalmic artery.

(c) The ophthalmic artery itself may enlarge and send branches to the orbital roof.

(d) The recurrent meningeal artery is a branch of the ophthalmic artery which passes through the superior orbital fissure and may enlarge to supply a sphenoidal meningioma.

(7) Absence of early arteriovenous shunting.

(8) Association of plain x-ray meningioma signs.

(a) Hyperostosis.

(b) Prominent vascular channels.

(c) Tumor calcification.

(d) Enlargement of foramen spinosum—not as reliable.

2. Intracerebral inferior frontal mass (e.g. glioma).
   a. No meningioma signs.
   b. Anterior cerebral branches are not entirely displaced away from the anterior fossa floor as they are in extracerebral tumors.
   c. Elevation of anterior cerebral and pericallosal arteries is not taut, but is wavy and irregular.
   b. Pericallosal genu forms a wide angle because of frequent extension of glioma to the corpus callosum.
   e. On AP view, angular shift does not occur; anterior cerebral artery does not reach midline as a taut arch but runs horizontally.
   f. On AP view, shift is either absent or round, depending on bilaterality or eccentricity of location of the mass.
   g. Angiographic glioma signs—the glioblastomas tend to present the most pathological tumor vessels of the gliomas.
      (1) There are many pathological arteries of supply which may be of "corkscrew" type.
      (2) Prominent early arteriovenous shunts are noted.
      (3) Drainage into deep veins is prominent.
      (4) Angiographic tumor cloud does not last long.
      (5) There may be no pathological vessels with only early venous filling.
      (6) Any glioma may present as an avascular mass on the angiogram; this is especially true of astrocytomas.

B. Pneumoencephalographic deformities
   1. Failure to fill the chiasmatic cistern (with filling of interpenduncular cistern)—early sign of an extracerebral subfrontal mass.
   2. Elevation of the floor of a single anterior horn—either extracerebral or intracerebral subfrontal mass.
   3. Medial dislocation and floor deformation of the ipsilateral anterior horn—either extracerebral or intracerebral unilateral subfrontal mass.
   4. Elevation of the floors of both anterior horns—usually an extracerebral mass.
   5. Nonfilling of both anterior horns—large subfrontal mass.
   6. Posterior displacement of the anterior wall (lamina terminalis) of the third ventricle—either extracerebral or intracerebral; compression of the infundibular recess of third ventricle.
   7. Occlusion of the foramen of Monro—large subfrontal mass with lateral ventricular hydrocephalus.
      a. Dilatation of both lateral ventricles with the smaller ventricle usually on the side of the mass, or
      b. Dilatation of a single lateral ventricle—the enlarged anterior horn is displaced to the side opposite the mass, or

c. Equally dilated, nondisplaced anterior horns—especially with large meningioma of the tuberculum sella.

8. Unilateral enlargement of an anterior horn may also occur with the following:
   a. Orbital and frontal encephalocele.
   b. Porencephalic anterior fossa cyst—post-traumatic.

Additional Diagnostic Clues in Frontobasal Syndromes

A. Plain x-rays, sellar, sinus and orbital views
   1. Pressure atrophy of the sella—this affects the dorsum sella, clinoids and sellar floor and is due to elevated intracranial pressure from any source. Pressure atrophy is most marked posteriorly and affects the dorsum and posterior clinoids first. The sella eventually enlarges.
   2. Posterior displacement of a calcified pineal by the frontal mass.
   3. Tumor calcification—this is commonly present in the oligodendroglioma on plain skull x-ray. However, a significant minority of astrocytomas, ependymomas and meningiomas also reveal calcification on plain films.
   4. Hyperostosis—usually most marked in the inner table, but may include the diploë and the outer table. This indicates a meningioma. "Spicule hyperostosis" can occur in locally invasive meningiomas or osteogenic sarcoma. The "blister sign" indicates a tuberculum meningioma with hyperostosis at the posterior ethmoid-sphenoid junction. Hyperostosis of the anterior clinoid indicates an inner ridge sphenoid meningioma. Hyperostosis of the orbital plate in olfactory meningiomas must be differentiated from osteoma of the orbital plate. The latter begins on the outer table and commonly involves the frontal or ethmoidal sinuses.
   5. Erosion of an anterior clinoid, unilaterally—usually due to an aneurysm or meningioma.
   6. "Ballooning" of the sella—pituitary adenoma, especially the chromophobe tumor, is the most common source and may extend subfrontally. The clinoids are "undercut" and pointed upwards. Destruction of the dorsum with retention of the posterior clinoids indicates an intrasellar tumor rather than pressure atrophy. Suprasellar calcification with or without sellar enlargement suggests craniopharyngioma. Less often, chromophobe adenomas may calcify. Sellar and parasellar calcification may occur in the wall of an aneurysm.
   7. Prominent vascular grooves on plain skull x-rays—indicate possibility of meningioma, arteriovenous malformation or chronic intracranial hypertension. When the enlarged grooves are middle meningeal and

the arterial branches are larger than their origin, meningioma is quite likely.

8. Suprasellar gas bubble—early and transient sign of post-traumatic pneumocephalus due to fracture in the anterior or middle fossa; occasionally due to neoplastic or infectious process with bone erosion.
9. Traumatic sinus fluid level—fracture in the anterior or middle fossa, seen on brow-up lateral.
10. Nontraumatic sinus fluid level—mucopus or mucocele.
11. Acute sinusitis (frontal, ethmoidal or sphenoidal)—uniform opacity with sharply defined sinus border.
12. Chronic sinusitis—opacity ("clouding") with poor definition of the sinus wall; frequent extension to other sinuses or "pansinusitis."
13. Expanding mucocele—most common in frontal sinus; opaque sinus with pressure erosion of sinus wall; erosion of bone is smooth with no scalloping; marginal sclerosis is common; extension to orbit and anterior fossa occurs; associated with recurrent sinusitis, infection ("mucopyocele") and occasionally with osteoma.
14. Osteoma—rounded bony mass usually involving frontal and ethmoidal sinuses; may be associated with sinus infection, frontal deformity and proptosis.
15. Neoplastic sinus erosion—nasopharyngeal carcinoma and lymphoepithelioma.
16. Orbital views.
    a. Bony defect.
        (1) Dorsolateral orbit—epidermoid.
        (2) Dorsomedial orbit—mucocele.
        (3) Orbital roof—encephalocele.
        (4) Optic foramen enlargement—optic nerve glioma.
        (5) Sphenoid bone defect—neurofibromatosis.
        (6) Orbital floor—carcinoma of maxillary antrum.
    b. Bony excess.
        (1) Neoplastic calcification—retinoblastoma.
        (2) Hyperostosis—meningioma.
        (3) Osteoma—orbital plate.
        (4) Pseudo-osteoma—fibrous dysplasia.

B. Electroencephalogram
1. Unilateral basal frontal mass lesion—unifrontal, frontotemporal or bifrontal high voltage slow activity (delta); EEG may be normal however.
2. Large subfrontal mass—bifrontal or bitemporal slowing; also seen with midline and brain stem lesions.

3. Large subfrontal mass with elevated intracranial pressure—generalized slow activity.
4. Subfrontal mass with seizure discharge—generalized spikes and sharp waves, nonfocal; "secondary bilateral synchrony" similar to spike-wave of petit mal may occur; focal spikes and sharp waves may occur most prominently in frontopolar, frontolateral or anterior temporal regions.

C. Brain scan
1. Basal meningioma—the brain scan is of great value in the diagnosis of any meningioma. It is especially helpful in the diagnosis of meningiomas in relatively silent regions such as the subfrontal area.
2. Glioblastoma multiforme—positive scan, often suggestive of extension to midline (corpus callosum).
3. Brain abscess—scan often positive.
4. Skull fracture with or without cerebral contusion—scan often positive.
5. Low-grade astrocytoma—readily missed on brain scan.

CHAPTER 3

FRONTOPOLAR SYNDROMES

Anatomical and Physiological Correlates

Sector: 2 and 3; prefrontal lobe, anterior to the coronal suture
Angiogram: Anterior Frontal
Pneumogram: Anterior and Superior Preforaminal

Neuroanatomy of the Frontal Pole

A. Afferents
1. Dorsomedial nucleus of dorsal thalamus—anterior thalamic peduncle.
2. Parietal, posterior temporal and occipital lobes, ipsilateral—long association tracts: superior and inferior fronto-occipital, superior longitudinal bundles.
3. Premotor, motor and basal frontal region, ipsilateral—short association tracts.
4. Temporal pole, ipsilateral—uncinate fasciculus.
5. Frontal, parietal and occipital lobes, contralateral—corpus callosum.

B. Efferents
1. Dorsomedial and lateral nuclei of dorsal thalamus—anterior thalamic peduncle.
2. Cerebral hemispheres—associational and commissural pathways listed above.
3. Putamen and globus pallidus—external capsule.
4. Red nucleus, substantia nigra, mesencephalic tegmentum—internal capsule.
5. Pontine nuclei and cerebellum—frontopontocerebellar tract, anterior limb of internal capsule.

Blood Supply of the Frontopolar Region

A. Arterial
1. Frontopolar artery, anterior cerebral.
   a. Arises distal to anterior communicating and orbital branches of the anterior cerebral artery.
   b. May arise from callosomarginal artery.
   c. Supplies medial and rostral surface of the frontal pole.
2. Orbitofrontal artery, middle cerebral.
   a. Arises distal to the anterior temporal branch of the middle cerebral artery.

b. Supplies the lateral surface of the frontal pole, and orbital surface of the basal frontal region.

B. Venous
1. Superficial frontal veins—enter the superior longitudinal sinus; earliest veins to fill on an angiogram.
2. Superficial middle cerebral (sylvian) vein—empties into sphenoparietal and cavernous sinuses.
3. Anterior cerebral vein—joins the basal vein (Rosenthal).

Infarction Syndromes of Arterial Occlusion in the Frontopolar Region

A. Occlusion of the frontopolar artery—occurs clinically in association with proximal anterior cerebral occlusion.
1. Contralateral grasp reflex.
2. Mental confusion.
3. Expressive dysphasia (major hemisphere).
4. Incontinence.
5. Contralateral leg paralysis and cortical sensory deficit.

B. Occlusion of the orbitofrontal artery—occurs clinically in association with cortical middle cerebral occlusion distal to perforating branches.
1. Contralateral face, arm and hand paralysis; leg paralysis if present is less severe.
2. Cortical sensory deficit in the paralyzed limb.
3. Expressive-receptive dysphasia—major hemisphere.

C. Occlusion of orbitofrontal artery alone
1. Expressive dysphasia—major hemisphere.
2. Facial weakness, contralateral.

Neurophysiology of the Frontopolar Region

A. Stimulation
1. Generally produces no detectable motor or sensory reaction.
2. May result in contralateral conjugate eye deviation—dorsolateral stimulation of "supplementary eye field."
3. Autonomic alterations—respiratory, cardiovascular, gastric motility—stimulation of anterior cingulate region on medial surface of frontal pole; similar to orbitofrontal stimulation.

B. Ablation
1. Unilateral prefrontal lobectomy, minor hemisphere—no clearly defined behavioral or neurological deficit.
2. Unilateral prefrontal lobectomy, major hemisphere—some diminution in spontaneity and fluency of speech may occur.
3. Bilateral prefrontal lobectomy, lobotomy or leucotomy of anterior

thalamic and associational tracts—severe behavioral deficits marked by apathy, inattention, inability to learn, impairment of recent memory, and stereotyped, undirected activity.

NEUROSURGICAL SYNDROMES OF THE FRONTOPOLAR REGION

Development

A. Traumatic—frontal smash syndrome—this is especially common with automotive trauma. There may be supraorbital, frontal boss or frontal sinus fracture. Frontal depressed fracture with acute coup contusion of the frontal poles, naso-oral hemorrhage, CSF rhinorrhea and pneumocephalus may occur. Frontal lobe laceration, acute frontal subdural (Fig. 24) or intracerebral hematoma may also be present. Contrecoup occipital polar contusion and traumatic brain swelling may complicate the picture. Cervical flexion—extension injuries and thoracic wall—pulmonary trauma may be associated.

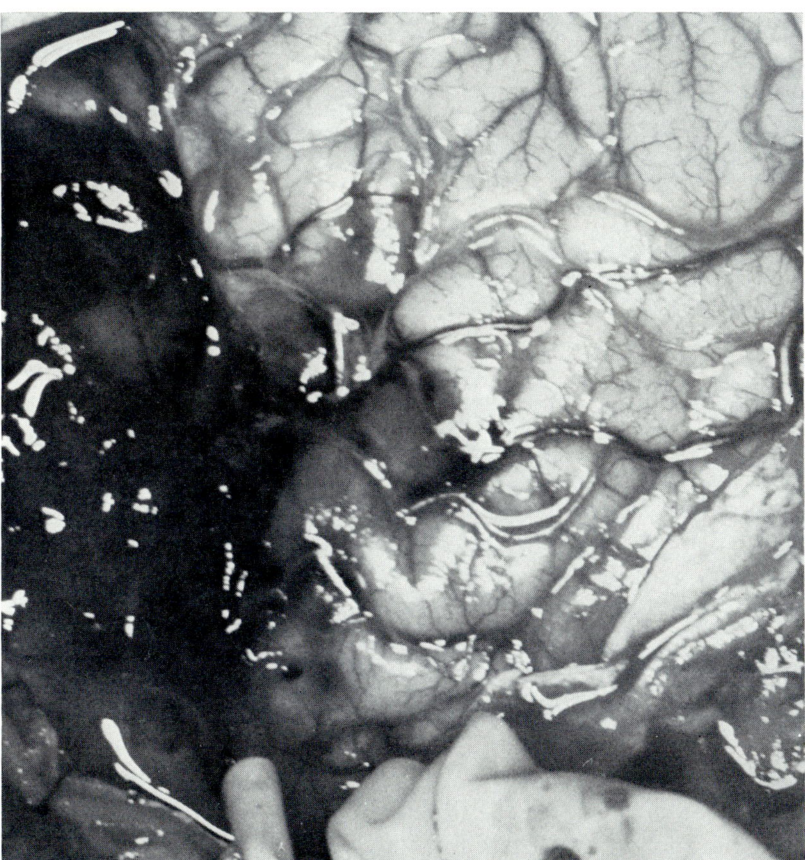

Figure 24. Acute frontal subdural hematoma. The solid clot of the acute subdural is associated with frontopolar and temporopolar contusion.

B. Anterior fossa extradural hematoma syndrome—this reveals slightly delayed signs following frontopolar trauma. Deterioration is often not as rapid as in the more common middle fossa extradural hematoma.

C. Acute obstructive hydrocephalus (Fig. 25)—rapidly dilating anterior horns in high-pressure hydrocephalus of various etiology may result in signs simulating a progressive frontopolar mass.

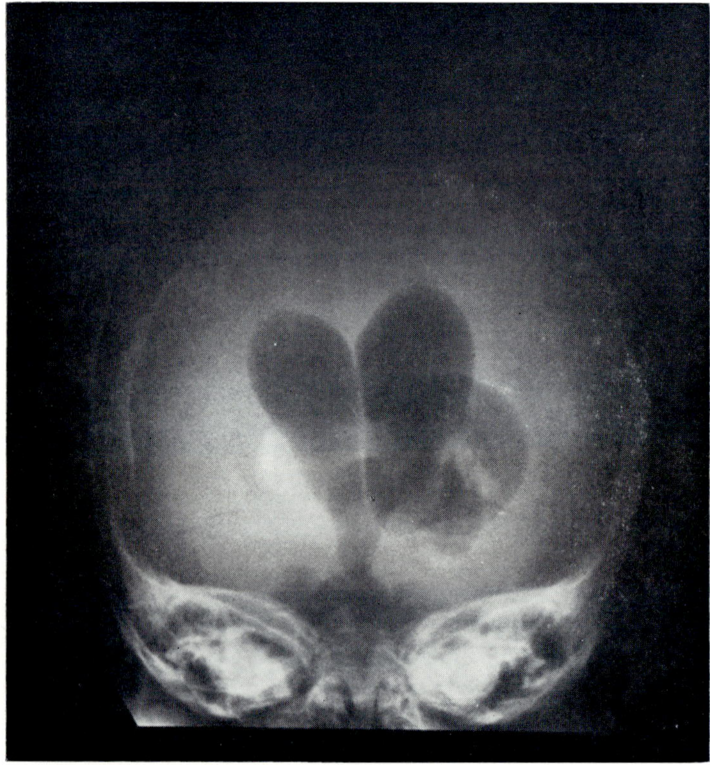

Figure 25. Hydrocephalus with frontal porencephalic cyst. The anterior horns are enlarged and their contours are rounded. Widening of the lateral angle of the anterior horn is often the earliest hydrocephalic sign. A porencephalic ventricular cyst is also present. The third ventricle is enlarged as well.

D. Osteomyelitis of the frontal bone—this is often the result of frontal sinusitis. There may be edema, erythema and tenderness over the forehead. There may be minimal signs of inflammation in patients receiving antibiotic treatment for sinusitis. Neurological deterioration indicates extension of infection to the brain (brain abscess, cerebritis), meninges (meningitis, subdural or epidural empyema) or major venous sinuses (sagittal sinus, cavernous sinus).

E. Frontopolar glioma (Fig. 26)—personality changes, mental aberrations and generalized convulsions of weeks or months duration may be historically obtained. There may be a short history of bifrontal or generalized headaches, vague visual disturbances and progressive obtundation. Memory disturbance and apathy may cloud historical facts which must be obtained from relatives.

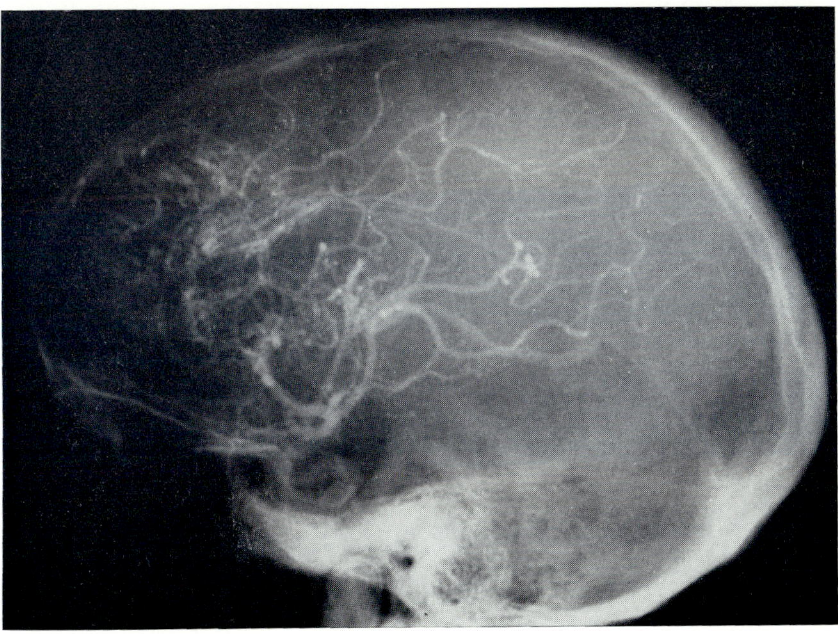

Figure 26. Frontal glioblastoma. Multiple pathological vessels of the type shown indicate glioblastoma.

F. Frontal parasagittal meningioma (Fig. 27)—the headaches are often of many months or years duration. Generalized seizures, progressive visual loss and mental abnormalities may also be historically present over many months.

G. Globular pterion meningioma—these outer sphenoidal tumors may produce focal cerebral seizures and eventual contralateral hemiparesis. With significant anterior fossa extension of the growth, there is subfalcial herniation of the ipsilateral frontal pole with compression of the opposite frontal pole.

H. Mucocele and osteoma of the frontal sinus—these may be silent, locally erosive or inflammatory in their manifestations.

I. Frontal encephalomeningocele—if not detected grossly in infancy, these may present later in life as an occult mass in the region of the nasion.

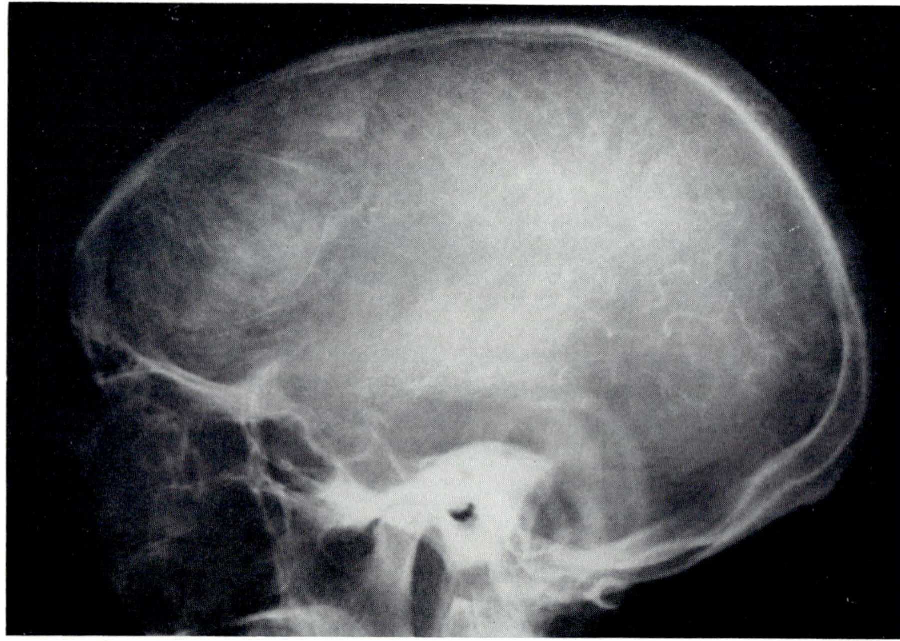

Figure 27. Frontopolar parasagittal meningioma. An angiographic "sunburst effect" is noted in the pronounced tumor cloud of this frontal meningioma.

Deficits of Frontopolar Syndromes

A. "Sign-silence"—especially common in unilateral, minor hemisphere lesions of intermediate or gradual development, in the absence of elevated intracranial pressure.

B. Behavioral signs of prefrontal syndrome—may be produced by the following:
   1. Bifrontal intracerebral lesion.
   2. Corpus callosum tumor.
   3. Unifrontal intracerebral mass of major hemisphere.
   4. Unifrontal intracerebral mass of minor hemisphere with elevated intracranial pressure.
   5. Midline extracerebral mass with mesial bifrontopolar compression.
   6. Lateral extracerebral mass with subfalcial herniation of ipsilateral frontal pole and bifrontopolar compression.
   7. Acute obstructive hydrocephalus with rapidly expanding anterior horns.
   8. Dementias and diffuse diseases of the cerebrum.

C. Neuropsychological signs
   1. Signs of visual inattention—frontal visual agnosia, inertia of gaze, easy

distractability, and apparent concentric contraction of visual fields due to inattention.

2. Impairment of recent memory; impaired voluntary and serial memorizing.
3. Frontal acalculia—general deterioration in calculation; may add and subtract but not multiply; perseverate calculation—subtraction of 7's from 100: 93,83,73; improper pronunciation of numbers.
4. Confusional episodes, disorientation in place and time, confabulation.
5. Apathy, lack of spontaneity, general slowing of intellectual process—especially in frontal pole of major hemisphere.
6. Apathetic-akinetic-abulic syndrome.

D. Ictal signs
1. Unconscious adversive seizure—loss of consciousness at the outset, with contralateral conjugate deviation of the eyes and head (Fig. 28) and posturing of contralateral arm.
2. Usually no aura; aura of desire to speak occasionally occurs.
3. Forced thinking syndrome of Penfield—a recurrent thought occurring as an aura to a generalized convulsion.
4. Psychomotor seizures—of temporal lobe type; parosmia usually unpleasant as in an uncinate seizure; pleasant olfactory hallucination—rare, but suggests anterior cingulate focus. Any olfactory hallucination should suggest the possibility of neoplasm.

E. Motor signs—lesions strictly limited to the frontal pole-prefrontal region, without elevated intracranial pressure, do not result in motor paresis or paralysis. However, voluntary motor control is impaired. The smaller the impairment, the more complex must be the motor task required to elicit the deficit. The "higher motor deficit" of the frontal pole consists of the following:
1. Difficulty with serial, alternate or novel motor tasks.
2. Difficulty with conflict motor tasks—verbal and visual instruction conflict is presented to the patient.
3. Verbal-motor disconnection—especially in major hemisphere lesion.
4. Motor perservation—repeated and often stereotyped motor response.
5. Motor reaction to irrelevant stimuli—random eye movements, disturbed search movements.
6. Ataxia limited to the contralateral leg—early sign of frontal pole lesion; tandem-walking shows awkward use of the contralateral foot.
7. Bilateral frontal ataxia—may be a late sign of a frontal mass; dysdiadochokinesis, dysmetria, and scanning speech are not components of frontal ataxia; cerebellar ataxia may eventually be produced by late effects of a frontal mass (cerebellar compression, displacement, herniation).

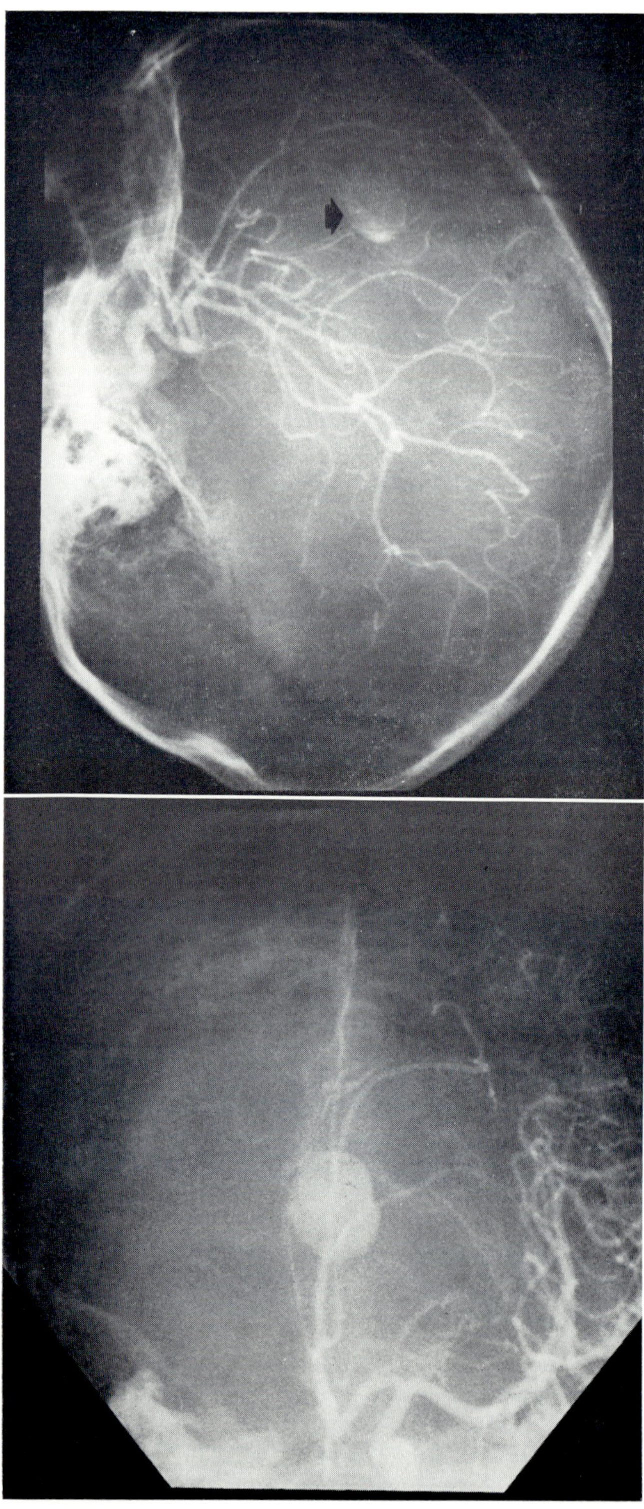

8. Tremor of the ipsilateral hand.
9. Homolateral motor syndrome—ipsilateral hemiplegia especially with the frontopolar extracerebral mass; due to posterior displacement of of the hemisphere and contralateral compression of the cerebral peduncle at the tentorial edge.
10. Loss of the superficial abdominal reflex, contralateral—may be an early sign, occurring in the absence of the Babinski sign; may be associated with a hyperactive deep (stretch) abdominal reflex.
11. Tonic plantar reflex, ipsilateral—slow tonic flexion of toes with slow release; may be an early sign of frontopolar mass; may occur in the absence of Babinski or grasp reflexes.
12. Plantar flexor reflexes, contralateral—quick toe flexion to percussion of the ball of the foot (Rossolimo sign) or dorsum of the foot (Mendel-Bechterew sign).

F. Signs of extension into regions adjacent to the frontal pole.
   1. Mesial cingulate extension.
      a. Akinetic mutism—bilateral anterior cingulate involvement.
      b. Autonomic signs—tachypnea, tachycardia.
      c. Leg weakness, unilateral or bilateral.
      d. Left-sided motor apraxia—anterior callosal extension.
      e. Variations in level of consciousness.
   2. Posterior premotor and motor extension.
      a. Grasp reflex—contralateral.
      b. Hoffmann sign—contralateral.
      c. Babinski sign—contralateral.
      d. Apraxia of gait, "magnetic apraxia" of the foot to the floor, "star-gait" (zig-zag).
      e. Inability to stand and walk—"astasia-abasia."
   3. Inferolateral frontal extension.
      a. Buccofacial apraxia.
      b. Facial weakness, contralateral.
      c. Expressive aphasia or dysphasia—major hemisphere.

G. Cranial nerve signs in frontopolar lesions.
   1. Papilledema—tends to occur late and may be absent despite elevated intracranial pressure.
   2. Anosmia and optic atrophy—basal frontal extension.
   3. Other cranial nerve signs—due to elevated intracranial pressure (uni-

Figure 28. Pericallosal aneurysm— lateral *(top)* and *AP (bottom)*. This unusual aneurysm presented with intracranial hemorrhage in a child of six years of age. Intracerebral hematoma was evident around the aneurysm sac. Adversive movements and deep coma occurred with the hemorrhage.

lateral or bilateral abducens palsy) and transtentorial herniation (ipsilateral oculomotor palsy).

H. Trauma signs
   1. Palpable supraorbital or depressed frontal fracture.
   2. Anterior sagittal sinus laceration.
      a. Compound midline frontal fracture with venous hemorrhage.
      b. Closed head injury with depressed midline frontal fracture.
   3. Traumatic sagittal sinus thrombosis—usually associated with linear fracture crossing the sinus; signs of elevated intracranial pressure and and intracerebral hemorrhage.
   4. Frontal sinus—anterior fossa fracture.
      a. Naso-oral hemorrhage and CSF rhinorrhea.
      b. Periorbital ecchymosis, swelling and subcutaneous emphysema.
   5. Coup frontopolar contusion.
      a. Depressed consciousness—traumatic brain swelling.
      b. Adversive early seizures.
      c. Acute subdural hematoma—often associated; tearing of superficial bridging veins and cortical laceration; progressive coma without lucid interval; transtentorial herniation syndrome (see below).
   6. Anterior fossa extradural hematoma syndrome.
      a. Prolonged "lucid interval"—hemorrhage due to a peripheral anterior meningeal arterial tear; bleeding and brain compression occur at a slower rate than in the more common middle (temporal) fossa extradural; the latter presents with either a rapidly progressive coma and no lucid interval, or with a brief lucid interval.
      b. Gradually increasing stupor.
      c. Initially slight contralateral central facial weakness due to frontal cortical compression.
      d. Transtentorial herniation syndrome.
         (1) Increasing coma.
         (2) Generalized increase in tone ("Gegenhalten"), especially in legs; often with stiff neck.
         (3) Contralateral hemiparesis, ipsilateral dilated pupil, noisy respiration, arterial hypertension, and bradycardia constitute the typical pattern.
         (4) Fixed pupil (s), extraocular palsy, decerebrate posture.
         (5) Eventual medullary collapse—hypoventilation, thready tachycardia, hypotension.
   7. Signs of associated flexion-extension neck injury—cervical spinal cord syndrome.
      a. Quadriplegia.

b. High sensory level.
c. Respiratory paralysis.
d. Abdominal distension.
e. Urinary retention.
f. Hypotension.

I. Syndrome of the parasagittal meningioma of the anterior third of the sagittal sinus
1. Long history of headaches, bifrontal or generalized.
2. Advanced chronic papilledema and secondary optic atrophy.
3. Generalized seizures—not as common as symptoms of visual loss.
4. Behavioral signs of bilateral frontopolar compression.

J. Syndrome of the parasagittal hyperostosing meningioma of the bregma
1. Visible or palpable bony midline mass most commonly at the bregma (union of sagittal and coronal sutures) .
2. Bony hyperostosis is excessive in comparison to size of the meningioma.
3. Tumor spreads down the falx bilaterally—eventually occludes the sagittal sinus.
4. Generalized seizures.
5. Unilateral globular extension of tumor—late signs of elevated intracranial pressure and paralysis greatest in the contralateral leg.

K. Syndrome of the frontal brain abscess (Fig. 29A-D) .
1. Frontal pole—common site of brain abscess; secondary to direct extension or retrograde infection via emissary veins from the following:
   a. Acute or chronic frontal sinusitis, with or without the following:
      (1) Osteomyelitis of frontal bone.
      (2) Extradural empyema.
      (3) Subdural empyema.
   b. Frontal fracture; penetrating injury with foreign body; CSF rhinorrhea.
   c. Frontal sinus obstruction and secondary infection—mucocele, osteoma.
2. Early signs of infection—fever, chills.
   a. Often not present unless primary focus (frontal sinusitis or osteomyelitis) is active.
   b. Headache, vomiting and generalized convulsions may occur in the early phase—"cerebritis."
3. Later signs of frontopolar mass.
   a. Elevated intracranial pressure—papilledema is common; abducens palsy; stupor.
   b. Frontal behavioral deficits.

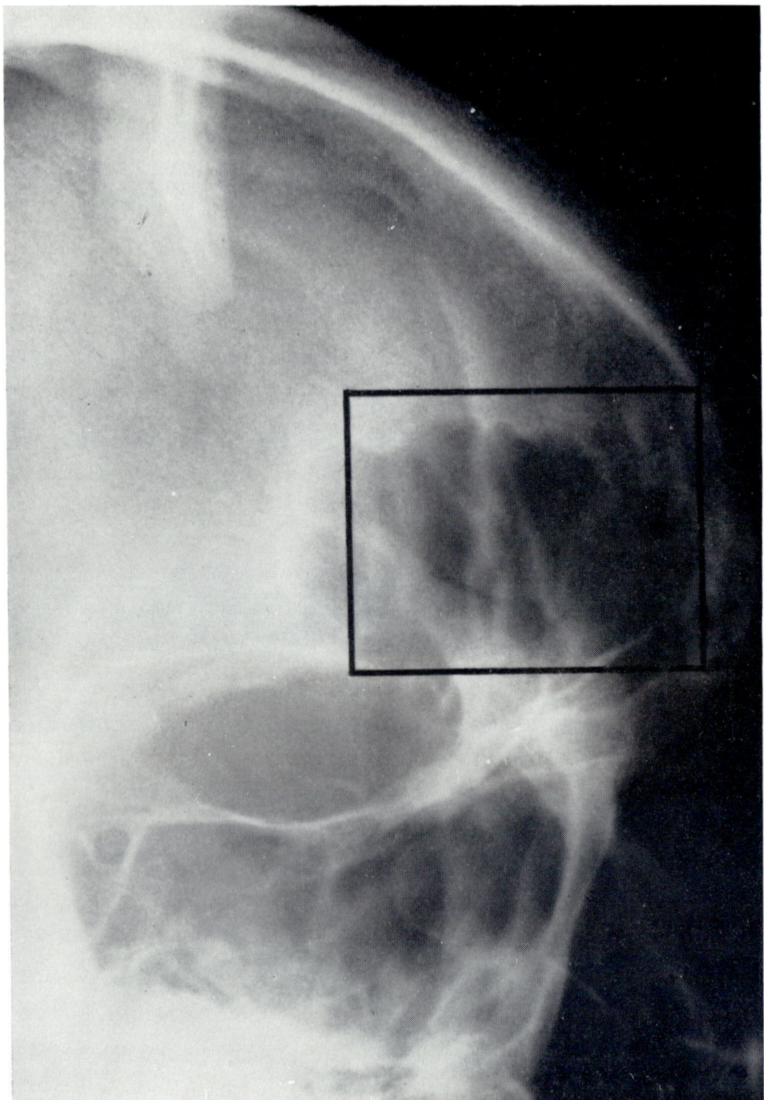

Figure 29 A.

Figure 29. *(A)* Frontal sinus fracture with frontal brain abscess. A stellate fracture in the frontal sinus is enclosed within the rectangle. *(B)* A rounded frontal shift of the pericallosal artery across the midline is seen in the AP arteriogram. *(C)* By virtue of the sinus fracture, air was present within the abscess cavity and can be seen within the frontopolar abscess in the lateral arteriogram. Middle and anterior cerebral arteries are caudally displaced while the carotid siphon is depressed *(D)* The relative avascularity of the frontal mass is best seen in the lateral venous phase.

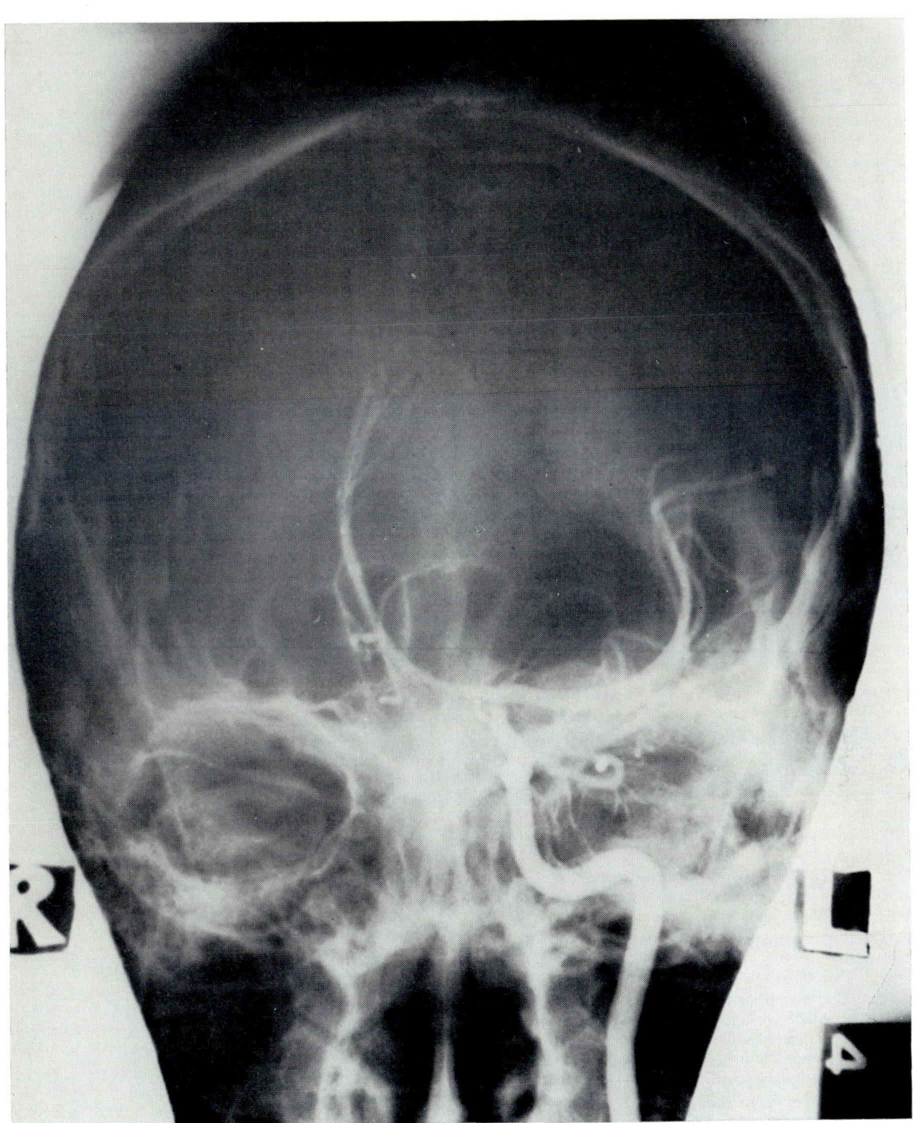

Figure 29 B.

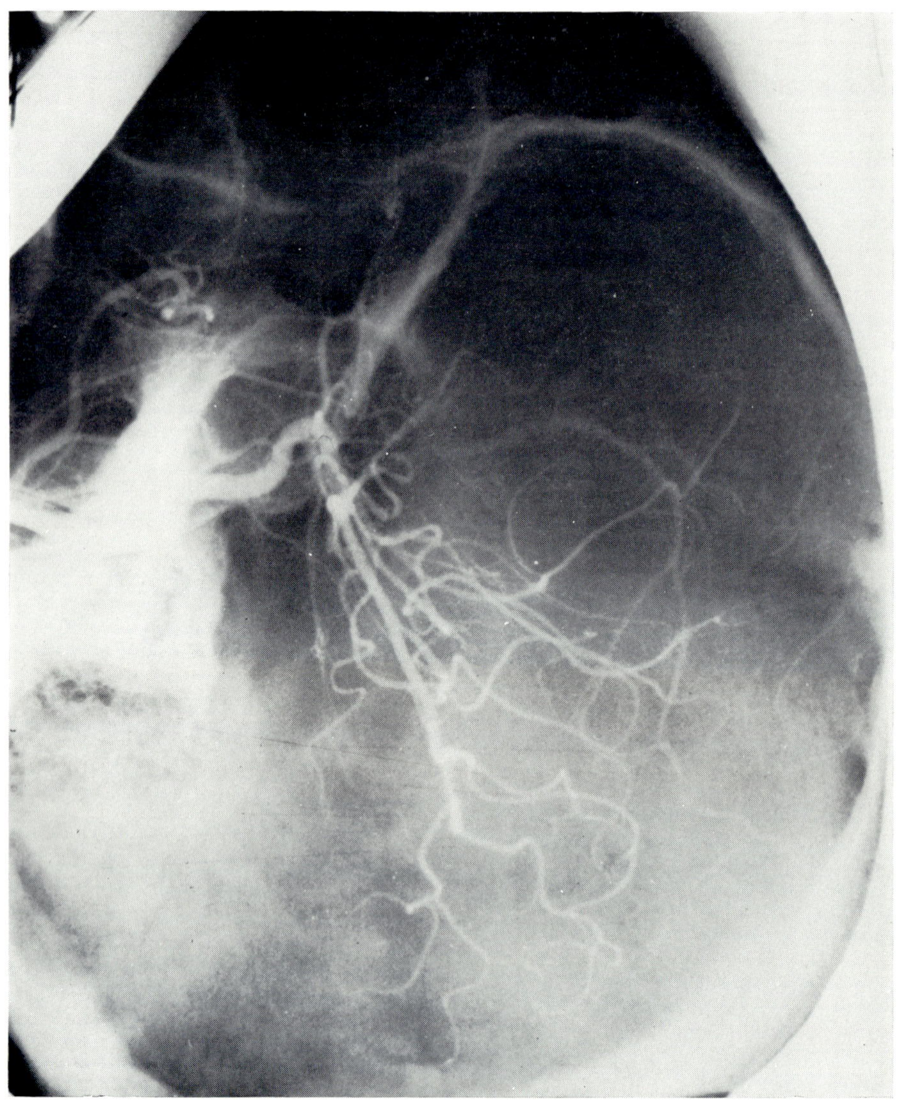

Figure 29 C.

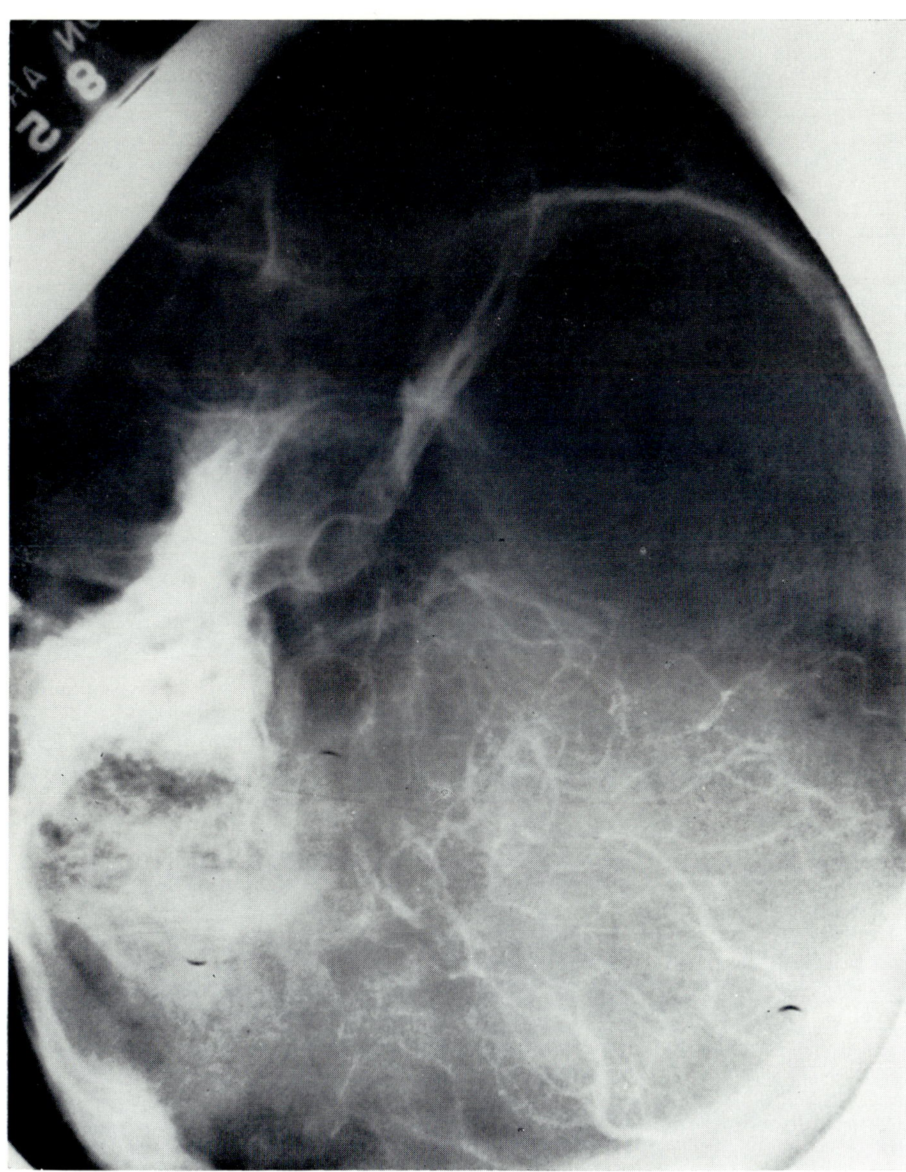

Figure 29 D.

c. Generalized seizures.
d. Often normal or subnormal temperature.

L. Satellite syndromes
1. Syndrome of frontal osteomyelitis.
a. Frontal bone—the most common site of osteomyelitis of skull vault.
b. The area of involved skull may be inconspicuous.
c. Postsinusitis, post-traumatic, postsurgical etiologies.
d. Clinical signs—edema of forehead, tenderness, erythema, periorbital swelling, and fever.
e. Clinical signs usually precede X-ray changes.

2. Frontal epidural abscess syndrome.
a. Localized to frontal region by adherence of dura to inner table at the coronal suture.
b. Severe frontal headache, with history of frontal sinusitis is typical.
c. Paucity of neurological signs.

3. Subdural empyema syndrome.
a. Not localized; spreads widely through subdural space.
b. History of frontal sinusitis is common.
c. Headache, chills and fever are typical in acute empyema.
d. Papilledema is common.
e. Syndrome of cerebral thrombophlebitis.
(1) Severe headache.
(2) Generalized or focal convulsions.
(3) Hemiparesis.
(4) Secondary to sinusitis, dental infection, meningitis, subdural empyema or septic venous sinus thrombosis.

4. Syndrome of cavernous sinus thrombosis.
a. Secondary to infection arising in the following:
(1) Central facial triangle—apex at frontal sinus, base along upper lip to nasolabial folds.
(2) Orbit.
b. Sudden onset with fever and chills; unilateral eye pain rapidly becoming bilateral; first division pain in forehead.
c. Acute papilledema, exophthalmos, periorbital edema, chemosis, diplopia and oculomotor palsy—bilateral, due to extension through the circular sinus.
d. Acute meningitis.

5. Syndrome of superior sagittal sinus thrombosis.
a. Septic.
(1) Infection within the central facial triangle, frontal osteomye-

litis, epidural or subdural empyema, extension from cavernous or lateral sinus infection.

(2) Fever, headache, papilledema; intracranial hemorrhage secondary to sinus and cortical venous obstruction; generalized attacks or jacksonian seizures beginning in the foot; paraplegia or hemiplegia; aphasia; pulmonary embolism and lung abscess may occur secondarily.

b. Nonseptic.

(1) Infantile (dehydration) nonseptic sinus thrombosis—edema of forehead, dilated fontanelle veins, convulsions.

(2) Anemia, polycythemia, leukemia, hypercoagulopathy, or hypotension may be associated.

(3) Gradual occlusion by parasagittal meningioma (adult)—may be silent.

(4) Acute traumatic occlusion—elevated intracranial pressure, intracerebral hemorrhage and focal deficits.

6. Syndrome of the nasofrontal mass of childhood.

a. Nasofrontal encephalomeningocele.

(1) May be occult, with slight widening of the root of the nose with a normal skin cover.

(2) May gradually enlarge with growth of the child and mimic solid tumor (firm, nonpulsatile).

(3) Rupture, CSF leak, meningitis.

(4) Marked hypertelorism, microphthalmia, microcephaly, and hydrocephalus—with gross nasofrontal encephalomeningocele.

b. Nasal glioma of infancy.

(1) Noninvasive developmental anomaly, usually extranasal over the bridge of the nose.

(2) May be intranasal and intracranial through a cribriform defect.

(3) CSF rhinorrhea, meningitis.

c. Angioma and dermoid—may present as a nasofrontal mass in infancy.

d. Common nasal polyp—rare under age five.

e. Primary olfactory neuroblastoma.

(1) Rare under the age of ten (in contrast to adrenal neuroblastoma of infancy occurring rarely after age five).

(2) May occur in an adult with a history of nasal polypectomy.

(3) Invasive with epistaxis, sinusitis, invasion of frontal bone and anterior fossa, penetration of dura, extension of tumor to the frontal pole; also frontopolar brain abscess may be associated.

(4) Invasion of orbit, maxillary antrum and distant metastasis.

Deformities (Angiographic and Pneumographic) of the Frontopolar Syndromes

A. Angiographic deformities
  1. Extracerebral frontopolar mass (e.g. meningioma).
    a. Posterior displacement (lateral view).
      (1) Anterior cerebral artery, proximal segment.
      (2) Pericallosal artery, flattening or reversal of genu.
      (3) Middle cerebral artery, proximal segment.
      (4) Internal cerebral vein, anterior segment.
    b. Midline shift (AP view).
      (1) Anterior cerebral artery, round shift.
      (2) Pericallosal artery, round shift, with posterior pericallosal returning to midline; a false anterior shift may result from slight rotation of the head.
      (3) Frontopolar artery, proximal segment.
      (4) Falx sign—hooking and depression of anterior cerebral artery by the falx as it returns to the midline after frontal shift.
      (5) No shift—midline extracerebral polar mass.
    c. Angiographic meningioma signs.
      (1) Prominence of frontopolar artery, sometimes more obvious than anterior cerebral.
      (2) Enlargement of superficial veins to the sagittal sinus—some parasagittal meningiomas.
      (3) Poor and delayed filling of frontal veins—any large frontal mass, extra or intracerebral.
      (4) Occlusion of anterior sagittal sinus.
      (5) Usual angiographic and plain skull meningioma signs—extracerebral blood supply, arterial "sunburst," homogenous tumor cloud, peripheral zone of increased density, hyperostosis.
  2. Intracerebral frontopolar mass (e.g. glioma).
    a. No meningioma signs.
    b. More prominent displacement of major arterial trunks due to associated cerebral edema may be present.
    c. Angiographic glioma signs.
      (1) Prominent arteriovenous drainage into deep veins.
      (2) Displacement of lenticulostriate arteries.
      (3) Widening of pericallosal genu due to extension into the corpus callosum.
      (4) Arteriovenous shunt with early veins, or just avascular mass.

B. Pneumoencephalographic deformities.

1. Amputation of anterior horn—foreshortened, truncated anterior horn; "mushroom deformity"; most common pneumographic frontopolar sign.
2. "Silver-fork deformity"—depression of the roof of the ipsilateral ventricle, due to subfalcial herniation, not to superior mass.
3. Depression of anterior horn—entire anterior horn inferiorly displaced by superopolar frontal mass.
4. Displacement of anterior horns and septum away from polar tumor.
5. Inequality of size of anterior horns, larger anterior horn usually contralateral; dilatation is not prominent.
6. Irregularity of anterior horn—suggests intracerebral mass (glioma) especially when bilateral.
7. Separation of anterior horns—either anterior parasagittal meningioma or invasion of septum by glioma.
8. Associated narrowing of temporal horn—any large frontal mass.
9. Deformities and shift of superior longitudinal fissure, cistern of corpus callosum, and cingulate sulcus—any frontopolar mass.
10. Late signs of large frontopolar mass with elevated pressure—posterior displacement of third ventricle and ambient wing cisterns (posterior border of pulvinar in lateral view).

Additional Diagnostic Clues in Frontopolar Syndromes

A. Plain skull x-rays

1. Posterior displacement of a calcified pineal by a frontal mass is often present. Pineal shift across the midline, if present, is less than angiographic anterior cerebral shift to the opposite side.
2. Benign hyperostosis frontalis interna—the hyperostosis is usually minimal in the midline and not associated with excessive vascular channels. The hyperostosis may be irregular or sheetlike. It is usually symmetrical and occasionally extends to other portions of the caudal calvarium. It should be differentiated from the hyperostosis of the anterior parasagittal meningioma.
3. Enlarged bregmatic veins—normal variant to be differentiated from parasagittal meningioma which may produce enlarged middle meningeal arterial channels.
4. Frontal sinus trauma—fracture of the posterior wall may be associated with visible herniation of the frontal pole into the sinus air shadow; pneumocephalus; "spontaneous ventriculogram"; depressed fracture often appears white and fragmented.
5. Frontal sinus infection—sinusitis; associated osteomyelitis of the frontal bone is indicated by irregular mottling and bone erosion.

6. Frontal sinus mass—mucocele; osteoma (see Ch. 2).
7. Nasofrontal defect—encephalomeningocele or tumor.

B. EEG

1. Unilateral frontopolar mass—unifrontal or frontotemporal high voltage slow activity (delta).
2. Midline frontopolar mass—bifrontal or bitemporal slow activity.
3. Seizure discharge—spikes and sharp waves may be focal or generalized; "secondary bilateral synchrony" suggests either mesial or subfrontal locus, mimicking brain stem origin.
4. Exceptionally slow focal frontal or frontotemporal activity—suggests brain abscess; often with widespread abnormality in addition to focal slowing; suggestive, but nondiagnostic.

C. Brain scan.

1. High uptake in parasagittal meningioma, glioblastoma and arteriovenous malformation.
2. Often positive in frontal abscess and may be positive in frontal osteomyelitis.
3. Often negative in low-grade, relatively avascular tumors.

CHAPTER 4

FRONTODORSAL SYNDROMES

Anatomical and Physiological Correlates

Sector: 4; the precentral motor region of the parasagittal and dorsal convexity

Angiogram: Anterior Suprasylvian

Pneumogram: Supraforaminal

Neuroanatomy of the Frontodorsal Region

A. The motor components
   1. Rolandic motor—in the depths of the central fissure and along the precentral gyrus.
      a. Parasagittal—paracentral lobule (cortical representation—leg).
      b. Dorsal—high (trunk-arm) and middle (hand-fingers) convexities.
      c. Lateral—low (face-vocalization) convexity; considered in Chapter 5 with frontolateral syndromes related to speech.

   Note: The central fissure is identified by the position of the rolandic artery. The "rolandic point" lies 2 cm posterior to the midpoint of the sagittal sinus. The central fissure has three segments: (1) mesial segment—a notch within the paracentral lobule, (2) dorsal segment—the "superior genu" or upper two-thirds of the central fissure which is concave rostrally, and (3) lateral segment—the "inferior genu" or lower third which is convex rostrally. The "rolandic operculum" lies within the central fissure at the juncture of the dorsal and lateral segments. The "motor strip" is obtained by electrostimulation producing focal motor responses at threshold intensity. The physiological motor strip may not always exactly correspond to the anatomical precentral gyrus.

   2. Premotor—immediately rostral to the rolandic motor cortex; the premotor region is not clearly demarcated from the frontal pole, which it joins in the vicinity of the coronal suture.
   3. Supplementary motor—the mesial parasagittal region rostral to the rolandic motor (leg) area of the paracentral lobule.
   4. Frontal oculomotor—posterior portion of the middle frontal gyrus, superior to the frontolateral region of Broca.

B. Afferent frontomotor pathways
   1. Thalamocortical.
      a. Ventral lateral nucleus (VL)—to entire frontomotor region.
      b. Ventral anterior nucleus (VA)—to premotor region.

2. Associational.
    a. Frontopolar, parietal and temporal—ipsilateral.
    b. Occipital eye field—to frontal oculomotor field, ipsilateral.
3. Commissural.
    a. Premotor region—bilateral connections to rolandic motor cortex.
    b. Parietal—callosal connections to the contralateral frontomotor region, in addition to ipsilateral projections.

C. Efferent frontomotor pathways
1. Corticospinal (pyramidal) tract—includes fibers of diverse origin, notably descending frontomotor and postcentral projections. The corticobulbar and "aberrant pyramidal tracts" do not enter the medullary pyramids and are therefore not strictly pyramidal; they arise from the frontolateral region and are considered in Chapter 5.
    a. Internal capsule—the corticospinal tract occupies the posterior limb, caudal to the corticobulbar tract (rostrocaudal sequence—face, arm, trunk, leg).
    b. Cerebral peduncle—the corticospinal tract occupies the central zone, lateral to the corticobulbar tract (mediolateral sequence—face, arm, trunk, leg).
    c. Pons—the corticospinal tract lies in bundles separated by the pontine nuclei and transverse pontine fibers.
    d. Medulla—motor decussation.
        (1) Crossed corticospinal tract—the majority of fibers of the lateral corticospinal tract (arm medial to leg).
        (2) Uncrossed corticospinal tract—a minority of fibers remaining in the ipsilateral corticospinal tract (leg).
        (3) Direct corticospinal tract—a small component of fibers forming the ipsilateral anterior corticospinal tract (neck and trunk) eventually crossing at cervicothoracic levels.
2. Frontal oculomotor projections.
    a. Occipital eye fields—ipsilateral inferior fronto-occipital fasciculus.
    b. Frontopontine tract—oculomotor projections from the frontal eye field join the descending frontopontine tract.
        (1) Internal capsule—near the genu.
        (2) Upper midbrain—in the most medial third of the cerebral peduncle.
        (3) Lower midbrain—rostral pons—majority cross (rostral to the facial decussation).
        (4) Pontine gaze center—contralateral; this in turn projects to the adjacent abducens nucleus and opposite oculomotor nucleus via the medial longitudinal fasciculus.

3. Corticothalamic—reciprocal innervation of the ventral lateral nucleus; also frontomotor projections to the center median nucleus.
4. Corticostriate.
   a. Rolandic motor—projects bilaterally upon the caudate-putamen complex.
   b. Premotor—projects ipsilaterally upon caudate and putamen.
   c. Supplementary motor—projects to the ipsilateral caudate head.
5. Corticoincertal, corticonigral, corticorubral and corticotegmental—descending frontomotor fibers to the core structures of the mesencephalic-diencephalic junction.

Blood Supply of the Frontodorsal Region

A. Arterial
   1. Ascending frontal arteries, middle cerebral—these are cortical branches which arise distal to the origin of the orbitofrontal artery.
      a. Prerolandic branch—supplies the premotor and oculomotor region.
      b. Rolandic branch—supplies the rolandic region. Both arteries supply the frontodorsal and frontolateral convexity cortex.
   2. Subcortical lenticulostriate branches, middle cerebral—supply the anterior two-thirds of the posterior limb of the internal capsule (i.e. corticospinal tract) .
   3. Callosomarginal artery, anterior cerebral—this is the cortical branch supplying the supplementary motor and paracentral motor and sensory regions for the leg and foot on the mesial surface. It also supplies adjacent superior frontal gyrus along the vertex.

B. Venous
   1. Superficial frontal (rolandic) veins—to the superior sagittal sinus.
   2. Superficial middle cerebral (sylvian) vein—to the sphenoparietal and cavernous sinuses.
   3. Greater anastomotic vein of Trolard—communicates with the following:
      a. Superior sagittal sinus.
      b. Superficial middle cerebral vein.
      c. Lesser anastomotic vein of Labbé—in turn communicates with the lateral sinus.
   4. Subcortical lenticulostriate veins—drain into the deep middle cerebral vein, which, with the anterior cerebral vein, forms the basal vein of Rosenthal.

Infarction Syndromes of the Frontodorsal Region

A. Occlusion of the ascending frontal arteries—usually occurs with cortical middle cerebral occlusion distal to the perforating branches.

1. Contralateral hemiplegia, most severe in the face, arm and hand.
2. Cortical sensory deficits in the paralyzed limbs.
3. Expressive-receptive dysphasia—major hemisphere.

B. Occlusion of lenticulostriate arteries
1. Contralateral capsular hemiplegia of face, arm, hand and leg of equal severity.
2. Contralateral hemisensory deficit.
3. Contralateral homonymous hemianopia.
4. Aphasia, major hemisphere.

C. Occlusion of callosomarginal artery—paracentral lobule infarction
1. Contralateral leg paralysis.
2. Contralateral cortical sensory deficit in the leg.
3. Incontinence is common (but also occurs with other infarctions).

Neurophysiology of the Frontodorsal Region

A. Stimulation
1. Rolandic motor cortex.
   a. Low threshold stimulus—discrete movements of the contralateral distal extremity (e.g. movement of an individual finger) are most characteristic.
   b. Gross axial and proximal extremity movements have lesser rolandic "cortical representation."
   c. Standard sequence—foot and ankle, then leg movements occur with mesial parasagittal stimulation; upon the dorsal convexity, proceeding inferiorly along the precentral gyrus, trunk, arm, wrist, hand and individual finger movements are produced; there is thus an inverted representation of the trunk and upper extremity.
   d. Reversal of sequence—stimulation of the frontolateral (in contrast to frontodorsal) rolandic convexity is associated with an erect representation of the face, in which the upper face and eyes are superior to the large region devoted to the mouth and tongue just above the sylvian fissure; sequence reversal from an inverted to an erect pattern occurs at the frontodorsal-frontolateral junction.
   e. Vocalization—occurs on stimulation of the frontolateral rolandic region (see Ch. 5).
   f. Discrete movements of analogous type can also be obtained on postcentral rolandic stimulation of parietal cortex.
2. Premotor cortex.
   a. Higher threshold stimulation required.
   b. Slower, more complex movements of the opposite half of the body occur.

   c. Head and eyes turn to the opposite side with arm elevation, elbow flexion and leg extension.
3. Supplementary motor cortex.
   a. High threshold.
   b. Rostrocaudal sequence—head, arm, leg.
   c. Slow movements of the opposite extremities with frequent bilateral responses.
   d. Speech arrest.
   e. Pupillary dilatation and tachycardia.
4. Frontal oculomotor cortex.
   a. Conjugate lateral deviation of the eyes to the opposite side; occasionally to the same side.
   b. Inferior stimulation—conjugate vertical deviation upward.
   c. Superior stimulation—conjugate vertical deviation downward.
   d. Pupillary dilatation and opening of eyelids.
5. Stereotactic stimulation of corticospinal fibers in the internal capsule.
   a. The corticospinal tract in man occupies the middle portion of the posterior limb, between the ventrobasal complex of the thalamus and the lenticular nucleus.
   b. Rostrocaudal sequence (face, arm, trunk, leg) in the capsule is similar to that of the cortex (obliquity of the rolandic fissure with face most rostral) .

B. Ablation
1. Rolandic motor cortex, sparing the premotor region.
   a. Contralateral hypotonic paralysis, especially for fine, discrete movements.
   b. Babinski sign—contralateral.
   c. Absence of spasticity.
2. Premotor cortex, sparing rolandic motor cortex.
   a. Contralateral hypertonic paresis of skilled movement.
   b. Spasticity and hyperactive deep tendon reflexes.
   c. Forced grasping.
3. Supplementary motor cortical ablation.
   a. Contralateral bradykinesia with minimal paralysis.
   b. Apraxia of gait.
   c. Forced grasping.
4. Frontal oculomotor cortical ablation.
   a. Transient contralateral horizontal gaze palsy.
   b. Vertical conjugate gaze remains intact.
5. Pedunculotomy—central third.

a. Contralateral partial hemiparesis with some preservation of finger movement.
b. Contralateral Babinski sign.

6. Transection of medullary pyramid.
   a. Contralateral hypotonic hemiplegia with permanent loss of discrete finger movement.
   b. Contralateral Babinski sign.

NEUROSURGICAL SYNDROMES OF THE FRONTODORSAL REGION

Development

A. Syndrome of acute craniocerebral vertex trauma
   1. Acute bilateral frontodorsal cerebral contusion—immediate paraplegia or triplegia (hemiplegia opposite the side of the greatest injury, with ipsilateral weakness confined to the leg); focal motor seizures are common.
   2. Traumatic middle sagittal sinus thrombosis—usually associated with vertex fracture, which may or may not be depressed (Fig. 30); progressive development of paraplegia, hemiplegia or triplegia, intracerebral hemorrhage and brain swelling as a result of acute venous obstruction.

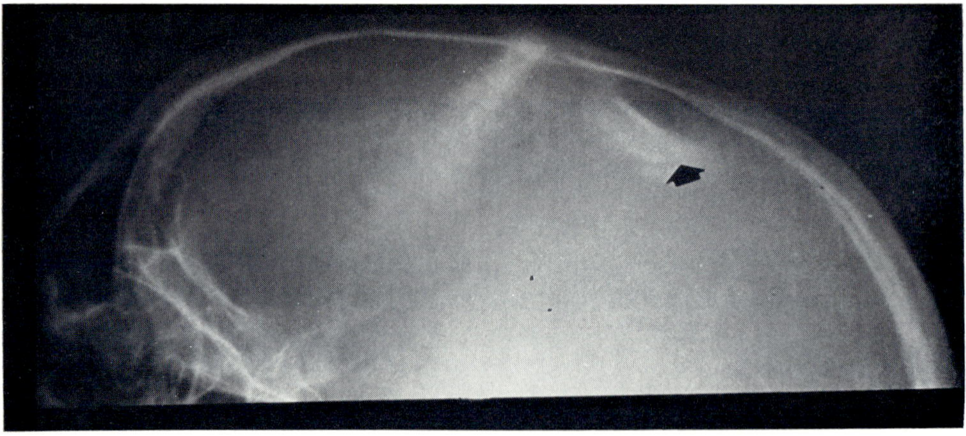

Figure 30. Depressed fracture of the cranial vertex. This high convexity frontodorsal depressed fracture lies in the region between the coronal suture and the central fissure of Rolando. Fracture lines on plain skull x-ray may appear black, gray or white.

   3. Parasagittal subdural hematoma—associated with tearing of cortical bridging veins to the sagittal sinus; major portion of hematoma along the falx, with progressive crural monoplegia of the opposite leg.

B. Syndrome of acute intracapsular hemorrhage—rapidly developing contralateral flaccid hemiplegia usually associated with coma, conjugate deviation of the eyes to the side of the clot, and chronic systemic hypertension.

C. Syndrome of the deep frontomotor glioma (Fig. 31)—progressive contralateral hemiparesis preceding the onset of generalized and focal motor seizures; progressive increase of intracranial pressure; seizures are common in astrocytoma and oligodendroglioma; fluctuating development of signs suggests a cystic glioma; rapid progression of signs suggests glioblastoma; sudden appearance of marked signs suggests intraneoplastic hemorrhage.

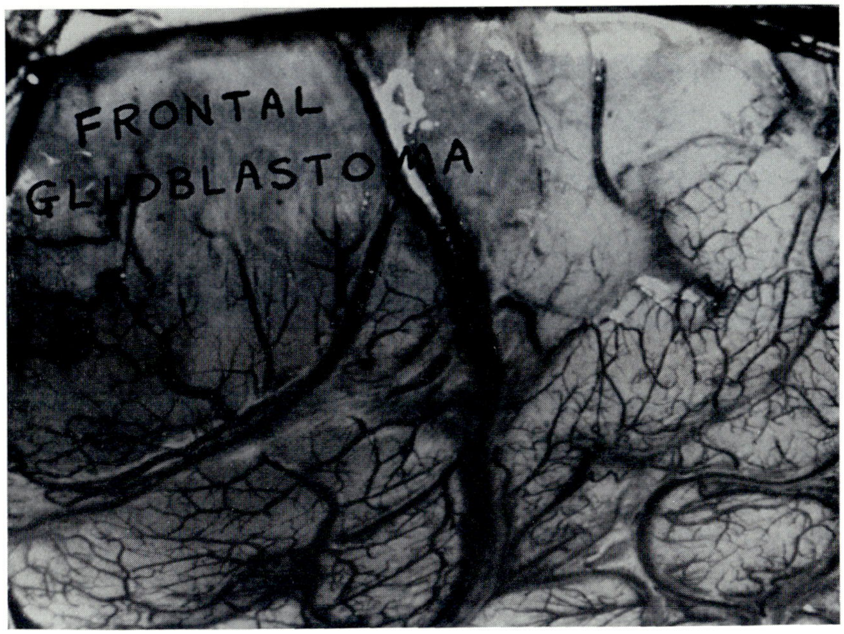

Figure 31. Frontodorsal glioblastoma. This frontal tumor is associated with marked pial invasion and vascular abnormality in the frontodorsal region.

D. Syndrome of the parasagittal meningioma of the central third of the sagittal sinus (Fig. 32).—focal jacksonian seizures beginning in the opposite foot may precede paralysis by months or years; slowly developing crural monoplegia of the opposite leg or paraplegia most marked distally occurs; occasionally isolated brachial monoplegia of the opposite arm occurs in prerolandic central-third meningiomas. The meningioma may arise from the falx well below the superior sagittal sinus (Fig. 33).

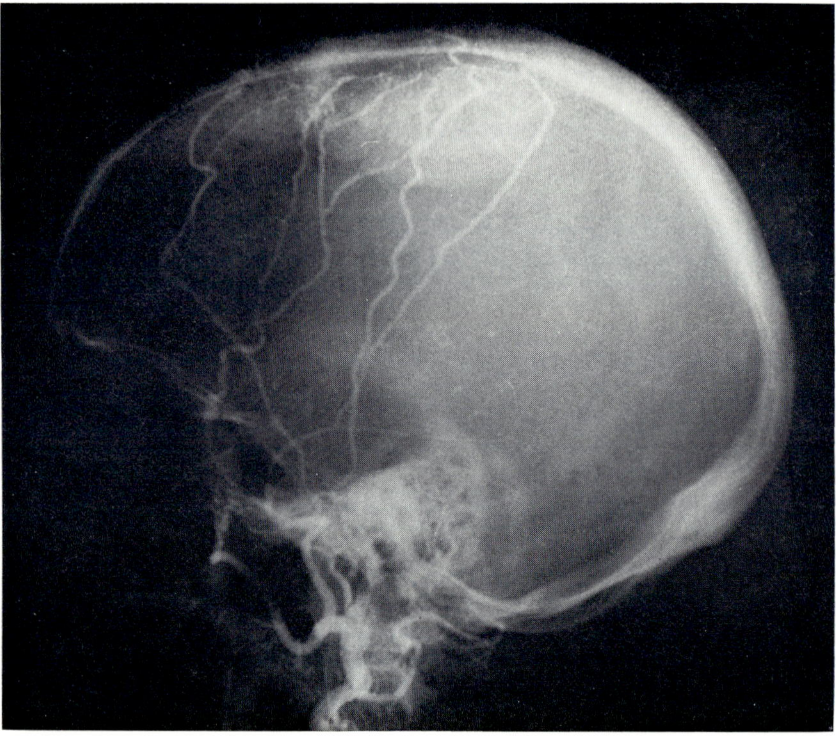

Figure 32. Frontodorsal parasagittal meningioma. External carotid supply to the parasagittal tumor cloud is prominent.

Deficits of the Frontodorsal Syndromes

Lesions involving the frontodorsal cortex or its subcortical pathways present a mixture of motor signs. Basic principles in central motor diagnosis are as follows:

1. The predominant motor deficit of the clinical mixture has the greatest localizing value.
2. The deeper the lesion, the more profound is the paralysis.
3. Deep subcortical lesions produce hemiplegias; monoplegia indicates a more superficial lesion.
4. Paralysis of rapid onset is flaccid early and spastic later; permanent flaccidity suggests thalamic or parietal extension.
5. Paralysis of gradual onset tends to be spastic from the beginning, especially as a result of lesions rostral to the precentral gyrus.
6. Cortical lesions tend to have focal motor seizures early and paralysis later (this does not apply to acute cortical lesions, in which case both seizures and paralysis are early signs).

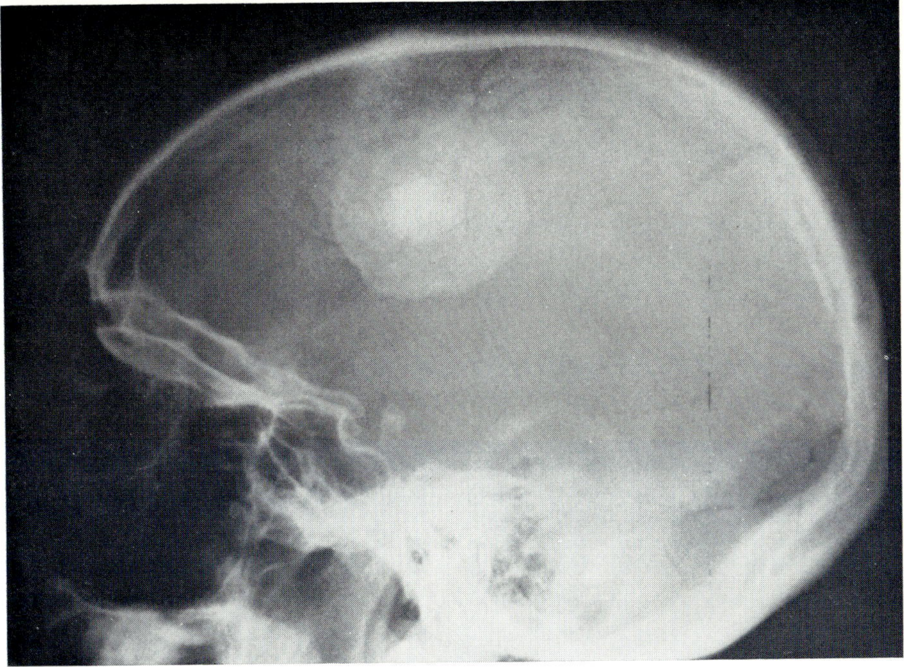

Figure 33. Falx meningioma. Tumor calcification deep in the interfrontal fissure indicates this midline frontodorsal meningioma arising from the falx at the inferior longitudinal sinus.

7. Deep subcortical lesions are usually associated with paralysis that precedes the onset of seizures.
8. Cortical lesions tend to produce dissociation with preservation of automatic and loss of voluntary movements.
9. Deep subcortical lesions produce more complete paralysis without dissociation.
10. Reverse-dissociation may occur in deep subcortical lesions with thalamolenticular extension (e.g. paralysis of spontaneous emotional expression exceeds that for voluntary movement) .

A. Rolandic motor deficits
   1. Paralytic signs.
      a. Brachial monoplegia—dorsal convexity rolandic lesion.
         (1) Paralysis of the opposite arm, most marked for discrete hand and finger movements.
         (2) Pseudoradial palsy—weakness most marked in the extensors of the hand and fingers, but including the small hand muscles.
         (3) Isolated digit palsy—especially the thumb and index finger; lower dorsal (middle convexity) region.

b. Crural monoplegia—mesial parasagittal rolandic lesion.
   (1) Paralysis of the opposite leg, most marked for distal foot and toe movements.
   (2) Decreased rate of "toe-tapping" and loss of all voluntary toe movement.
   (3) Pseudoperoneal palsy—weakness is most marked in dorsiflexion of the ankle, although plantar flexion is also impaired.
   (4) The above signs of rolandic foot paralysis may be minimal during walking.

c. Cortical hemiplegia—dorsomesial rolandic lesion.
   (1) Unequal paralysis of the opposite arm and leg, usually most marked for hand and finger movements.
   (2) Resembles the unequal distribution of centrum semiovale hemiplegia; the latter is commonly associated with apraxia.
   (3) Differs from the global hemiplegias occurring with capsular and brain stem lesions, in which both arm and leg are more equally and profoundly involved.

d. Faciobrachial paralysis—dorsolateral rolandic lesion.
   (1) Paralysis of the opposite lower face and arm with sparing of the leg.
   (2) Acute lesions lead to transient tongue deviation to the paralyzed side, with inability to point the tongue toward the side of the lesion.
   (3) Acute lesions may result in jaw deviation to the paralyzed side upon opening the mouth.
   (4) Faciobrachial paralysis of rolandic origin is maximal in the opposite face, hand and fingers; in contrast, faciobrachial paralysis greatest in the opposite face and shoulder suggests occlusion of Heubner's artery.

e. Central facial palsy.
   (1) Weakness of the opposite lower face, without any extremity weakness, occurs with lesions in the frontolateral rolandic, opercular, frontopolar, frontobasal and temporopolar regions; it may be the sole motor sign.
   (2) It is often associated with deficits in expressive speech when the lesion is situated in the dominant hemisphere (see Ch. 5).

f. Paracentral paraplegia—bilateral involvement of the mesial paracentral lobules.
   (1) Weakness of both lower extremities, most marked distally.
   (2) Bladder and rectal symptoms may occur.
   (3) Mimics spinal paraplegia; in the latter, sphincter disturbances are more extreme.

(4) Pontine paraplegia consists of flaccid lower extremities with hypertonus of the upper extremities.

g. Paracentral triplegia.

(1) Bilateral involvement with cortical paraplegia and hemiplegia combined.

(2) Greatest weakness is in the leg of the hemiplegic side.

2. Reflex signs of rolandic motor lesions.

a. Babinski sign—the most constantly present clinical sign of a corticospinal lesion; however, it may occur with lesions at any level from the frontomotor cortex to the L_5 segment of the spinal cord.

b. "Babinski equivalents"—less constant signs in which dorsiflexion of the great toe results from pressure beneath the external malleolus (Chaddock), stroking along the tibia (Oppenheim), squeezing the calf (Gordon), pinching the Achilles tendon (Schaefer), or downward snapping of the fourth toe (Gonda).

c. Deep tendon reflexes.

(1) Depressed on the opposite side in acute lesions associated with flaccid paralysis; return before the onset of spasticity, to become hyperactive with the evolution of spasticity.

(2) Exaggerated on the opposite side in slowly developing lesions associated with progressive spasticity.

d. Superficial abdominal reflexes.

(1) Depressed on the opposite side.

(2) May be associated with hyperactive deep abdominal (stretch) reflex opposite the lesion on percussion below the costal margin.

(3) Often associated with a depressed cremasteric reflex opposite the lesion.

e. Clonus.

(1) Sustained regular beats at the ankle, patella or wrist opposite the lesion.

(2) Like the other reflex signs, clonus occurs with cerebral, brain stem or spinal lesions.

3. Ictal signs of rolandic motor lesions.

a. Focal jacksonian motor seizure—gross clonic movements contralateral to the side of the lesion.

(1) Thumb and index finger—the most common site of onset; dorsal convexity.

(2) Corner of the mouth—next in frequency; lateral convexity.

(3) Foot, usually great toe—least of the three sites in frequency; mesial parasagittal.

b. Spread of motor ictus.

(1) May remain localized and continuous—"epilepsia partialis continua."

(2) "Jacksonian march"—spread occurs from the distal limb proximally; spread from this point to a second limb begins proximally and spreads distally; a slow rate of spread is more apt to remain confined to one limb.

(3) Consciousness—retained for a relatively long period; loss of consciousness accompanies rapid spread with bilateral motor convulsion.

c. Focal motor seizures and paralysis.

(1) Preictal paralysis—if present, it is magnified immediately postictally.

(2) Ictal paralysis—a rapidly appearing local paresis of transient duration may be the only ictal sign, occurring in the absence of convulsive movement.

(3) "Todd's postictal paralysis"—temporary weakness of convulsed parts following the ictal phase.

d. Focal motor seizures and brain tumor.

(1) The seizure may be the only sign of a brain tumor.

(2) The closer the tumor to the central fissure of Rolando, the higher the incidence of focal motor seizures.

(3) The focal motor seizures may be falsely localizing if the tumor is associated with elevated intracranial pressure and brain shift.

(4) Mixed jacksonian attacks, in which the distribution of the convulsive movement does not follow the usual pattern, suggest brain tumor rather than some other lesion.

(5) Epilepsia partialis continua is uncommon with brain tumors, occurring more often in atrophic and postencephalitic cases.

(6) Unusually prolonged Todd's postictal paralysis suggests the presence of a brain tumor.

(7) Focal paresis preceding the development of seizures favors a deep subcortical glioma.

(8) Generalized seizures preceding focal motor seizures also favors a deep subcortical glioma.

(9) Variability of the site of focal onset in an individual patient can occur with either a glioma or a meningioma.

(10) Seizures are most common in the slowly growing astrocytomas and meningiomas. While they are somewhat less common in the more rapidly advancing glioblastoma, when seizures do begin they tend to occur at more frequent intervals in these cases.

B. Premotor and supplementary motor deficits—the clinical signs of lesions of the dorsal premotor and mesial supplementary motor regions are similar in many respects and may be conveniently grouped together.
   1. Motor Signs.
      a. Paralysis.
         (1) Acute lesions produce transient paresis of the contralateral limbs with impairment of skilled movement.
         (2) Gross motor power is relatively preserved.
         (3) Paresis limited to the leg suggests mesial rather than dorsal convexity involvement.
      b. Spasticity.
         (1) Spasticity is prominent in premotor-supplementary motor lesions, diminishing as the lesion approaches the rolandic fissure; postcentral parietal lesions are typically flaccid.
         (2) Spasticity may precede paralysis in slowly developing premotor lesions.
      c. Apraxia.
         (1) Motor ("kinetic") apraxia—characteristic of a premotor lesion.
            (a) Clumsiness in the performance of purposeful movements of the hand in the absence of gross paralysis.
            (b) Left frontomotor lesions produce either bilateral or right-sided apraxia; right frontomotor lesions produce left-sided apraxia.
            (c) Lack of use of the apraxic limb resembles "parietal neglect," but other parietal signs are absent.
         (2) "Magnetic" apraxia—characteristic of supplementary motor lesions.
            (a) Apraxia of gait—the patient's feet stick to the ground during the initiation of movement.
            (b) Unilateral foot movements are superior to bilateral foot movements.
            (c) Motor perseveration—inertia of all foot movements is followed by stereotyped repitition of the movement once begun.
            (d) Star gait—deviation toward the unilaterally apraxic leg which takes a shorter step results in a zig-zag, star-shaped gait.
   2. Reflex signs of premotor and supplementary motor lesions.
      a. Tonic reflexes.
         (1) Forced grasping—most marked in the opposite hand, especially when the patient is turned on his side with the lesion down.
         (2) Grasp reflex of the foot—pressure on the ball of the great toe

results in prolonged clenching of paper held between tightly adducted toes.

(3) Bulldog reflex—involuntary grasping and holding of an object placed between the teeth.

(4) Tonic plantar reflex—slow tonic flexion of the toes in response to stimulation of the sole, with slow release; ipsilateral to the lesion.

(5) Tonic spasms of fingers and toes—persistent digit spasm ipsilateral to the lesion.

(6) Tonic diagonal rigidity—hypertonus of the ipsilateral leg and opposite arm.

b. Exaggerated flexor reflexes.

(1) Hyperactive plantar flexor reflex—rapid flexion of the toes in response to tapping the ball of the foot ("Rossolimo sign") or the dorsolateral foot ("Mendel-Bechterew sign"); contralateral to the lesion.

(2) Hyperactive finger flexor reflex—rapid flexion of the fingers to volar ("Rossolimo of the hand") or dorsal ("Mendel-Bechterew of the hand") percussion; contralateral to the lesion.

(3) Hoffmann sign—flexion and adduction of the thumb and flexion of the index finger in response to snapping the nail of the extended middle finger; contralateral to the lesion.

(4) Exaggerated Mayer's sign—hyperactive adduction and opposition of the thumb in response to firm flexion of the middle finger; contralateral to the lesion.

(5) Exaggerated Leri's sign—hyperactive flexion at the elbow in response to forced flexion of the fingers and wrist; contralateral to the lesion.

(6) Diagonal flexion reflex—flexion of the wrist and fingers results in flexion of the opposite leg.

(7) Crossed flexion reflex—flexion of the hip, knee and ankle results in similar flexion of the opposite leg.

3. Ictal signs—conscious adversive seizures.

a. Premotor seizures.

(1) Turning of head, eyes and body precedes loss of consciousness, in contrast to the unconscious adversive seizure of the frontal pole lesion.

(2) Head and eyes, then arm and trunk turn opposite to the lesion, rarely toward it.

(3) No sensory aura occurs.

(4) The contralateral arm and leg are postured, the arm raised and flexed, the patient appearing to look at his extended hand;

the leg is usually extended; clonic-tonic convulsive movement of these extremities occurs with falling to the side opposite the lesion.

b. Supplementary motor seizures—similar to the premotor conscious adversive seizure except for the following:
   (1) A sensory aura may occur: either a nonspecific body sensation or numbness of the opposite foot.
   (2) Speech arrest may occur during the conscious phase.

C. Frontal oculomotor deficits
   1. Acute unilateral lesion of the frontal oculomotor field or its pathways above the brain stem.
      a. Gaze palsy—transient weakness of conjugate gaze contralateral to the lesion; most marked in coma of sudden onset; gaze palsy is on the same side as the coexisting hemiplegia.
      b. Conjugate deviation—to the side of the lesion, occurring with stupor and coma; the patient looks toward the destructive cerebral lesion.
      c. The alert patient may have no visual complaints (e.g. diplopia does not occur) and conjugate gaze may appear normal except for the following:
         (1) Dissociated paralysis of voluntary conjugate gaze—inability to look to the opposite side on command, while optically induced reflex movements (e.g. pursuit, convergence) are intact.
         (2) Latent gaze palsy—weakness in conjugate gaze to the opposite side present only on attempted lid closure.
         (3) Spasticity of conjugate gaze—conjugate deviation to the opposite side on forced lid closure.
         (4) Gaze paretic nystagmus—coarse horizontal nystagmus on conjugate gaze to the side opposite the lesion.
         (5) Oculocephalic test—head turning toward the lesion may induce conjugate deviation toward the gaze paretic contralateral side.
         (6) Pseudohemianopia—loss of visual attention to the side opposite a frontal lesion, usually associated with a conjugate gaze palsy; normal visual fields on perimeter and tangent screen testing.
      d. Ocular seizures—secondary to a frontal oculomotor focus; the patient looks away from the irritative cerebral lesion.
         (1) Ocular turning precedes head turning.
         (2) No visual aura.
         (3) Oculocephalic turning is usually followed by generalized convulsion with loss of consciousness.
         (4) Oculocephalic contraversive seizure—ictus limited to head and eyes without spread to the extremities or loss of consciousness.

(5) Seizure nystagmus—transitory, but it may be the only ictal sign; head and eyes deviate to the side of the quick component.

2. Acute bilateral cerebral lesions of the frontal oculomotor pathways.
   a. Persistent rather than transitory loss of voluntary gaze to one or both sides; reflex movements are intact although following movements may be slow and irregular.
   b. Oculomotor apraxia—random eye movements with apraxia of head movement; gives erroneous impression of blindness.
   c. Pseudo-ophthalmoplegia—loss of all voluntary gaze movements, both horizontal and vertical, with pseudobulbar palsy; convergence and following movements persist.
   d. Spasm of ocular fixation—involuntary pursuit of a target following ocular fixation; associated palsy of voluntary gaze.
   e. Ocular bradykinesia—appearance of ocular immobility with paucity of blinking, ocular lag on head turning, and loss of voluntary gaze.

3. Level of the lesion in conjugate gaze palsy.
   a. Frontal cortical oculomotor field (e.g. acute cortical contusion).
      (1) Weakness of voluntary conjugate gaze is transient; gaze palsy and extremity weakness are on the same side (opposite the lesion).
      (2) Motor deficit is most marked in the hand opposite the lesion.
      (3) Ocular seizures are common.
   b. Frontopontine oculomotor tract in the internal capsule (e.g. hypertensive intracapsular hemorrhage).
      (1) Gaze palsy and extremity weakness are more pronounced and associated with stupor or coma.
      (2) Motor deficit is a dense hemiplegia involving the opposite face, arm and leg.
      (3) Conjugate deviation of the eyes and head to the side of the destructive lesion is prominent.
   c. Frontopontine oculomotor decussation (e.g. acute midbrain lesion).
      (1) Bilateral paralysis of conjugate horizontal gaze.
      (2) Paralysis of conjugate vertical gaze.
      (3) Paralysis of convergence.
   d. Pontine gaze centers (e.g. acute pontine lesion).
      (1) Permanent horizontal gaze palsy, usually bilateral.
      (2) Conjugate vertical gaze and convergence are spared.
      (3) Unilateral pontine lesion—ipsilateral conjugate gaze, abducens and facial palsy with contralateral hemiplegia; the gaze palsy

and extremity weakness are on opposite sides in contrast to cerebral lesions.

(4) Head and eyes are usually not deviated; when conjugate deviation occurs, it is toward the side opposite the lesion; when head rotation is present, it is opposite to the direction of eye deviation.

(5) Oculocephalic test—head turning will not overcome a pontine gaze palsy; in contrast, conjugate deviation to the gaze paretic side may occur with head turning in cerebral lesions.

4. Localizing value of ocular seizures.
   a. Frontodorsal irritative lesion—oculocephalic turning without a visual aura may occur alone; it may be followed by a jacksonian motor march; it may be followed by a generalized convulsion with loss of consciousness.
   b. Frontopolar irritative lesion—unconsciousness precedes adversive oculocephalic turning to the opposite side; adversive turning appearing late in the course of a generalized seizure does not have the same localizing significance.
   c. Parieto-occipital irritative lesion—visual aura precedes conjugate deviation to the opposite side; occipitopolar lesions are less apt to be associated with generalized convulsions than are more rostral lesions.
   d. Temporal lobe irritative lesion—psychomotor seizures are often accompanied by irregular conjugate gaze shifts as though responding to formed visual stimuli; associated with automatisms, olfactory, visual and auditory hallucinations.
   e. Grand mal—upward slightly divergent ocular movements, widely separated eyelids, pupillary dilatation and sluggish light reflexes are common ocular signs.
   f. Petit mal—relative ocular immobility with a direct forward stare, with or without frequent blinking.

Deformities (Angiographic and Pneumographic) of the Frontodorsal Syndromes

A. Angiographic deformities due to anterior suprasylvian parasagittal meningiomas.
   1. Depression (lateral view).
      a. Pericallosal artery, middle segment.
      b. Internal cerebral vein.
      c. Relatively less or minimal depression of middle cerebral group—the angiographic sylvian point is not depressed by frontal parasagittal tumors but is by the parietal parasagittal mass.

2. Midline shift (AP view).
   a. There may be no shift or marked shift of the midline pericallosal vessels depending on eccentricity and size of tumor.
   b. There may merely be a "triangular or V-shift" of small size of the pericallosal artery under the falx; this is usually distal.
   c. There is lateral displacement of the callosomarginal artery away from the midline.
3. Occlusion of the superior sagittal sinus—may be evident on the angiogram; collateral venous channels with retrograde flow may be present.
4. Angiographic meningioma signs—arterial sunburst, persistent tumor cloud and extracerebral arterial supply to the tumor via meningeal and scalp arteries.

B. Angiographic deformities with parasagittal intracerebral gliomas—these may be difficult to separate from parasagittal meningiomas because the pericallosal artery and internal cerebral vein may be depressed in the lateral view in either case. Midline shift of the pericallosal artery is also variable with parasagittal gliomas. However, the following points differentiate the intracerebral lesion:
1. On the lateral view, the pericallosal and the callosomarginal arteries diverge due to gliomatous expansion of the cingulate gyrus.
2. On the AP view, the callosomarginal artery is not displaced laterally away from the midline.
3. There are no angiographic meningioma signs and no sagittal sinus occlusion occurs.
4. There may be early and prominent deep venous drainage and arteriovenous shunts.
5. The tumor may appear to be avascular.

C. Angiographic deformities with frontodorsal convexity suprasylvian meningiomas.
1. Depression (lateral view).
   a. Sylvian triangle, upper border.
   b. Closure of the carotid siphon.
2. Midline shift (AP view).
   a. Square shift of pericallosal artery across the midline.
   b. Shift of the internal cerebral vein across the midline.
3. Angiographic meningioma signs (see A,4 above).

D. Angiographic deformities with frontodorsal convexity glioma
1. Depression (lateral view).
   a. Sylvian triangle, with separation of opercular vessels and depression of the angiographic sylvian point (parietal region) by tumor extension or edema.

b. Closure of the carotid siphon.
c. Depression of the internal cerebral vein—deep cerebral extension, invasion of corpus callosum or edema.

2. Midline shift (AP view) .
   a. Square shift of the pericallosal artery across the midline.
   b. Shift of the internal cerebral vein across the midline.
   c. Lateral displacement of the sylvian vessels indicates deep intracerebral extension.
3. Angiographic glioma signs (see B, 4 and 5 above) .

E. Pneumographic deformities with the frontodorsal mass
   1. Localized depression in the roof of the lateral ventricle above the region of the foramen of Monro indicates a superior frontodorsal mass. The roof may be concave or flat. The localized deformity may be unilateral or bilateral. The usual source of this deformity is the parasagittal meningioma.
   2. A lateral cerebral or extracerebral mass can also produce a unilateral deformity of the ventricular roof by compression of the roof beneath the lower border of the falx, beneath which it herniates. In this instance, the flattening of the roof is not as localized as in the parasagittal mass. The shift across the midline tends to be greater when due to the lateral mass than when the result of a parasagittal tumor. The latter can also produce septal and third ventricular shifts, but may alternatively produce no shift of the midline. The lateral mass, in addition to subfalcial flattening of the ventricular roof, is apt to deform the temporal horn. This is spared by the parasagittal mass. In addition, the lateral mass can only flatten the roof of the ipsilateral ventricle. Bilateral roof deformities indicate parasagittal tumor.
   3. Congenital coarctation of the lateral ventricular wall is incidental, unilateral, and not associated with shift or other ventricular deformity.
   4. Widening of the cingulum, callosum or septum is suggestive evidence of glioma.
   5. On the AP view a "double shadow" can be seen through the frontal horn due to depression of the roof of the supraforaminal portion of the ventricle. If shift is present, the apex of the septum is always shifted at least as much, if not more than its base by the superiorly situated tumor.

Additional Diagnostic Clues in Frontodorsal Syndromes

A. Plain skull x-rays
   1. Shift of a calcified pineal—this may be depressed, posteriorly dis-

located, shifted across the midline or not shifted at all by a frontodorsal mass.

2. Pressure atrophy of the dorsum sella and posterior clinoids due to chronic intracranial hypertension is common in parasagittal meningiomas, but also occurs in the gliomas including the glioblastoma.
3. Local hyperostosis, hypervascularity and tumor calcification in the parasagittal region indicates meningioma. Ipsilateral or bilateral enlargement of middle meningeal channels may occur.
4. Frontoparietal convexity meningiomas are somewhat less common than the parasagittal form and are indicated by similar local changes on plain skull x-rays, with more prominent midline shift of the pineal to the opposite side.
5. Depressed fracture in the frontodorsal region is common following cranial vertex trauma.

B. EEG

1. Parasagittal tumors of the central third (rolandic-parietal) of the sagittal sinus often escape EEG diagnosis. Both meningiomas and gliomas in the central parasagittal region are less apt to result in slow (delta) activity than tumors in other cerebral sites.
2. EEG asymmetries tend to be minimal in central-parasagittal tumors.
3. Slow activity due to a rolandic tumor tends to be in the less diagnostic theta range (4-7 cycles per second). When delta activity due to a frontodorsal mass lesion does occur, in may be most prominent over the parietotemporal leads.
4. Vertex rhythms occur normally which widen the limits of rolandic electrographic variability.

C. Brain scan

The brain scan has particular value in both central-parasagittal and rolandic-parietal diagnosis.

1. The parasagittal meningioma almost always produces a positive scan.
2. The central glioblastoma commonly produces a positive scan.
3. The middle cerebral arteries in the rolandic-parietal region constitute the main terminus of carotid blood flow. This general region is thus the most common site for metastatic tumors to the brain. Metastatic carcinoma commonly produces a positive scan and multiple or bilateral deposits are often indicated by scanning techniques.
4. The arteriovenous malformation is most common within the middle cerebral distribution and produces a high rate of positive scans.
5. Cerebral infarction most commonly occurs within middle cerebral territory and may mimic brain tumor. The initial scan is often negative at the time of acute infarction, becoming positive in most cases

within ten to thirty days. The patient is often clinically improving during the phase in which the scan has become positive, which is unlike the behavior of most brain tumors. Most scans revert to negative after six months in cerebral infarction.

6. The chronic subdural hematoma commonly occurs over the cerebral convexity. It presents often with a fluctuating spastic hemiparesis suggesting frontodorsal compression. A positive scan with increased uptake adjacent to the calvarium is the "subdural pattern." While scans are commonly positive in chronic subdurals (i.e. neovascular membranes), they are often negative in more acute cases. The subdural pattern can be simulated by metastatic carcinomatosis of the meninges, granulomatous meningitis or with dural invasion by glioblastoma, oligodendroglioma or medulloblastoma.

CHAPTER 5

FRONTOLATERAL SYNDROMES

Anatomical and Physiological Correlates

Sector: 2, 3, 4, lower frontal convexity; includes Broca's region in the posterior part of the inferior frontal convolution and frontal operculum; also includes the precentral gyrus adjacent to the inferior third of the rolandic fissure ("face")

Angiogram: Lateral frontal

Pneumogram: Lateral foraminal

Neuroanatomy of the Frontolateral Region (Figs. 34 and 35)

A. Frontolateral regions related to speech

1. Classical Broca's area—inferior frontal convolution.
   a. Pars opercularis.
   b. Pars triangularis.

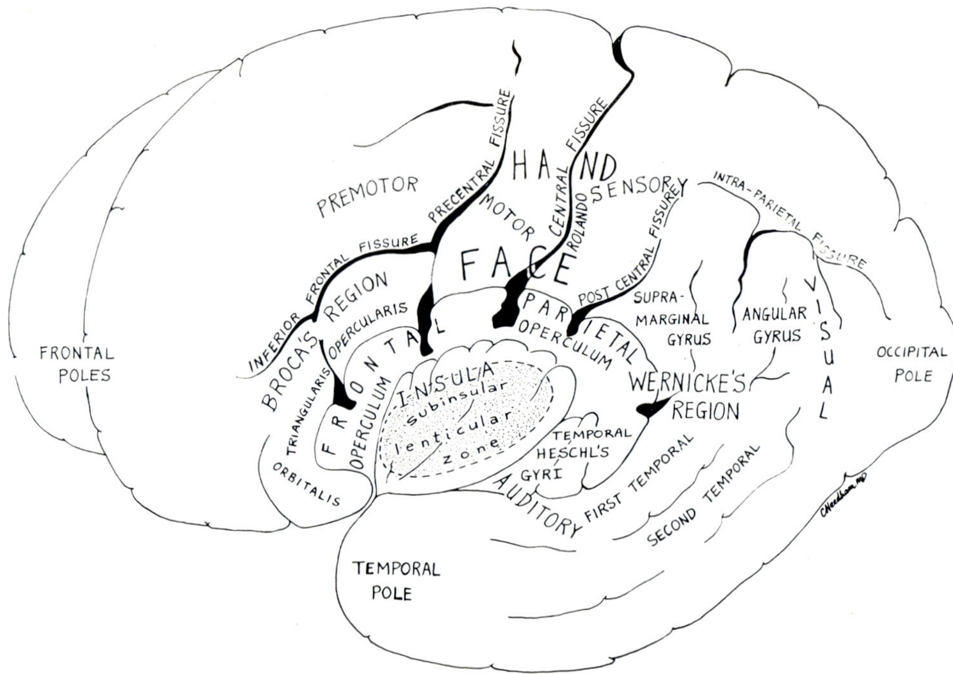

Figure 34. The dominant hemisphere for speech. A lateral view indicates Broca's and Wernicke's areas, in addition to associated opercular, subinsular and cortical regions of importance in the comprehension and expression of language.

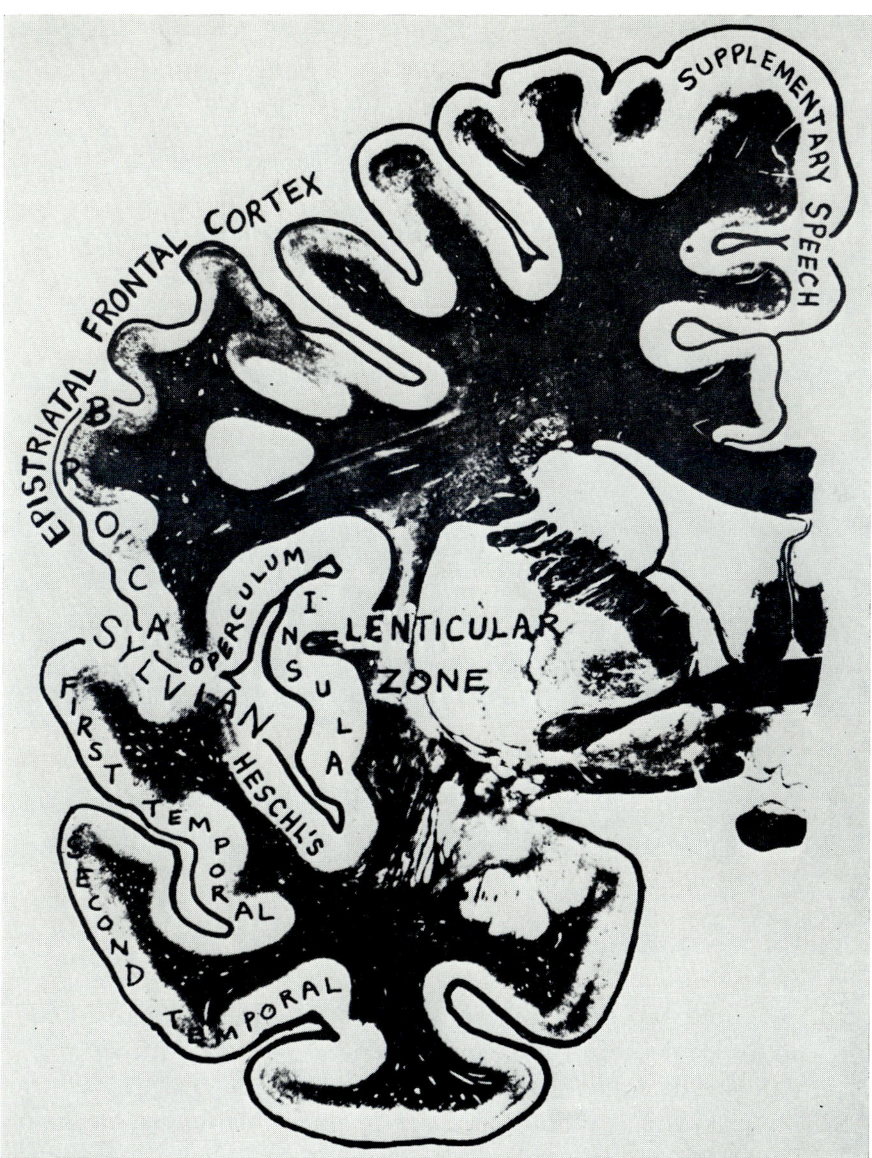

Figure 35. The lenticular, epistriatal and supplementary speech zones. A coronal view depicts frontal, temporal and subcortical regions associated with speech. Broca's area lies adjacent to epistriatal frontal cortex related to expressive speech. Penfield's supplementary speech area of the parasagittal region is noted. Heschl's primary auditory cortex of the temporal operculum relates to the first and second temporal convolutions for receptive speech. Marie's subinsular lenticular zone is a subcortical connection path between motor and sensory speech regions.

2. Epistriatal frontal cortex—other than classical Broca's area.
   a. Adjacent posterior part of middle frontal convolution—joins the inferior part of the frontal oculomotor field.
   b. Precentral face area—rostral to the inferior genu of the rolandic fissure.
   c. Adjacent insula of Reil.
3. Lenticular zone of Marie—subcortical isthmus pathway from parietotemporal speech areas.

B. Afferent frontolateral pathways
   1. Thalamocortical—ventral lateral nucleus (VL).
   2. Associational—frontal, parietal and temporal.

C. Efferent frontolateral pathways
   1. Corticobulbar tract—arises from the frontolateral precentral and opercular region and descends in close proximity to the corticospinal tract; it is clinically considered a pyramidal component although it does not enter the medullary pyramid. It is distributed to the cranial nerve motor nuclei of the brain stem and has both ipsilateral and contralateral terminations. It includes both direct corticobulbar and "aberrant pyramidal" tracts which descend in the medial lemniscus to cranial motor nuclei. Bilateral terminations include the oculomotor, trigeminal, facial (upper face) and ambiguus nuclei. Chiefly contralateral terminations include abducens, facial (lower face) and hypoglossal nuclei.
      a. Internal capsule—corticobulbar fibers are rostral to corticospinal within the posterior limb.
      b. Cerebral peduncle—corticobulbar fibers are medial to corticospinal within the central third.
      c. Midbrain corticobulbar fibers—to the oculomotor nuclei.
      d. Midbrain aberrant pyramidal tract—enters the medial lemniscus to the oculomotor, abducens and spinal accessory nuclei.
      e. Pontine corticobulbar fibers—to the trigeminal nuclei.
      f. Pontine and pontobulbar aberrant pyramidal tracts—in the medial lemniscus to trigeminal, facial, ambiguus and hypoglossal nuclei.
      g. Medullary corticobulbar fibers—to the ambiguus and hypoglossal nuclei.
   2. Corticothalamic tract—reciprocal innervation of the ventral lateral nucleus.
   3. Associational tracts—to parietotemporal speech areas.
   4. Corticostriate and corticotegmental—to caudate, putamen and brain stem tegmentum.

Blood Supply of the Frontolateral Region

A. Arterial—middle cerebral branches
  1. Lenticulostriate subcortical branches.
  2. Cortical branches.
    a. Insular branches.
    b. Orbitofrontal branches.
    c. Ascending frontal branches—prerolandic and rolandic arteries.

B. Venous
  1. Superficial frontal veins—drain frontolateral cortex; to sagittal sinus and superficial middle cerebral vein.
  2. Superficial middle cerebral (sylvian) vein—drainage of operculum and convexity cortex; to sphenoparietal and cavernous sinuses.
  3. Deep lenticulostriate veins—drainage of lenticular zone; to the deep cerebral venous system via deep middle cerebral vein to the basal vein of Rosenthal.

Infarction Syndromes of Arterial Occlusion Resulting in Speech Deficits

A. Dominant middle cerebral occlusion—the "artery of aphasia"
  1. Proximal middle cerebral occlusion.
    a. Mixed expressive-receptive speech deficit; total aphasia or coma if acute occlusion occurs.
    b. Contralateral hemiplegia, hemisensory deficit, hemianopia.
  2. Distal orbitofrontal occlusion.
    a. Predominantly expressive dysphasia.
    b. Contralateral facial weakness.

B. Dominant carotid occlusion
  1. Signs similar to proximal middle cerebral occlusion.
  2. Ipsilateral monocular blindness, transient or permanent; ipsilateral retinal pallor.
  3. Carotid bruit—partial occlusion.
  4. Diminution or loss of carotid pulsation—in the neck and peritonsillar fossa by palpation.
  5. Increased pulsation of ipsilateral superficial temporal artery—occlusion of internal carotid in the neck with patency of external carotid.

C. Dominant proximal anterior cerebral occlusion—if acute, infarction and associated brain swelling may produce the following:
  1. Expressive dysphasia.
  2. Mental confusion or coma.
  3. Right hemiplegia.
  4. Left apraxia.

5. Grasp reflex.
6. Incontinence.

Neurophysiology of Motor Speech in Man

A. Electrostimulation
   1. Broca's area—speech arrest.
   2. Lower motor strip—speech arrest and crude vocalization.
   3. Supplementary motor area of Penfield—speech arrest.

B. Excision and lobectomy
   1. Excision of Broca's area—expressive aphasia.
   2. Excision of supplementary motor area—transient expressive dysphasia.
   3. Prefrontal lobectomy, minor hemisphere—no objective speech deficit.
   4. Prefrontal lobectomy, major hemisphere, sparing Broca's area—decrease in spontaneity and fluency of speech may occur.

C. Carotid amytal speech test
   1. Transient dysphasia (both expressive and receptive) if major hemisphere receives the amytal as a result of carotid injection in the alert patient. Dysnomia is marked.
   2. Following initial momentary confusion upon the injection of amytal, dysphasia and dysnomia do not occur on the minor hemispheral side.
   3. Contralateral transient hemiplegia, hemisensory deficit and hemianopia are readily detected when either side receives amytal.

D. Hemisphere disconnection—section of corpus callosum
   1. Major hemisphere (left hemisphere of the right-handed patient) is the "talking hemisphere."
   2. Minor hemisphere is expressively aphasic and almost entirely agraphic.
   3. Minor hemisphere is able to respond nonverbally to its limited language comprehension.

NEUROSURGICAL SYNDROMES OF THE FRONTOLATERAL REGION

Development of a Major Hemisphere Expressive Speech Deficit

A. Syndrome of traumatic lateral convexity contusion, laceration or intracerebral hematoma—the sudden onset of aphasia or dysphasia is noted if the patient is not already comatose. Contralateral, usually right-sided hemiparesis and focal motor seizures are common. Local signs of coup scalp and cranial trauma in the region of the pterion may be noted. An acute epidural or subdural hematoma may be associated with the underlying contusion, with or without evidence of associated fracture. Progressive impairment of consciousness indicates extracerebral or intracerebral hematoma or brain swelling. Contracoup parieto-occipital trauma may result in contusion of the opposite frontolateral region and temporal pole against the pterion and sphenoid ridge.

B. Syndrome of acute spontaneous intracerebral hemorrhage—this is usually the result of chronic systemic hypertension. Acute hemorrhagic infarction may result from middle cerebral thrombosis or embolism. A ruptured aneurysm or arteriovenous malformation or intraneoplastic hemorrhage may produce a similar picture. A coagulopathy may be etiological. A global aphasia (or coma) is common, with a dense hemiplegia, hemisensory defect and hemianopia on the opposite (usually right) side. Head and conjugate eye deviation to the left are common.

C. Syndrome or acute carotid occlusion (Fig. 36)—this may occur suddenly as a result of neck trauma or basal skull fracture. It may be the result of internal carotid or carotid bifurcation occlusion by thrombus at the site of an atheromatous plaque. Carotid occlusion as a result of embolus, arteritis, cervical abscess or as a complication of angiography may occur. Global aphasia (or coma) is common and is associated with ipsilateral (usually left) monocular blindness and retinal pallor. There is reduced or absent ipsilateral carotid pulsation with or without a bruit. Contralateral (usually right) hemiplegia, hemisensory deficit and hemianopia are notable.

D. Syndrome of the temporal lobe abscess—a predominantly expressive dysphasia may result by mass effect upon the adjacent frontolateral operculum. A predominantly receptive dysphasia may be produced by involvement of Wernicke's region (posterior superior temporal gyrus). Middle ear, or mastoid infection and lateral sinus thrombosis may be associated. A relatively rapid uncal transtentorial syndrome with progressive coma and hemiparesis may result.

E. Syndrome of the temporal glioma—a glioblastoma may produce a progressive dysphasia of a few weeks duration followed by a relatively rapid uncal-transtentorial herniation syndrome.

F. Frontolateral glioma syndrome (Fig. 37)—clonic contractions of the right half of the face (pseudo facial tic) with a progressive, chiefly motor dysphasia, apraxia of the tongue and right central facial palsy occurs with the Broca glioma. Duration of symptoms tends to be greater before transtentorial herniation than with the temporal glioma.

G. Sylvian or outer sphenoid ridge globular meningioma—these extracerebral tumors grow to large size before detection in most instances. Speech deficits may be absent or late in appearance. Focal cerebral seizures with speech arrest and postictal dysphasia may be noted (as in dominant

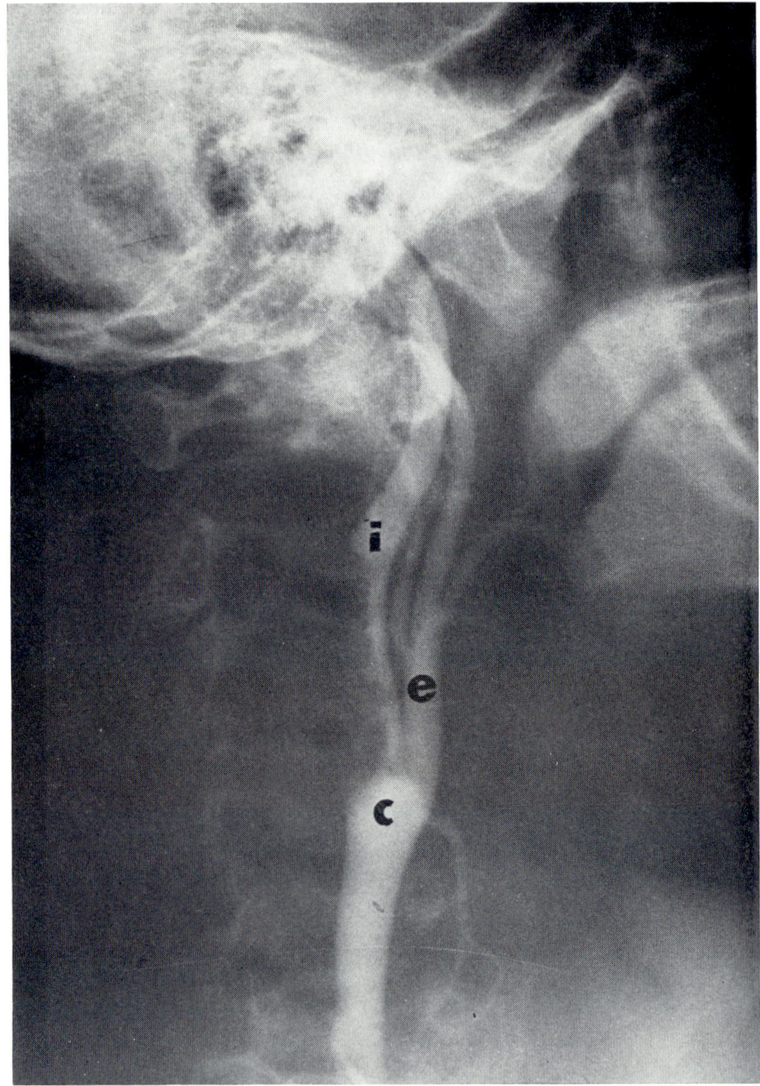

Figure 36. Carotid thrombosis. Occlusion of the internal carotid artery beginning at the bifurcation is present. The patent external carotid is identified by its many branches in the neck. Internal carotid branches, in contrast, are intracranial rather than cervical.

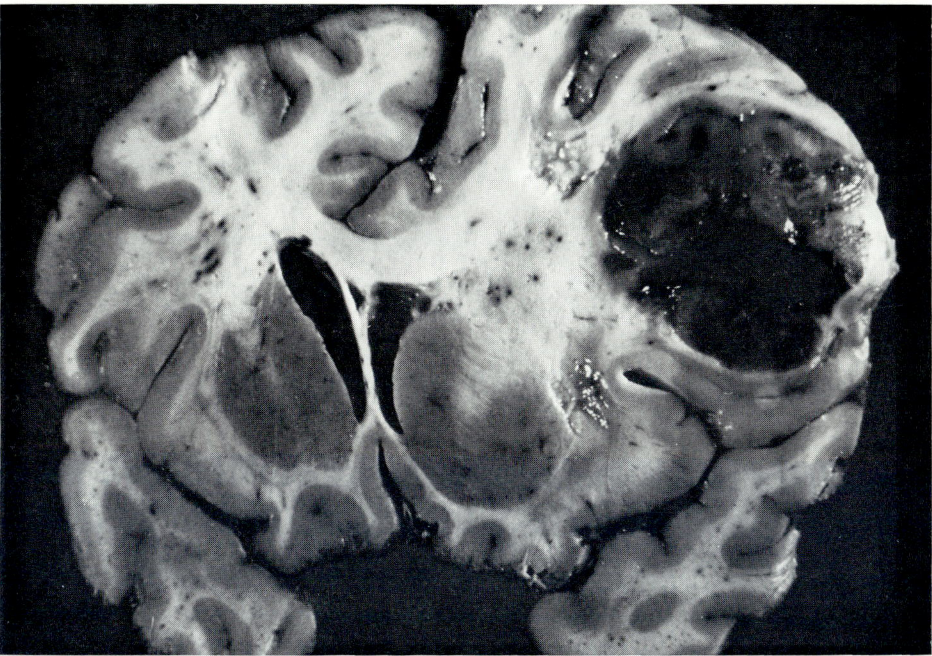

Figure 37. Frontolateral glioblastoma. The bulk of the tumor is frontolateral. The white matter deep to the gross tumor is expanded, suggesting deep extension and edema. Note the contralateral shift and deformity of both anterior horns.

gliomas). Generalized attacks with an aura of a desire to speak sometimes occur. Contralateral facial or faciobrachial weakness of spastic type and chronic papilledema may occur. Marked hyperostosis of the orbit with proptosis and a prominent temporal boss is more common in pterional meningiomas en plaque than in globular forms.

H. Chronic subdural hematoma—this may produce a late or fluctuating speech deficit associated with a fluctuating, or progressive, spastic right hemiparesis. There may be no definite history of trauma and the general course may mimic a brain tumor, stroke or progressive dementia.

Deficits of the Frontolateral Syndrome

Cerebral Speech Disorders

A destructive lesion within the territory of the left middle cerebral artery characteristically results in the language disorder broadly termed "aphasia." This is true of virtually all right-handed patients and two-thirds of left-handed patients. The communication blockade usually involves both the comprehension and expression of spoken and written language. Acute left-sided carotid or middle cerebral occlusion, central intracerebral hemorrhage, or contusion of the intra- and parasylvian cortex produces a total or relatively complete global aphasia. This acute paralysis of language is typically accompanied by a total ("dense") flaccid right hemiplegia. When these events occur with coma, as is often the case, the aphasia is masked during the comatose phase. Global aphasia must be differentiated from "mutism," a speechless akinetic state associated with altered consciousness (e.g. "coma vigil"). The responsible lesion in akinetic mutism is anterior cerebral, diencephalic or upper brain stem in situation, involving the orbitofrontal, septal, hypothalamic or mesencephalic "core" of the brain. "Anarthria" is a speechless state resulting from paralysis of the labial, glossal, pharyngeal, laryngeal and respiratory muscles of articulation. It is a nonlanguage disorder in which the comprehension of speech is intact. "Dysarthria" is the more common partial articulatory disorder presenting as "slurred speech," assuming bulbar, pseudobulbar, extrapyramidal, cerebellar and myasthenic forms. The responsible lesions in these nonaphasic, nonlanguage disorders are bilateral. In contrast, the cerebral language deficit of complete aphasia or partial dysphasia is the result of a unilateral, and always cerebral, lesion. Hysteria is an occasional source of total speechlessness.

Dominant cerebral lesions resulting in partial language disorders, the "dysphasias," present a spectrum of difficulties in the expression and comprehension of speech. The dysphasias are typically "mixed" to a greater or lesser degree, the deficiencies being both motor and sensory. Responsible lesions are often nonacute but progressive as in suprasylvian, retrosylvian or infrasylvian gliomas or in intrasylvian meningiomas. Acute vascular or traumatic lesions of limited extent similarly may produce partial communication deficits. There is rostrocaudal localizing value in the specific character of the dysphasia. Two major forms, expressive and receptive, occur. Dominant frontolateral lesions produce an expressive dysphasia (conversation is markedly reduced; comprehension is relatively intact; what little is spoken is correct but poorly pronounced). Dominant parietotemporal lesions result in receptive dysphasia (comprehension is severely disturbed; conversation is excessive and filled with erroneous words reflecting misunderstanding of language). Two less common dysphasias are also notable for their localizing significance. Lesions of the dominant frontoparietal operculum produce conduction dysphasia (comprehension of spoken and written language is relatively good; reading aloud and verbal expression are impaired by the use of erroneous words; pronunciation is intact). Lesions of the dominant temporal lobe result in nominal dysphasia (marked inability to name objects while comprehension and conversation are otherwise relatively intact). The parasylvian region primarily involved can be identified as follows:

1. Expressive dysphasia—sectors 2, 3, 4.
2. Receptive dysphasia—5, 6, 7.
3. Conduction dysphasia—sectors, 4, 5.
4. Nominal dysphasia—sectors 6, 7.

Lesions whose effects are confined to the nondominant hemisphere or to the frontal pole, temporal pole or occipital pole of the dominant hemisphere typically spare speech. Compression of adjacent structures may produce misleading or "false-localizing" signs (e.g. expressive dysphasia resulting from a mass lesion of the temporal pole with transsylvian compression of Broca's area). As a lesion progresses, the identities of the discrete dysphasias merge with one another. Diffuse lesions or tumors with significant brain edema also result in loss of definition of the cerebral speech disorder. Thus, localizing diagnosis in late cases is often impaired; it is also compounded by the false-localizing signs which may accompany elevated intracranial pressure. However, the clinical usefulness of specific speech deficits remains unsurpassed when they are detected in the individual patient. For convenience of description the separate dysphasias are discussed as follows:

1. Expressive dysphasia—Chapter 5, "Frontolateral Syndromes."
2. Conduction dysphasia—Chapter 6, "Parietal Syndromes."
3. Receptive dysphasia—Chapter 7, "Caudal Cerebral Syndromes."
4. Nominal dysphasia—Chapter 8, "Temporal Lobe Syndromes."

Frontolateral Syndrome of Expressive Dysphasia

Expressive or "motor" dysphasia is the clinical expression of a dominant frontolateral lesion. The lesion may directly involve the cortex or it may "disconnect" the frontolateral cortex from parietotemporal and subcortical inputs. While speech deficits have been lateralized to the left hemisphere in virtually all truly right-handed patients, two-thirds of the left-handed or ambidextrous also have left hemispheral speech dominance. Right hemisphere lesions presenting as speech deficit (crossed aphasia syndrome) are thus restricted to a significant minority of left-handed or ambidextrous patients. It is most important to obtain historical evidence of handedness in all neurosurgical patients. Detection of "sinistral signs" of left-handedness or ambidexterity becomes particularly important in the following:

1. The comatose patient with no available history.
2. The confused or uncooperative patient.
3. The alert patient with signs pointing to a left hemisphere lesion (e.g.

right hemiplegia and right homonymous hemianopia) who presents no speech deficit.

Sinistral signs bear upon the issue of cerebral lateralization, and are thus elemental to any consideration of the signs of speech deficit which more narrowly indicate cerebral localization.

Sinistral Signs

A. Sinistral signs in the alert patient indicating occult left-handedness or ambidexterity.
   1. Use of the left eye in sighting a rifle.
   2. Use of the left foot in kicking a football or in hopping.
   3. Use of the left hand in "mirror writing," the script produced being reflected legibly by a mirror.
   4. Asymmetrical prayer sign—the dorsal wrist angle is more obtuse on the left with the hands opposed in the attitude of prayer.
   5. Upper thumb sign—the left thumb is superior with the hands clenched and fingers interdigitating.
   6. Upper forearm sign—the left forearm is superior when arms are folded across the chest.

B. Sinistral signs in the comatose patient
   1. Arm-flexion sign—the left humeroradial angle is more obtuse when both upper limbs are flexed at the elbow.
   2. Nail-width sign—the left fingernail is wider than the right when the fifth digits are compared.
   3. Developmental smallness of the right hemiface, right hand or right foot—left hemisphere may still be dominant for speech, although these findings increase the possibility of right-sided speech representation.
   4. Wristwatch sign—if the wristband has a buckle, it is ordinarily applied to the opposite wrist by the preferred hand.

Deficits of the Frontolateral Syndrome of Expressive Dysphasia

A. Soft signs of early impairment—partial or slowly progressive lesion.
   1. Slight hesitancy of speech.
   2. Purposefully slow speech to avoid incorrect word usage.
   3. Trouble finding the appropriate word.
   4. Slow enunciation of words.
   5. Right facial weakness most apparent during speech.
   6. General conversational speech otherwise reasonably intact.
   7. General comprehension appears normal.

B. Signs of moderate impairment
   1. General reduction of total amount of speech.

2. Able to repeat more words than can be spontaneously pronounced.
3. While spontaneous pronunciation is poor, objects may be correctly named.
4. Frontal dysnomia—the patient may have difficulty naming common objects. When the examiner supplies false names for the object, the patient will make negative gestures or say No. The patient will write the correct name. The patient's writing ability is the key to his "inner speech" if he has severe verbal expressive aphasia.
5. Frontal dyslexia—the patient often understands what is read, but reading aloud is severely impaired; he has difficulty remembering a series of words, and frequently looks back to the beginning of the sentence.
6. Frontal dysgraphia—the patient can copy correctly and can write single words, but he writes poorly to dictation; errors in spelling words and in transfer from printed word to script occur.
7. Buccofacial apraxia—unable to protrude tongue or smile on request despite the absence of weakness; "voluntary-automatic dissociation" occurs in which involuntary buccofacial movements are unimpaired.
8. Right brachiofacial paresis is commonly associated.
9. Cortical dysarthria—conversational speech is markedly impaired not only by its general reduction, but also by poor pronunciation of what is spoken.
10. Comprehension, while superior to conversation, is impaired chiefly due to poor recall of long spoken phrases (poor word-memory).
11. Reduction of gestures associated with speech.

C. Signs of severe impairment—usually due to sudden vascular insult (infarction or hemorrhage), or direct trauma.
   1. Almost total reduction of speech—Yes or No responses.
   2. Motor agraphia—similar reduction in written language.
   3. No gestures.
   4. Defective understanding of both spoken and written language.
   5. Right hemiplegia.

D. Chief differential points distinguishing predominantly expressive (frontal) dysphasia from predominantly receptive (temporoparietal) dysphasia.
   1. General reduction of speech.
   2. Cortical dysarthria, buccofacial apraxia.
   3. Comprehension usually better than conversation.

E. Crossed aphasia syndrome—speech deficit due to a right hemisphere lesion.
   1. Practically never occurs in the truly right-handed person.

2. Occurs in one of three left-handed or ambidextrous patients.
3. Associated lateralizing signs in the left-handed aphasic patient.
   a. Alexia—strongly favors a left hemisphere lesion.
   b. Agraphia—generally favors a left hemisphere lesion.
   c. Motor apraxia—generally favors a left hemisphere lesion.
   d. Acalculia or constructional apraxia—either the right or left hemisphere.

F. Signs suggesting supplementary motor speech syndrome—parasagittal.
   1. Uncommon, but can occur with parasagittal meningioma of the middle third of the superior longitudinal sinus, especially when complicated by focal cerebral seizures.
   2. Expressive dysphasia occurring with jacksonian seizures beginning in the foot.
   3. Weakness of one or both legs.
   4. Urinary incontinence.

Deformities (Angiographic and Pneumographic) of the Frontolateral Syndrome

A. Angiographic deformities
   1. Extracerebral frontolateral mass (e.g. anterior intrasylvian meningioma).
      a. Elevation (lateral view)—middle cerebral branches of the anterior part of the sylvian triangle.
      b. Depression (lateral view).
         (1) Middle cerebral branches of the posterior part of the sylvian triangle.
         (2) Carotid siphon.
      c. Midline shift (AP view).
         (1) Anterior cerebral artery.
         (2) Internal cerebral vein—not exceeding anterior cerebral shift.
      d. Meningioma signs—extracerebral vascular supply, hyperostosis, characteristic tumor cloud which persists.
   2. Intracerebral frontolateral mass (e.g. glioma of frontal operculum).
      a. Depression (lateral view)—middle cerebral branches in the anterior part of the sylvian triangle.
      b. Midline shift (AP view)—same as in extracerebral lesion.
      c. Glioma signs—prominent arteriovenous drainage into deep veins, displacement of lenticulostriate arteries, widening of pericallosal genu due to callosal extension.

B. Pneumographic deformities (extracerebral or intracerebral mass)

1. Marked contralateral displacement of both anterior horns, with subfalcial herniation, is characteristic.
2. Lateral wall of ipsilateral anterior horn is displaced medially, and the roof of this horn is flattened by subfalcial herniation.
3. Lateral ventricular angle of ipsilateral anterior horn is narrowed.
4. Anterior horns are unequal, the smaller horn being ipsilateral.
5. Narrowing of ipsilateral temporal horn.
6. Obliteration of ipsilateral sylvian cistern.

Additional Diagnostic Clues in Frontolateral Syndromes

A. Plain skull x-rays
  1. Intracranial or extracranial carotid calcification—atherosclerosis.
  2. Contralateral and posterior displacement of calcified pineal-frontolateral mass.
  3. Hyperostosis and increased vascular markings—pterional or greater sphenoidal wing—globular or en plaque meningiomas.
  4. Calcification over lateral convexity—can occur in chronic subdural hematoma.
  5. Fracture in region of the pterion may be associated with frontolateral contusion or laceration.
  6. Fracture in region of the pterion with contralateral pineal shift—middle meningeal tear with acute epidural hematoma until proven otherwise.

B. EEG
  1. Difficult to completely differentiate a vascular from neoplastic lesion on the basis of EEG.
  2. Generalized slowing largely lateralized to one hemisphere—suggests carotid occlusion.
  3. Generalized bilateral slowing upon unilateral carotid compression—suggests occlusion of opposite carotid.
  4. Generalized reduction of all EEG activity on the side of the lesion—suggests subdural hematoma.
  5. Reduction of background activity and focal slowing maximal in lateral frontal or anterior temporal regions—suggests either mass lesion (frontolateral, intrasylvian or anterior temporal) or middle cerebral occlusion.
  6. Focal slowing in subarachnoid hemorrhage—suggests either associated hematoma or vasospasm or arteriovenous malformation.

C. Brain scan
  1. Usually positive in sylvian and sphenoidal meningiomas, glioblastomas and arteriovenous malformations.

2. Commonly positive in metastatic carcinoma and may indicate multiple deposits.
3. May be negative early and positive later in cerebral infarction.
4. Often positive in chronic subdural hematoma with neovascularization of subdural membranes.

CHAPTER 6

PARIETAL SYNDROMES

Anatomical and Physiological Correlates

Sector: 5; the retrorolandic region behind the central fissure and above the posterior sylvian fissure. The parietal lobe is situated beneath the caudal half of the parietal bone. The sagittal suture is the midline union of the two parietal bones. This suture and the parietal bones begin at the coronal and end at the lambdoid suture. A point midway along the sagittal suture is the "rolandic point," corresponding to the apex of the central fissure. The rostral portion of the parietal bone overlies the precentral and premotor regions of the frontal lobe, while the caudal half overlies the parietal lobe.

Angiogram: Posterior Suprasylvian

Pneumogram: Postforaminal

Neuroanatomy of the Parietal Lobe

The frontal lobe of preceding chapters is relatively well demarcated from the remainder of the cerebral convexity by the rolandic and sylvian fissures. This remaining half of the cerebral convexity consists of the following three general regions:

1. Retrorolandic (parietal).
2. Retrosylvian (caudal).
3. Infrasylvian (temporal).

The retrorolandic parietal lobe is the subject matter of this chapter. The subcortical white matter of this region is situated above the uppermost fibers of the optic radiation. Lesions whose effects are limited to the retrorolandic parietal lobe characteristically spare the visual fields. The retrosylvian and infrasylvian regions are set forth in the next two chapters. The subcortical white matter of both the caudal cerebral and temporal areas contains the optic radiation. Subcortical lesions adjacent to the atrium and occipital horn of the lateral ventricle (caudal cerebral), or adjacent to the temporal horn, readily interrupt the geniculocalcarine pathway in its passage to the primary visual cortex of the mesial occipital pole. Thus, the presence or absence of visual field deficit, plus the character of the deficit if present (i.e. hemianopia, quadrantanopia), constitutes a practical clinical reason for subdividing the posterior hemisphere in this manner. This usefulness is amplified when employed in conjunction with angiographic and pneumographic correlates.*

A. Afferents

1. Ventral posterior medial nucleus (VPM) of the dorsal thalamus—to the lower postcentral gyrus and parietal operculum (face).
2. Ventral posterior lateral nucleus (VPL) of the dorsal thalamus—to the upper postcentral gyrus (arm) and posterior paracentral gyrus (leg); the last is most lateral in VPL.
3. Pulvinar and lateral thalamic nuclei—to the superior parietal lobule.
4. Rolandic motor cortex—short association fibers.
5. Other parietal regions—short association fibers.
6. Frontal, temporal, occipital and cingulate regions—longer association fibers including the superior and inferior longitudinal bundles.
7. Contralateral parietal cortex—via corpus callosum.

B. Efferents

1. Corticothalamic fibers to VPM, VPL, pulvinar and lateral thalamic nucleus.
2. Short and long association fibers to the rolandic motor cortex and frontal, temporal and occipital regions; callosal fibers to opposite parietal cortex.
3. Parietal pyramidal fibers—descend with the corticospinal system to motor centers in the brain stem and spinal cord.

**Note:* The traditional division of the merging posterior parietal, posterior temporal and occipital areas into separate lobes involves the construction of imaginary lines. The "parieto-occipital sulcus" is prominent on the mesial surface of the hemisphere but extends only a short way over the lateral convexity. The "preoccipital notch" is an inferior caudal depression at the edge of the hemisphere in the region where the transverse sinus begins to curve downward to become the sigmoid sinus. Construction of an imaginary line from the parieto-occipital sulcus superiorly to the preoccipital notch inferiorly delimits the occipital lobe. A second imaginary line has traditionally been employed from the caudal end of the posterior ramus of the sylvian fissure to the previously constructed parieto-occipital line. This delimits the parietal lobe above from the posterior temporal region below. The construction of artificial lines commends itself primarily on the basis of clinical and radiological usefulness. In actual fact the posterior parietal, posterior temporal and occipital regions are not distinct on inspection of the lateral surface of the brain. The parietal supramarginal gyrus is continuous with the first temporal, and the parietal angular gyrus is continuous with the second temporal convolution (Fig. 34). Posterior parietal and temporal gyri are continuous with occipital gyri. The term "caudal cerebral" is employed for this posterior parietal-temporal-occipital region of confluence for reasons of ease of terminology and clinicoradiological usefulness. The parietal contribution to the caudal cerebral region lies in the vicinity of the angular gyrus. The uppermost fibers of the optic radiation lie deep to the white matter of the angular gyrus, while the more rostral bulk of the parietal lobe—i.e. the retrorolandic portion, lies superior to the visual radiation.

Blood Supply of the Parietal Lobe (Retrorolandic)

A. Arterial
  1. Middle cerebral branches.
    a. Anterior parietal branch—to the postcentral gyrus.
    b. Posterior parietal branch—to the supramarginal gyrus and superior parietal lobule (lateral surface) .
  2. Anterior cerebral branches.
    a. Paracentral branch of the callosomarginal artery—to the paracentral lobule.
    b. Anterior and posterior internal parietal branches of the distal pericallosal artery—to the superior parietal lobule (mesial surface).
  3. Posterior cerebral branches.
    a. Posteromedial central branch—to the posterior third of the posterior limb of the internal capsule; contains thalamocortical sensory fibers to the parietal lobe and lies caudal to the corticospinal component.
    b. Parieto-occipital branch—to the mesial surface in the region of the parieto-occipital fissure.

B. Venous
  1. Superior parietal veins—to the sagittal sinus.
  2. Greater anastomotic vein of Trolard—to the sagittal sinus, superficial middle cerebral vein and lesser anastomotic vein.
  3. Rolandic vein—to the sagittal sinus and superficial middle cerebral vein.
  4. Superficial middle cerebral (sylvian) vein—to the sphenoparietal sinus and cavernous sinus.
  5. Lesser anastomotic vein of Trolard—to the lateral sinus.
  6. Posterior vein of the corpus callosum—drains the mesial parietal lobe and enters the great vein of Galen.

Infarction Syndromes of Arterial Occlusion of the Parietal Region

A. Occlusion of the anterior and posterior parietal branches of the middle cerebral artery.
  1. Contralateral flaccid hemiplegia with hemisensory deficit most severe in face, arm and hand, and less severe in the leg.
  2. Predominantly receptive dysphasia which may later resolve into a conduction dysphasia—major hemisphere.
  3. Initial contralateral homonymous hemianopia which may clear.
  4. General lack of concern or "parietal neglect."

B. Occlusion of the callosomarginal artery—paracentral lobule infarction.

1. Contralateral leg paralysis.
2. Contralateral cortical sensory deficit in the leg.
3. Incontinence.

C. Occlusion of posterior cerebral artery branches to the parietal lobe—usually occurs as a result of more proximal posterior cerebral occlusion. This may complicate intracranial hypertension with transtentorial compression of the posterior cerebral artery as it passes around the midbrain to reach the tentorial edge.
   1. Contralateral homonymous hemianopia—occipital infarction; there may be bilateral cortical blindness if both posterior cerebral arteries are compressed.
   2. Alexia, visual agnosia—major hemisphere.
   3. Thalamic syndrome—with hemisensory deficit and spontaneous pain ("anesthesia dolorosa") due to vascular occlusion involving the thalamogeniculate branch of the posterior cerebral artery.
   4. If the posterior cerebral occlusion is the result of transtentorial compression by supratentorial mass, the above signs will be masked by the presence of coma; third nerve palsy and contralateral hemiplegia are commonly associated.

Neurophysiology of the Parietal Region

A. Stimulation
   1. The human postcentral sensory cortex, when stimulated electrically in the unanesthetized state, results in sensations of numbness or tingling or sense of movement in contralateral body parts.
   2. The sensory sequence is generally similar to the motor sequence of the precentral cortex.
   3. Both sensory and motor responses can be obtained from either pre- or postcentral electrostimulation. Sensory responses are more common postcentrally, while motor responses are more common precentrally.
   4. The inferior half of the postcentral gyrus, when stimulated, results in sensations localized to the face or mouth. The face is represented in an upright fashion with large lips, and the tongue and pharynx are represented below it.
   5. The superior half of the postcentral gyrus, when stimulated, results in sensations largely localized to contralateral extremities whose distal parts have the greatest representation.
   6. A reversal of sequence, also present in the motor region, exists at a midpoint between the upper and lower portions of the postcentral gyrus. The trunk and extremities are thus oriented in a direction opposite the upright orientation of the face.

7. The convex dorsal surface of the postcentral gyrus constitutes the region representing the hand and fingers. Representation of an enlarged thumb lies immediately above the upper face. Proceeding toward the vertex, the proximal arm, trunk and proximal leg are represented. Sensations localized to the foot or genitalia may be elicited upon stimulation of the paracentral lobule on the mesial surface of the hemisphere.

B. Ablation

Extirpation experiments in animals reveal variable deficits upon parietal excision.

1. Contralateral hypotonia and hyporeflexia.
2. Contralateral poverty of movement out of proportion to the degree of paralysis.
3. Contralateral muscle atrophy.
4. Ataxia.

NEUROSURGICAL SYNDROMES OF THE PARIETAL LOBE

Development

A. Acute parietal contusion syndrome—the contralateral paralysis is flaccid with hyporeflexia, yet the distribution is cortical with relative sparing of one extremity. In contrast, the flaccid paralysis of deep capsular type presents an equally profound weakness of both extremities on the hemiplegic side. Focal cerebral seizures are common in cortical contusion and may be entirely motor, although hemiparesthesiae on the opposite side may be reported. If the patient is alert, a profound parietal hemisensory deficit may be elicited.

B. Syndrome of acute craniocerebral vertex trauma—see Chapter 4. The parietal lobe forms the caudal border of the central third of the sagittal sinus. Trauma to the cranial vertex is commonly frontoparietal with a mixture of sensorimotor deficits.

C. Metastatic carcinoma to the brain—in the older age group, the brain tumor suspect is particularly apt to harbor a metastatic deposit (s) . The most common source is carcinoma of the lung. Occasionally, the pulmonary primary will not be obvious at the time of clinical intracranial metastasis. Pulmonary carcinoma may present as a pseudoabscess of the brain with a necrotic, inflammatory intracerebral mass. All brain tumor suspects must have a chest x-ray. The primary site may involve any organ system. The metastases are usually multiple, but frequently present neurological deficits suggesting a single mass lesion. In a significant minority a single deposit may be the only central nervous system (CNS) lesion. Metastatic carcinoma may involve the craniocerebral-spinal axis at any level. The majority of cerebral metastases however are parietal, parietofrontal or parietotemporal. This results directly from the fact that the middle cerebral artery tree is the major recipient of carotid blood flow. Metastatic carcinomas are said to be more common on the left side, but this may be due to resultant speech deficit and consequent earlier diagnosis. Metastatic disease less often involves the vertebrobasilar system with production of a posterior fossa mass. Cranial and meningeal involvement also occur. The patient with metastatic carcinoma to the brain commonly presents with obtundation or confusion with some degree of hemiparesis. Brain edema characteristically accompanies cerebral metastases. Edema reaches a peak within three to four days in most instances. Progressive obtundation and increasing neurological deficit typically are noted during this period. Stupor may mask the presence of cortical discriminatory sensory loss. The latter may become more obvious upon reduction of brain swelling as a result of steroid therapy. The patient often does not appear to be appropriately concerned and may even neglect an obvious deficit.

D. Multifocal tumor syndrome—in addition to metastatic carcinomas, there are other sources of the multifocal mass syndrome. Glioblastoma accounts for the vast majority of primary gliomas in the older age group also subject to metastatic disease. Glioblastoma may be multifocal, may give evidence of subpial spread, dural invasion and CNS metastases. Medulloblastoma may occasionally occur in the young adult, although it is more common in childhood. It also tends to spread widely in the CNS and may invade the dura. Oligodendroglioma similarly may spread intraventricularly or may invade the leptomeninges. Pinealomas and choroid plexus papillomas also give rise to CNS metastases. Diffuse meningeal involvement is characteristic of CNS melanoma. The primary source may be occult, ocular or meningeal. Amelanotic melanomas may simulate glioblastoma. Malignant melanoma may be simulated by the benign melanotic meningioma of the posterior fossa which is rare. Primary reticulum cell tumor of the brain is a malignant neoplasm which is often multifocal, presenting as an acute encephalopathy. Multifocal cerebral abscesses may complicate bacteremia or meningitis and may present a similar clinical picture usually with signs of systemic toxicity.

E. Syndrome of the parasagittal meningioma of the central third of the sagittal sinus—see neurosurgical syndromes of the frontodorsal region. A marked sensory ataxia with impaired position sense in the legs, complicated by a slowly progressive paraparesis should suggest parietal compression, the bulk of the tumor being postrolandic. Focal jacksonian sensory or sensorimotor seizures may precede the paralysis by months or years.

The Parietal Lobe Syndrome

Parietal signs are among the most subtle and complex. The patient is characteristically unconcerned about his disability. His responses typically vary (Fig. 38). It is clinically useful to delimit the rostral retrorolandic (parietal) syndrome from a caudal retrosylvian (parieto-temporo-occipital) syndrome.

A. Parietal lobe syndrome (this chapter).
   1. Parietal hemiparesis.
   2. Parietal hemisensory deficit.
   3. Jacksonian sensory seizures.
   4. Conduction aphasia.

B. Caudal cerebral syndrome (next chapter)
   1. Central hemianopia.
   2. Complex disorders of recognition (including receptive aphasia).
   3. Visual seizures.

Deficits of the Parietal Syndrome

A. Parietal hemiparesis—while a lesion entirely confined to the parietal lobe does not produce paralysis, postcentral parietal lesions typically also involve the rolandic motor system. This rostral boundary region is formed by corticospinal (frontodorsal) and corticobulbar (frontolateral) descending tracts. These are joined by postcentral parietal fibers. Combined involvement of these frontoparietal systems leads to the following:
   1. Hypotonic hemiparesis opposite the lesion—the motor disability greatly exceeds the degree of paralysis.
   2. Muscular wasting—most marked in the affected hand and appears earlier than "atrophy of disuse"; wasting may even precede paralysis and is not accompanied by fasciculations.
   3. Impaired position sense of the affected limb—may be associated with abnormal postures of the involved extremity.
   4. Associated "astereognosis"—inability to identify objects placed in the affected hand; may be accompanied by poverty of palpatory movements.
   5. Abnormal plantar response in the affected foot—the normal flexion reflex may be totally lost; the Babinski sign is most common; "Babinski-extinction" may occur in which dorsiflexion of the great toe is extinguished by double simultaneous plantar stimulation.
   6. Anosognosia—unawareness of left hemiplegia associated with a right

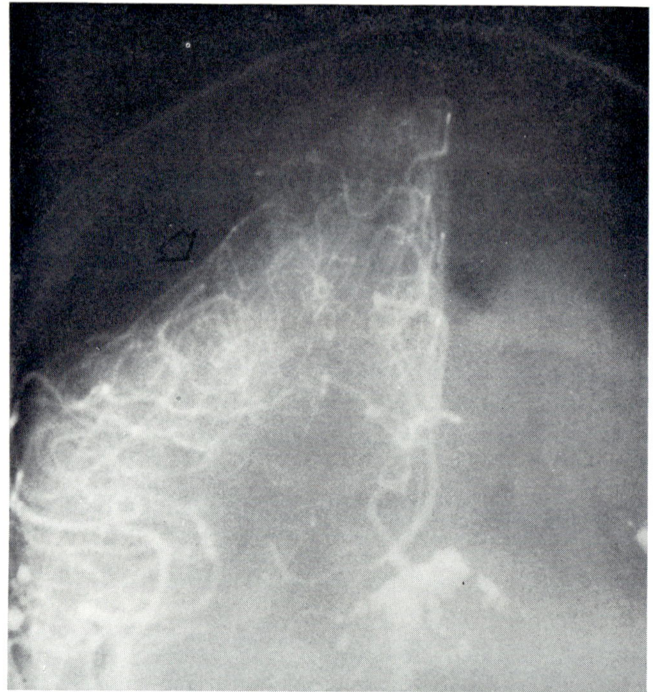

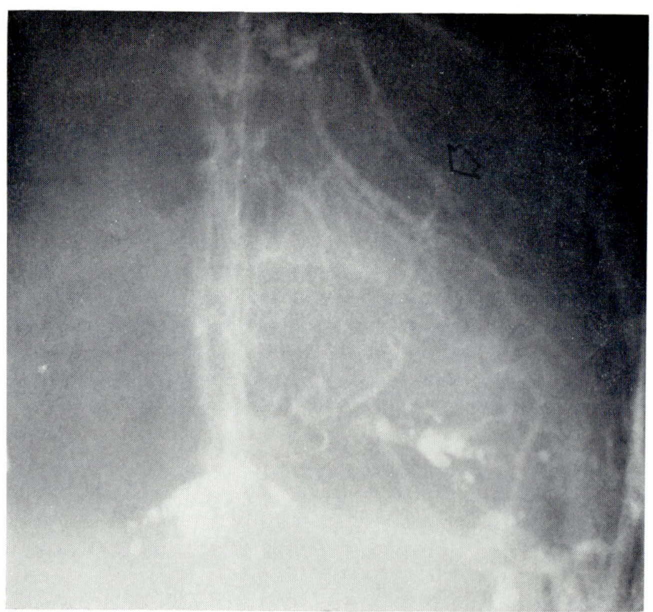

parietal lesion (e.g. the normally subordinate left hand, now deprived of strength and postural sensibility, is ignored by the patient).

B. Parietal hemisensory deficit—this includes both cutaneous (superficial) and postural (deep) contralateral sensory impairment.
   1. Parietal cutaneous signs—these consist of hemihypesthesia and a variety of tactile discriminatory signs.
      a. Parietal hemihypesthesia—diminished pinpoint and touch opposite a parietal lesion.
         (1) The patient is unaware of this defect.
         (2) The sensory loss is never complete (i.e. anesthesia does not occur).
         (3) The partial loss is most marked and most common in the hand (volar surface).
         (4) In the lower extremity, the sensory impairment is most marked in the foot.
         (5) The transition to normal sensation is gradual.
         (6) The deficit may be limited to the extremities; if the impairment includes the face and trunk, the midline of the face and trunk are spared.
         (7) Hypesthesia is often transient; it is more marked and more extensive with deeper lesions than with cortical lesions.
      b. Tactile discriminatory signs—these are not well tested in the presence of gross hypesthesia in which the primary sensation of touch is disturbed. They may be evident following transient hypesthesia. They are most typical of parietal cortical disturbance.
         (1) Tactile inattention—on bilateral simultaneous touch, the stimulus opposite the lesion is not felt; this is an early sign and may be the sole sign of parietal disease; it is most marked in the hands.
         (2) Two-point discrimination—inability to identify duality of touch opposite the lesion, an equal separation of the points being recognized as two on the side of the lesion.

Figure 38. Bilateral subdural hematomas—arterial (*top*) and venous (*bottom*) phases. Bilateral subacute subdural hematomas thickest over the parietal lobes resulted in paraparesis in a forty-year-old man. No history of trauma was given on admission, the patient being unable to walk or stand for several days. A rather variable sensory level over the trunk and an inappropriate lack of concern regarding his disability were the sole parietal signs in this alert patient. Motor and sensory signs resolved following evacuation of these subdurals. Intracranial Pantopaque® is present as a result of a myelogram done on admission. The myelogram was entirely negative. Relatives, and later the patient himself, recalled that he had fallen, sustaining a minor blow to the head, a number of days before.

(3) Three-point touch—inability to identify the duality of touch occurring only with a simultaneous third stimulus to the normal hand.
(4) Tactile localization—the patient with "atopognosis" is unable to accurately localize a stimulus; the faulty response is usually proximal to the target point.
(5) Tactile perseveration—the patient describes the sensation of continued contact in its absence.
(6) Tactile allochiria—the stimulus is referred to the opposite normal hand; the reverse may occur.
(7) Tactile agnosia (astereognosis) —this is the inability to identify objects by touch.
   (a) This includes the related tactile misidentification of the shapes, sizes, textures, and weights of objects; a given weight is lighter in the affected hand ("abarognosis").
   (b) Like the other tactile discriminatory activities, the primary sensations must be relatively intact; thus, the inability to identify letters written on the skin ("graphanesthesia") is a parietal sign only in the presence of peripheral sensation.
   (c) Astereognosis is often accompanied by poverty of palpatory movements as a result of unilateral neglect; there is usually an associated defect in postural sense.

2. Parietal postural signs—these are the deficits in "deep sensibility" in which recognition of passive movement is impaired.
   a. The more rostral the parietal lesion, the greater the deficiency in position sense.
   b. Unawareness of the direction of movement and associated hypotonus may produce peculiar postures in the affected limb.
   c. Pseudoathetosis—irregular wandering movements of the affected fingers.
   d. Parietal sensory ataxia—disturbed position sense resulting in motor incoordination opposite a parietal lesion.
      (1) Most marked for finger movements.
      (2) The ataxia increases with eye closure.
      (3) Ataxic paraparesis—occurs with bilateral paracentral lobule involvement resulting in impaired position sense in both legs.
      (4) Pseudocerebellar ataxia—uncommon form of incoordination of the limbs opposite a parietal lesion with intact position sense; related to parietal neglect or spatial disorientation.
   e. Parietal drift—slow drooping of the fingers of the outstretched limb opposite a parietal lesion; deficiencies in position sense are most marked distally.

f. Postural-vibratory dissociation—while postural abnormality is common with parietal cortical lesions, vibratory sense is relatively intact; impaired vibratory sense due to a cerebral lesion indicates thalamic involvement.

C. Jacksonian sensory seizures—contralateral focal sensory seizures occur with irritative rostral parietal lesions.
   1. Quality of abnormal sensation.
      a. Paresthesias are most common, usually numbness or tingling; dysesthesias of unpleasant burning or coldness rarely described as pain occur occasionally.
      b. Sensation of movement without actual movement occurs as a focal ictal event.
   2. Site of origin.
      a. Hand, thumb or index finger most common.
      b. Tongue and perioral region on one side.
      c. Hand, tongue and lips together.
      d. Foot least common.
   3. Spread of ictus.
      a. Sensory march—the paresthesia spreads proximally after remaining confined to a single limb.
      b. Sensorimotor march—the paresthesia may precede a jacksonian motor march as a recurring sensory aura.
      c. Generalized convulsion—may or may not follow the sensory ictus.
   4. Postictal phase—the parts involved in the sensory seizure may reveal transient postictal hemisensory loss.
      a. Diminished two-point discrimination.
      b. Astereognosis.
      c. Impaired position sense.

D. Conduction aphasia (dysphasia for partial deficits)—this speech defect is characteristic of lesions of the dominant frontoparietal operculum. The deficit is intermediate between frontal Broca's expressive aphasia and caudal Wernicke's receptive aphasia.
   1. Points of similarity between expressive and conduction aphasia.
      a. The comprehension of spoken language is good (comprehension is poor in receptive aphasia).
      b. Comprehension of written material is also good, but reading aloud is impaired (receptive aphasia is associated with alexia; both comprehension and ability to read aloud are poor).
   2. Points of similarity between conduction and receptive aphasia.
      a. Repetition sign—the patient cannot correctly repeat the words he hears (in expressive aphasia, the patient can repeat more words than he can spontaneously pronounce).

b. Paraphasia—the patient substitutes the wrong word for the proper one; he is often unaware of his errors.
c. Parietal dysnomia—the patient frequently misnames objects and is unconcerned by his errors (in expressive aphasia, objects are often named correctly although poorly pronounced; "frontal dysnomia" indicates that while the patient is unable to name the object, he can write the correct name).
d. Articulation is relatively intact.

Deformities (Angiographic and Pneumographic) of the Parietal Syndromes

A. Angiographic deformities due to posterior suprasylvian parasagittal meningiomas.
 1. Depression (lateral view).
  a. Pericallosal artery, distal segment.
  b. Internal cerebral vein.
  c. Angiographic sylvian point.
 2. Midline shift (AP view).
  a. A "triangular or V-shift" of the distal pericallosal under the posterior falx is most often seen.
  b. No shift, or more massive subfalcial herniation may be noted depending on size and eccentricity of the parasagittal mass.
  c. Lateral displacement of the callosomarginal artery away from the midline.
 3. Occlusion of the superior sagittal sinus in the parietal region—collateral venous channels and retrograde flow may occur. Sinus occlusion may be partial with narrowing or it may be complete. The parasagittal meningioma may of course have no effect at all upon the sagittal sinus. Vertex hyperostosis or invasive epidural tumor growth may displace the sinus downward.
 4. Angiographic meningioma signs with an arterial sunburst, persistent tumor cloud and extracerebral arterial supply—irregular and enlarged meningeal arteries derived from the occipital arteries of the scalp may enter the tumor through enlarged parietal foramina.

B. Angiographic deformities due to posterior suprasylvian parasagittal gliomas.
 1. Separation of the pericallosal and callosomarginal arteries on the lateral view—this may be difficult to interpret at the distal ends of these arteries. In addition, certain parasagittal meningiomas may induce sufficient edema in the adjacent cingulate gyrus to widen it, simulating a glioma.

2. The callosomarginal artery is not displaced laterally from the midline on the AP view.
3. Early deep draining veins, arteriovenous shunts, brief persistence of tumor cloud or avascularity indicate a glioma. Demonstration of extracerebral blood supply to the tumor heavily favors meningioma. In unusual cases, glioblastomas which invade the dura or falx can develop extracerebral vascular supply.
4. Depression of the pericallosal artery, internal cerebral vein and angiographic sylvian point can occur with either intracerebral or extracerebral parietal parasagittal tumors. Midline shift may or may not occur with either.

C. Angiographic deformities due to metastatic intracerebral tumors.
   1. A variety of angiographic deformities are compatible with metastatic intracerebral tumors: avascularity, hypovascularity and occasionally hypervascularity with tumor vessels may be present.
   2. Evidence of multifocal deposits is common.
   3. Evidence of bilaterality is also common.
   4. Evidence of cerebral edema is prominent.
   5. Mass effect within the middle cerebral arterial distribution is particularly common and may be suprasylvian, retrosylvian, infrasylvian, or intrasylvian.
   6. When an avascular mass in the lateral intracerebral region with associated hemispheral edema does not shift the midline to the opposite side (absence of subfalcial hernia) in the older adult, metastatic bilateral carcinoma should be suspected, with contralateral edema preventing the expected shift.
   7. Evidence for only a single mass does not rule out metastatic carcinoma.

D. Pneumographic deformities due to parietal lesions.
   1. Postforaminal tumors in the parasagittal region, whether extra or intracerebral, depress the roof of the lateral ventricle behind the foramen of Monro and in front of the atrium.
   2. The lateral ventricular angle is depressed on the AP view, while midline shift of the ventricle is minimized by the width of the semirigid posterior falx. A "double shadow" can be seen, the lateral edge of the normal anterior horn being higher than its medial edge, while the roof of the depressed ventricular body is inclined the opposite way.
   3. Parietal and other posterior cerebral tumors commonly translate their mass effect to the deep cerebral draining veins of the diencephalon, basal ganglia and upper brain stem. This results in cerebral edema, more generalized ventricular compression and rostral herniations distant from the posterior tumor.

Additional Diagnostic Clues in Parietal Syndromes

A. Plain skull x-rays

1. Depression of a calcified pineal (lateral view)—most supratentorial tumors displace the pineal posteriorly and downward (i.e. the frontal half of the cerebrum is more commonly the site of tumor than the caudal half). The parietal tumor may only depress the pineal without other shift.
2. Pressure atrophy of the sella—indicates intracranial hypertension and probable tumor without pointing to the tumor site.
3. Radiolucencies and radiodensities of the parietal bones—since both parietal bones taken together constitute the major portion of the calvarium, they are a frequent site of abnormal bony lesions. Normal radiolucencies must be excluded.
   a. Parietal foramina—these are not ordinarily of pathological significance and may even be quite enlarged without indicating a tumor. Increased meningeal vascular grooves entering enlarged parietal foramina should raise the possibility of meningioma. Pacchionian granulations usually adjacent to the longitudinal sinus also account for normal radiolucencies. Diploic venous channels may result in local radiolucency of normal type between the inner and outer table.
   b. Hemangioma of the skull—usually involves the parietal bone of the adult producing a firm tender mass beneath the scalp. A circular or irregular radiolucency with bony spicules on tangent views indicates the site of the tumor.
   c. Metastatic carcinoma of the skull—irregular areas of diminished density which are multiple and discrete may result from various primaries. At times the lesion is solitary. Cranial metastases often are present without evident cerebral metastases and vice versa. Multiple myeloma typically produces multiple "punched out" lesions. Any part of the vault or base may be involved.
   d. Fibrous dysplasia of the skull—may produce a mixed density-lucency pattern of the vault with pseudo-osteomas, pseudo-hyperostosis and irregular cystic decalcified calvarial lesions. It may be monostotic in the skull with a single radiolucency. Increased density diffusely affecting the cranial base, with involvement of the orbits, sinuses and clinoids may occur. Children or adults may be affected.
   e. Eosinophilic granuloma of the skull—a radiolucent bone lesion with irregular margins, usually affecting young adults.
   f. Epidermoid—the radiolucent skull defect is surrounded by a sharp margin of increased density. Epidermoids may also occur intra-

cranially, especially in the cerebellopontine angle. They may present as a parasellar, intrapetrous or intraventricular mass. They occur in childhood or in adult life. The epidermoid of the calvarium usually begins between the tables and erodes them.

g. Osteoma—this characteristically begins in the outer table and is most common frontally. Involvement of the frontal or ethmoidal sinus is typical. Secondary sinusitis may be associated. Adolescents or adults are affected.

h. Hyperostosis of meningioma—begins in the inner table, but may extend to both tables and may produce a firm mass beneath the scalp. It occurs radiographically in a third of meningiomas. Since parasagittal meningiomas of the central third of the sagittal sinus constitute a common form, bony changes at the biparietal junction should be carefully noted. The hyperostosis may be associated with bone erosion and spicule formation simulating osteogenic sarcoma.

i. Osteochondroma of the skull—the lesion usually involves the cranial base and is mixed lucent-dense on x-ray and protrudes above the surrounding bone.

B. EEG

1. Parasagittal parietal tumors may escape EEG diagnosis (see Ch. 4, EEG).
2. Convexity parietal tumors, like rolandic tumors, may result in local theta rather than the slower more prominent delta rhythm. The delta focus of a parietal tumor may be more prominent in the temporal or temporoparietal leads.
3. Caudal parietal tumors may result in a diminished alpha rhythm on the side of the tumor.
4. Diminished alpha rhythm along with general reduction in all background activity is compatible with subdural hematoma over the convexity, the reduction being on the side of the subdural. Focal delta activity with slow waves, sometimes of reduced amplitude, may occasionally be seen in subdurals. Bilateral subdurals are readily missed due to symmetry of background activity. Frontal slowing (delta) may indicate brain stem compression (by subdural or other mass) and may occur prior to obtundation. Local depression of background rhythms is never pathognomonic, since it can also occur with infarction, hemorrhage or cerebral atrophy.
5. EEG study may be of value in screening known cases of carcinoma of the lung for cerebral metastases. However, the EEG may be occasionally negative with cerebral metastases. Focal delta activity is a positive sign, but multiple deposits are not usually recognized.

C. Brain scan

1. The brain scan is quite helpful in the diagnosis of rolandic-parietal tumors (see Ch. 4, Brain scan). The scan is commonly positive at the site of meningioma, glioblastoma, and metastatic carcinoma. Large midline uptake may indicate bilateral parasagittal meningioma or "butterfly" glioblastoma of the corpus callosum. Evidence of multiplicity is usually due to metastatic carcinoma, but may indicate CSF metastases of a primary brain tumor or "multifocal" glioblastoma. In unusual instances, multiplicity may indicate multiple meningiomas.
2. The scan is helpful in vascular lesions, being positive in most angiographically demonstrable arteriovenous malformations with or without hemorrhage. Small arteriovenous malformations, especially when deeply situated, may be missed. The scan is typically negative early and positive later in the usual ischemic infarction. Hemorrhagic infarction may result in an early positive scan.
3. The value of the brain scan in craniocerebral trauma is greatest in the detection of the chronic subdural hematoma, with a peripheral uptake on frontal projection. Lateral views may be negative. In acute head injury, the scan may be positive due merely to scalp contusion or skull fracture and therefore has a lesser value in the detection of acute intracranial hematomas. An acute subdural often produces a negative scan, although underlying cerebral contusion or overlying cranial or scalp trauma may result in a positive scan.
4. Metastatic carcinoma to the skull and various primary cranial tumors, skull defects and benign calvarial bone lesions (e.g. fibrous dysplasia) may result in a focal positive scan. A "subdural pattern" may be simulated.

CHAPTER 7

CAUDAL CEREBRAL SYNDROMES

Anatomical and Physiological Correlates

Sector: 6; the retrosylvian region; the confluent posterior temporal-parietal-occipital region surrounding the atrium of the lateral ventricle (Fig. 39)
Angiogram: Retrosylvian
Pneumogram: Periatrial

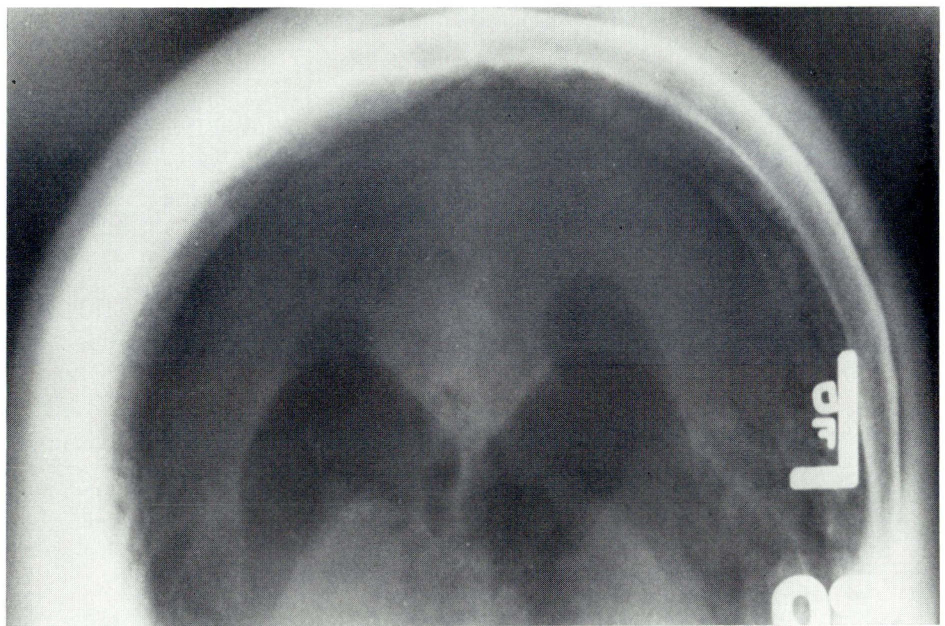

Figure 39. The caudal cerebral region—air study. The trigone or atrium of the lateral ventricle is the ventricular junction of the body and temporal and occipital horns. The trigone is the ventricular center for the caudal cerebral region (see Fig. 1, 3 and 5), which is considered "periatrial." The occipital horn is the most variable part of the ventricular system and may be absent. The occipital horn is commonly asymmetrical, the larger of the two usually being the left.

Neuroanatomy of the Caudal Cerebral Region

Neurosurgical lesions (i.e. tumors) of the caudal pole of the brain tend to involve not only the occipital lobe, but also the posterior parietal and posterior temporal regions. Anatomically they are continuous structures. For example, the parietal supramarginal, angular and postparietal gyri are continuous with the superior temporal, middle temporal and occipital convolutions, respectively. Functionally, the occipital visual areas are closely related to visual association areas in the posterior parietal lobe (i.e. angular gyrus) and receptive speech areas in the posterior part of the superior temporal gyrus (i.e. Wernicke's area) . The uppermost fibers of the optic radiation form the inferocaudal border of the parietal lobe, lying deep to the white matter of the angular gyrus. Thus a central hemianopia, combined with a retrosylvian mass on an angiogram, or a periatrial mass on a pneumogram, quite specifically characterizes this caudal cerebral region.

A. Afferents

1. Lateral geniculate nucleus of the dorsal thalamus—to the primary visual cortex (calcarine cortex) on the medial surface of the occipital pole, via the optic radiation.
2. Frontal, parietal, temporal and insular fibers—to the secondary (parastriate) visual cortex of the occipital pole and to the tertiary (preoccipital) visual cortex of the posterior parietal and posterior temporal region. Includes motor, sensory and auditory input.
3. Short association pathways—from the primary mesial visual cortex to secondary visual areas on the lateral surface.
4. Callosal pathways—through the posterior portion of the corpus callosum between visual association areas of each side.
5. Frontal eye fields to the occipital eye field of the opposite side.
6. Long and short association pathways from the occipital visual cortices and from parietotemporal regions to the angular gyrus.
7. Primary auditory region in the temporal operculum (Heschl's gyri) , temporal lobe, Broca's region, the insula and frontoparietal operculum, and occipital visual cortex—to Wernicke's area in the posterior portion of the superior temporal convolution. Wernicke's area is caudally continuous with the parietal angular gyrus and superiorly continuous with the parietal supramarginal gyrus.

B. Efferents

1. Short association fibers from the calcarine primary visual cortex to the parastriate secondary visual cortex.
2. Short and long association pathways—from the parastriate region to the preoccipital and angular visual cortices, and to frontal, parietal, temporal and insular regions; callosal pathways to contralateral visual association areas.
3. Corticotectal and corticomesencephalic paths—from the parastriate region to pretectal, tectal and tegmental brain stem centers; similar pathways exist from the preoccipital visual cortex ("occipital eye field") .

4. Corticocortical pathways—from the angular gyrus to parietotemporal regions and occipital eye fields.
5. Reciprocal efferents from Wernicke's region to widespread cortical regions frontally and caudally.

Blood Supply of the Caudal Cerebral Region

A. Arterial
   1. Middle cerebral branches.
      a. Parieto-occipital branch—to the angular gyrus, preoccipital and occipital regions of the lateral convexity.
      b. Posterior temporal branch—to Wernicke's region and the temporo-occipital cortex of the lateral convexity.
   2. Posterior cerebral branches.
      a. Calcarine branch—to the primary striate visual cortex on the mesial surface of the occipital pole.
      b. Posterior temporal branch—to the temporo-occipital cortex of the mesial convexity.
      c. Posterolateral central branch—to the lateral geniculate body, and to the optic radiation in the retrolenticular portion of the internal capsule.
B. Venous
   1. Parieto-occipital veins—to the posterior sagittal sinus.
   2. Inferior temporo-occipital veins—to the transverse sinus.
   3. Lesser anastomotic vein of Labbé—to the transverse sinus below and the superficial sylvian vein above.
   4. Internal occipital veins—to the great vein of Galen, in turn draining into the straight sinus.

Infarction Syndromes of Arterial Occlusion in the Caudal Cerebral Region

A. Occlusion of the angular artery—parieto-occipital branch, middle cerebral artery (Gerstmann's syndrome, dominant side).
   1. Finger agnosia.
   2. Right-left disorientation.
   3. Acalculia.
   4. Agraphia.
   5. Alexia—commonly associated.
B. Occlusion of the posterior temporal branch, middle cerebral artery—this may occur as part of a slightly more proximal cortical middle cerebral occlusion leading to a posterior parietotemporal infarction including Wernicke's area (dominant side).
   1. Aphasia.

2. Agraphia.
3. Alexia.

C. Occlusion of the posterior cerebral artery
1. Homonymous hemianopia.
2. Alexia and visual agnosia—dominant side.

Neurophysiology of the Caudal Cerebral Region

A. Primary (striate) visual cortex
1. Macular representation (central vision) is most caudal in the calcarine region; the cortical macular field is relatively extensive.
2. Peripheral retinal representation (peripheral vision) is most rostral in the calcarine region.
3. The inferior retina is represented upon the inferior lip of the calcarine fissure; the optic radiation serving the inferior retina passes in Meyer's loop around the temporal horn of the temporal lobe before proceeding caudally; these fibers serve the superior visual field.
4. The superior retina is represented upon the superior lip of the calcarine fissure; the optic radiation serving the superior retina passes directly back into the caudal cerebral region; these fibers serve the inferior visual field.
5. Semidecussation in the optic chiasm permits binocular contralateral homonymous representation of visual fields upon each calcarine cortex.
6. Bilateral destruction of the primary visual cortex leads to complete blindness and loss of visual awareness.

B. Secondary (parastriate) and tertiary (preoccipital) visual cortex
1. Lesions of these regions result in visual agnosias and impairment in reflex eye movement (i.e. following and fixation).
2. In addition to the functions of visual association, these regions and their descending corticotectal and corticotegmental pathways are necessary for the integrity of a normal opticokinetic response.
3. Electrostimulation of occipital visual cortices results in the experience of elemental bits and streaks of light and color without more detailed or familiar visual scenes.

C. Angular gyrus, Wernicke's region and surrounding parietotemporal cortex—considered "interpretive cortex," the integrity of which is necessary for the recognition of complex visual and auditory symbols, including those of written and spoken language. Lesions of this region result in a complex array of deficits in the visual-spatial-body-image sphere combined with severe communication block. The general deficit may be considered a profound "asymbolia."

NEUROSURGICAL SYNDROMES OF THE CAUDAL CEREBRAL REGION

Development

A. Syndrome of acute occipitopolar contusion—injury to the occipital poles may result in immediate and bilaterally complete central blindness. The blindness may resolve into homonymous hemianopia opposite the more severely traumatized pole with resolution of caudal cerebral edema. There may be an initial homonymous hemianopia, but quadrantanopia is uncommon in blunt trauma. It can occur in penetrating wounds. Laceration of the transverse or posterior sagittal sinus with intracerebral, subarachnoid or subdural hemorrhage may occur. Coma may be progressive due to the presence of clot and edema. The obtundation masks the evidence of blindness. Cortical blindness is associated with retention of light reflexes. The presence of clot and transtentorial herniation is associated with diminution and loss of the light reflex as a result of oculomotor palsy. Cerebral edema due to caudal cerebral contusion may be particularly profound due to translated compression effect upon deep central venous drainage in the region of the great vein of Galen. Massive edema without hematoma may itself induce central transtentorial compression with ultimate loss of light reflexes.

B. Syndrome of traumatic blindness—craniocerebral trauma may result in immediate or delayed, partial or complete blindness as a result of a variety of mechanisms. Coup damage to the occipital poles is a relatively uncommon source of traumatically occurring visual loss. Localizing principles in determining the site of visual pathway damage in trauma cases are as follows:

1. The presence of coma masks the evaluation of blindness and renders assessment of direct and consensual light reflexes of great importance.
2. The direct light reflex is completely lost on the side in which an optic nerve is completely severed. No consensual light reflex will be seen on the side opposite the severed optic nerve. The opposite eye must be shaded during the test.
3. Light reflexes are elicited bilaterally when the retina served by the normal optic nerve is stimulated. The reflex thus obtained from the side of a severed optic nerve is consensual (i.e. the oculomotor nerve to the blind eye remains intact).
4. Complete transverse section of the optic chiasm, in addition to bilaterally complete blindness, results in bilateral loss of direct and consensual light reflexes. This is identical to the result of section of both optic nerves. It contrasts to bilateral damage to the visual cortex

(cortical blindness) and bilateral lesions of the optic radiations (double hemianopia) in that these hemispheric (central) forms of blindness are associated with retention of direct and consensual light reflexes bilaterally.

5. Complete section of an optic tract, before it reaches the lateral geniculate, leads to retention of direct and consensual light reflexes bilaterally, provided the functionally intact portion of the retina of either eye is stimulated. It is difficult to avoid stimulation of functional retina due to intraocular reflection of light. Section of an optic tract is thus readily separated from section of an optic nerve in which the light reflex is lost.
6. Bilateral section of the optic tracts, beyond the lateral geniculate, as they approach the tectum (superior colliculus) produces bilateral loss of all light reflexes with the retention of vision. This is rare and is the direct opposite of bilateral cortical blindness.
7. Unilateral oculomotor involvement (usually by compression or stretching of the nerve or midbrain compression, ischemia or hemorrhage) produces loss of both the direct and consensual light reflex on the paralyzed side. This differs from unilateral optic nerve damage which also results in loss of the direct reflex, but in contrast spares the consensual reflex of the pupil of the blind eye. In oculomotor palsy sufficient to impair the light reflex, the trauma patient is commonly obtunded or comatose (transtentorial herniation) so that vision cannot be tested. The other signs of oculomotor palsy such as a dilated pupil, ptosis and extraocular palsy indicate the source of light reflex failure. Bilateral oculomotor involvement, noted later in transtentorial herniation, leads to bilateral loss of the light reflex.
8. In the confused or lightly obtunded patient whose visual field is difficult to assess, hemianopia may be suspected by the position in which the patient holds his head: he tends to turn his head away from the hemianopic side. This impression may be confirmed by menace testing of the visual field. The presence of a dense flaccid hemiplegia on the hemianopic side indicates involvement of the posterior capsular portion of the optic radiation (retrolenticular) on the opposite side.
9. Alert patients with subhemispheric (optic nerve, chiasm or optic tract) optic pathway lesions are usually quite concerned about the presence of their visual loss (i.e. their "visual consciousness" is intact). Alert patients with hemispheric (optic radiation, visual cortex) optic pathway lesions are often unconcerned or unaware of the presence of visual loss. This tendency increases as the occipital pole is approached (i.e. visual consciousness is impaired).

10. Visual loss is monocular rostral to the chiasm (unless of course, both optic nerves are involved) or binocular caudal to the chiasm.
11. Monocular blindness may be of ocular or optic nerve origin. Optic nerve involvement may be intra-orbital (retrobulbar), at the cranio-orbital junction (optic foramen), or intracranial (suprasellar). Monocular blindness may result from ophthalmic artery or carotid occlusion.
12. Binocular blindness (due to trauma) is usually intracranial in origin. Hemianopias of heteronymous type (usually bitemporal) implicate the chiasm and are unusual in acute trauma cases, but may be seen later as a result of post-traumatic arachnoiditis. Hemianopias of homonymous type are more common and implicate the optic radiation or visual cortex. Homonymous hemianopia of optic tract origin is less common.
13. Central visual acuity is most commonly impaired with ocular, optic nerve or chiasm involvement. Unilateral tract or hemispheral visual involvement tends to spare visual acuity.

Specific causes of the syndrome of traumatic blindness include the following:

1. Direct ocular injury—trauma to the cornea or lens; intraocular hemorrhage; traumatic retinal detachment. Retinal and preretinal hemorrhage can also result from intracranial-subarachnoid traumatic hemorrhage without direct ocular injury. If such hemorrhage in the preretina (subhyaloid and vitreous) lies in front of the macula, severe central visual loss occurs.
2. Retrobulbar hemorrhage with optic nerve compression and proptosis.
3. Hemorrhage into the optic nerve sheath with eventual optic atrophy.
4. Compression of the optic nerve (and ophthalmic artery) at the optic foramen—basal skull fracture or fracture of the anterior clinoid are often associated. Contrecoup contusion of the optic nerve at the foramen may occur with eventual optic atrophy.
5. Secondary optic atrophy consequent to papilledema of long standing may lead to blindness as a late consequence of trauma (e.g. traumatic subarachnoid hemorrhage with late communicating hydrocephalus).
6. Traumatic carotid occlusion—neck injury or basal skull fracture with acute monocular blindness as a result of retinal ischemia may occur. Central cerebral infarction with contralateral homonymous hemianopia may be noted.
7. Traumatic disruption of the optic chiasm—unusual, but can occur in transtemporal gunshot wounds or other penetrating injury.
8. Optochiasmatic arachnoiditis can be a late complication of traumatic

subarachnoid hemorrhage and can lead to progressive optic atrophy and visual loss. Visual field deficits may be bizarre.

9. An optic tract lesion due to trauma is most apt to be the result of transtentorial compression of the tract as it curves around the cerebral peduncle. A form of "transtentorial hemianopia" commonly obscured by the presence of coma, but detectable postoperatively (e.g. following evacuation of subdural hematoma) may be noted.
10. Occipital lobe infarction due to trauma constitutes another form of transtentorial hemianopia due to compression and stretching of the posterior cerebral artery as it courses around the peduncle to reach the tentorial edge. This is also commonly obscured by the presence of coma and may be detected postoperatively.
11. Traumatic intracerebral hematoma—intracapsular involvement of the retrolenticular optic radiation with resultant homonymous hemianopia may occur.
12. Temporal lobe contusion (or intratemporal hematoma)—may result in one of four patterns.
    a. Temporal pole contusion without any visual accompaniment.
    b. Temporal pole contusion with uncal herniation and compression of the optic tract or posterior cerebral artery (transtentorial hemianopia).
    c. Midtemporal contusion with involvement of Meyer's loop—superior quadrantanopia on the opposite side.
    d. Posterior temporal contusion (i.e. caudal cerebral) with contralateral hemianopia.
13. Parietal lobe contusion (or intraparietal hematoma)—may also result in one of four patterns.
    a. Retrorolandic parietal contusion with sparing of the optic radiation.
    b. Parietal mass with resultant transtentorial compression of the posterior cerebral artery.
    c. Parietal mass with edema extending into the upper optic radiation —may produce inferior quadrantanopia on the opposite side.
    d. Posterior parietotemporal or parieto-occipital (i.e. caudal cerebral) mass with contralateral hemianopia.
14. Occipito-polar contusion—may result in various patterns.
    a. Bilateral permanent cortical blindness.
    b. Bilateral cortical blindness with resolution into homonymous hemianopia opposite the more severely contused pole.
    c. Initial homonymous hemianopia opposite a contused occipital pole.

d. Quadrantanopia—uncommon in cerebral trauma; when it occurs it is more apt to be due to midtemporal involvement of Meyer's loop (i.e. where the optic radiation is more widely distributed than it is at the caudal pole).

e. Occipitopolar injury may result in an altitudinal (horizontal) hemianopia. Inferior horizontal hemianopia is the type seen (upper radiations and upper cortical damage). Superior horizontal hemianopia due to trauma tends to be obscured by associated intracranial hemorrhage and coma due to associated transverse sinus trauma.

15. Extracerebral hematomas.

a. The acute epidural and acute subdural hematomas are usually associated with progressive coma preventing detection of visual impairment. Light reflex loss accompanies third nerve palsy as a result of transtentorial herniation.

b. The patient harboring a chronic hematoma may be quite alert and visual fields should be carefully tested. A progressive hemiparesis is commonly associated, and the differential diagnosis commonly rests between chronic subdural, brain tumor and stroke. Demonstration of a hemianopia in such a patient is an important point in favor of an intracerebral rather than extracerebral mass. Subdurals of sufficient size to result in hemianopia (i.e. transtentorial hemianopia) commonly produce obtundation which prevents the detection of the field cut.

C. Syndrome of the caudal cerebral arteriovenous malformation (Figs. 40 and 41)—the majority of arteriovenous malformations clinically present with acute subarachnoid hemorrhage. Episodes of bleeding may be multiple. The majority of arteriovenous malformations are supratentorial. They are most often within the distribution of the middle cerebral artery. They are somewhat more common caudally than rostrally. Aneurysms are a much more common source of spontaneous subarachnoid hemorrhage, but these are uncommon in the caudal cerebral region. Seizures occur in a third of arteriovenous malformations as a presenting sign. Seizures with a visual aura implicate the caudal cerebral region. Progressive receptive dysphasia, dementia and hemianopia in a relatively young adult or adolescent may be due to arteriovenous malformation and may mimic a dominant caudal cerebral tumor. A slowly progressive hemiparesis also commonly occurs in the absence of hemorrhage. It usually results from repeated and additive episodes of ischemia and infarction related to progressively increasing arteriovenous cerebral shunt. Cases of infantile hemiplegia, especially with repeated episodes of men-

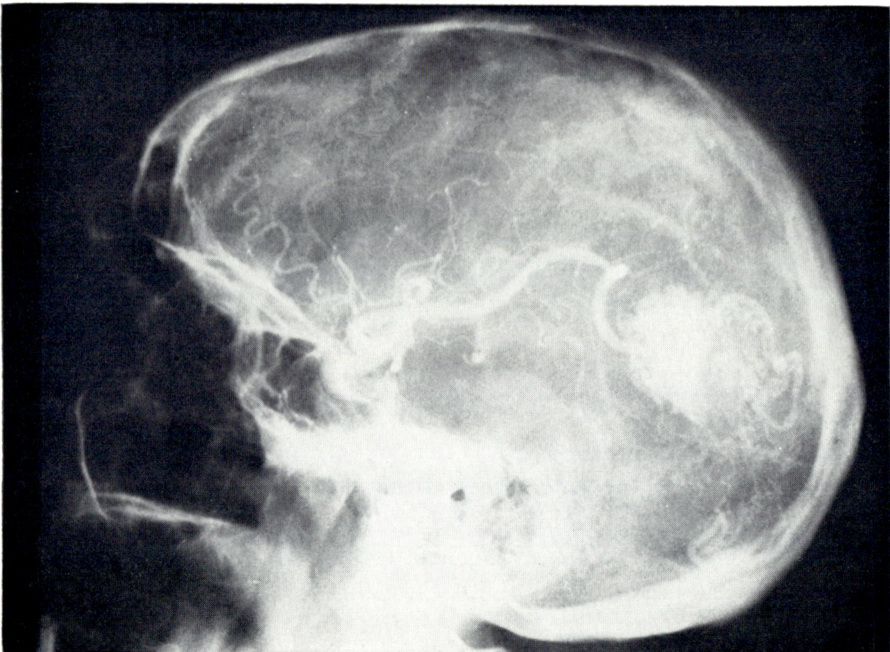

Figure 40. Caudal cerebral arteriovenous malformation (posterior parieto-occipital). A large middle cerebral feeding vessel passes caudally to the AVM.

ingitis, should be investigated for arteriovenous malformation with repeated bleedings simulating meningitis. Arteriovenous malformation may present in infancy with intracranial bruit and cardiac failure. Arteriovenous malformation (aneurysm) of the vein of Galen usually presents as hydrocephalus in infancy but may be occult until later life. Intracranial bruits in adult life are more common in carotid-cavernous fistula, extracranial arteriovenous malformation and vascular meningioma than in intracerebral arteriovenous malformation.

D. Sturge-Weber's disease (pial angiomatosis) —the patient often presents in childhood with a cutaneous angioma of the face in the trigeminal distribution and cerebral seizures. Progressive dementia is common, but subarachnoid hemorrhage occurs only in a small minority of cases. The capillary-venous malformation of pial angiomatosis is most often in the caudal cerebral region.

E. Caudal cerebral glioma syndrome—gliomas of the hemisphere are less common in the caudal portion of the brain than rostrally. An occipital glioma typically extends deeply in the white matter of the posterior parietal and posterior temporal regions and into the posterior limb of the internal capsule. Progressive dementia, hemianopia and hemiparesis

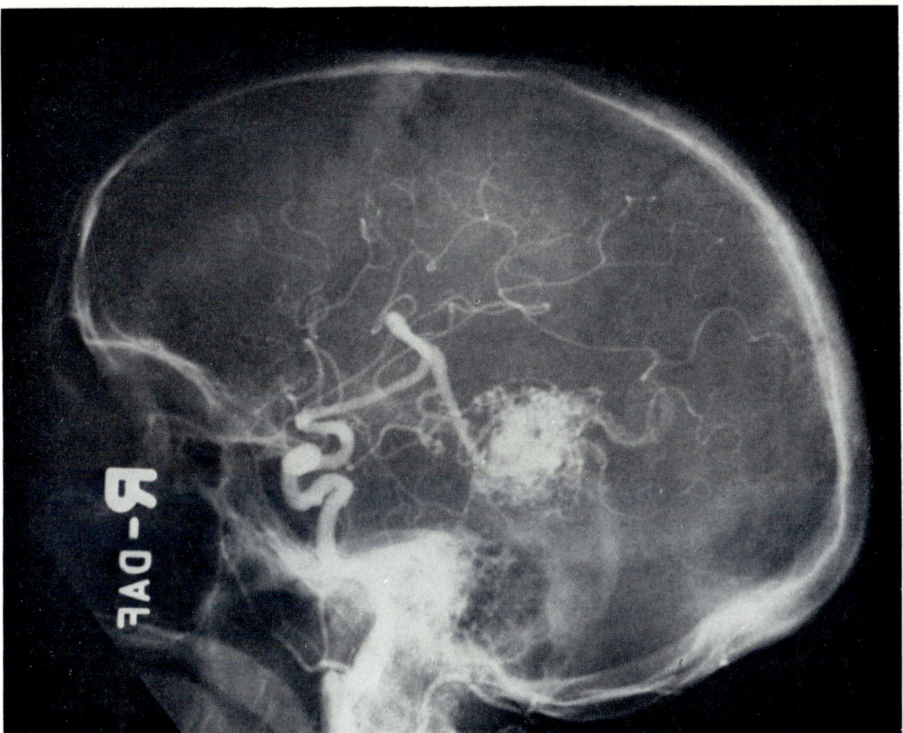

Figure 41. Caudal cerebral arteriovenous malformation (posterior temporal). Large middle cerebral and smaller carotid feeding vessels enter the AVM. Large, tortuous and early filling cerebral veins drain the malformation.

occur. Dementia is more prominent with dominant cerebral involvement, and dysphasia, dyslexia and dysgraphia may be marked. Headache may be occipital or frontal or generalized. Seizures, with or without visual aura, may occur.

F. Tentorial meningioma syndrome (Fig. 42A-F) —like gliomas, meningiomas are also relatively uncommon at the caudal pole of the brain. The tentorial meningioma at the time of diagnosis is usually of large size despite compression of primary visual areas. Chronic papilledema is usually present and cerebellar signs are common. The tumor may lie above or below or across the tentorium and to either side or through the posterior falx. It may occupy both supratentorial and subtentorial compartments at once. It may occlude the posterior sagittal sinus or the transverse sinus. It may compress and displace the vein of Galen and straight sinus. Symptoms include occipital, cervical or frontal headaches of long duration. Focal cerebral seizures with a visual aura of bright or flashing lights may precede other symptoms by months or years. Pro-

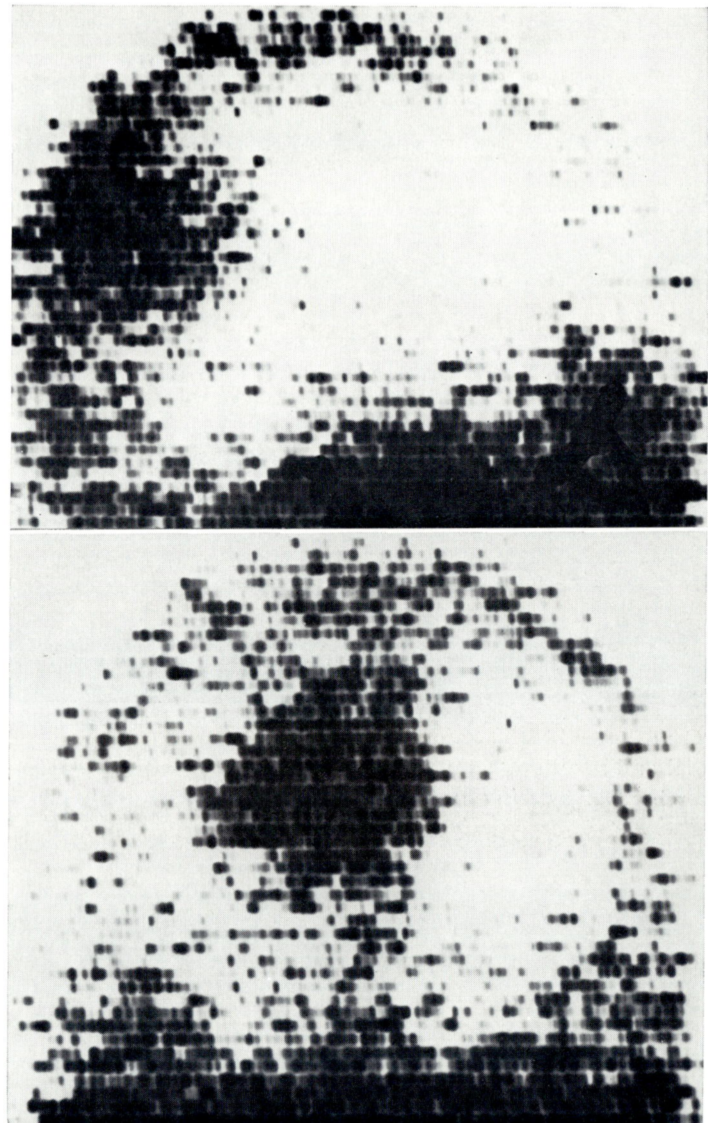

Figure 42. Tentorial meningioma. The lateral *(A)* and occipital *(B)* brain scans reveal the heavy uptake of this large tentorial meningioma. The lateral vertebral arteriograms in the early *(C)* and late *(D)* phases depict the abnormal tumor vessels and tumor cloud. The vertebral arteriograms in frontal projection show a different view of the same caudal extracerebral mass. *(E* and *F)*. Malignant cells were present within this unusual meningioma. A pea-sized daughter meningioma with separate dural attachment was adjacent to the main tentorial tumor at surgery in this previously nonoperated patient.

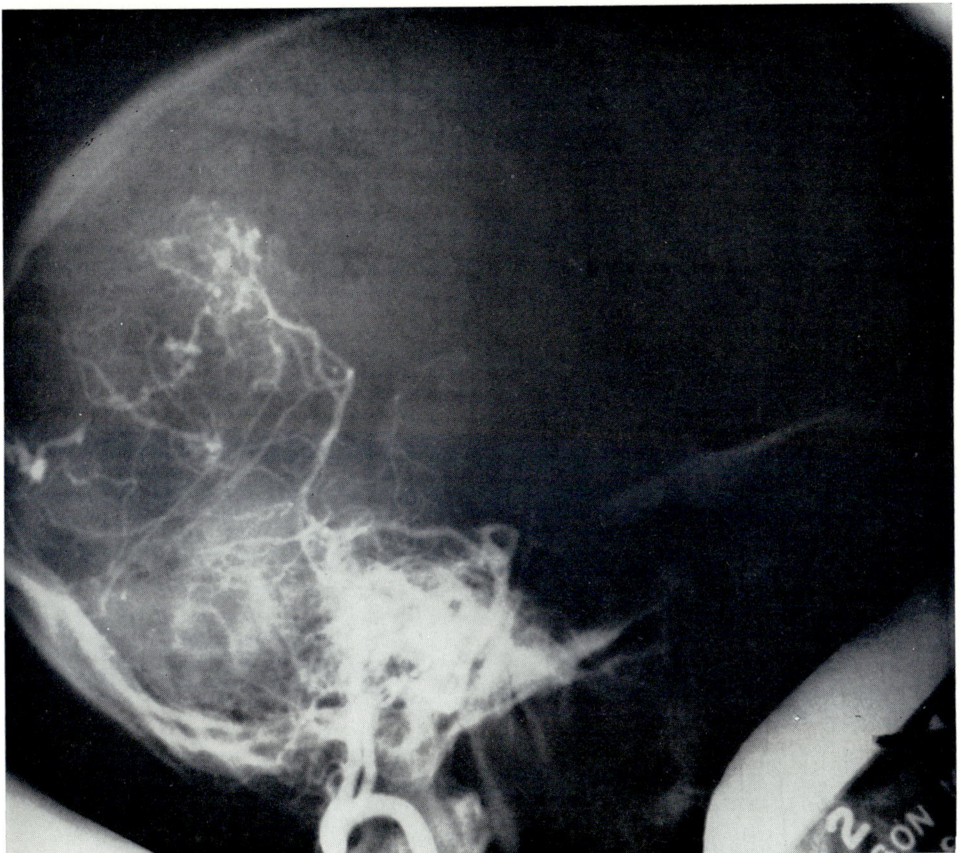

Figure 42 C.

gressive visual deterioration is common and occurs with secondary optic atrophy consequent to papilledema. Hemianopia is progressive and, unlike temporal tumors, if a quadrantanopia is detected, it usually involves the inferior fields. The usual field changes include homonymous hemianopia, peripheral field constriction and enlargement of the blind spot. Cerebellar signs include ataxia, hypotonia, hyporeflexia, and nystagmus. Intracranial hypertension due to the bulk of the tumor may be magnified by cerebral edema resulting from compression of the deep venous drainage of the brain, in the region of the vein of Galen. Venous sinus occlusion contributes to the intracranial pressure. Persistent vomiting, increasing headache and obtundation occur late. Palpable hyperostosis in the region of the occiput is occasionally present, along with marked increase in the prominence of scalp vessels.

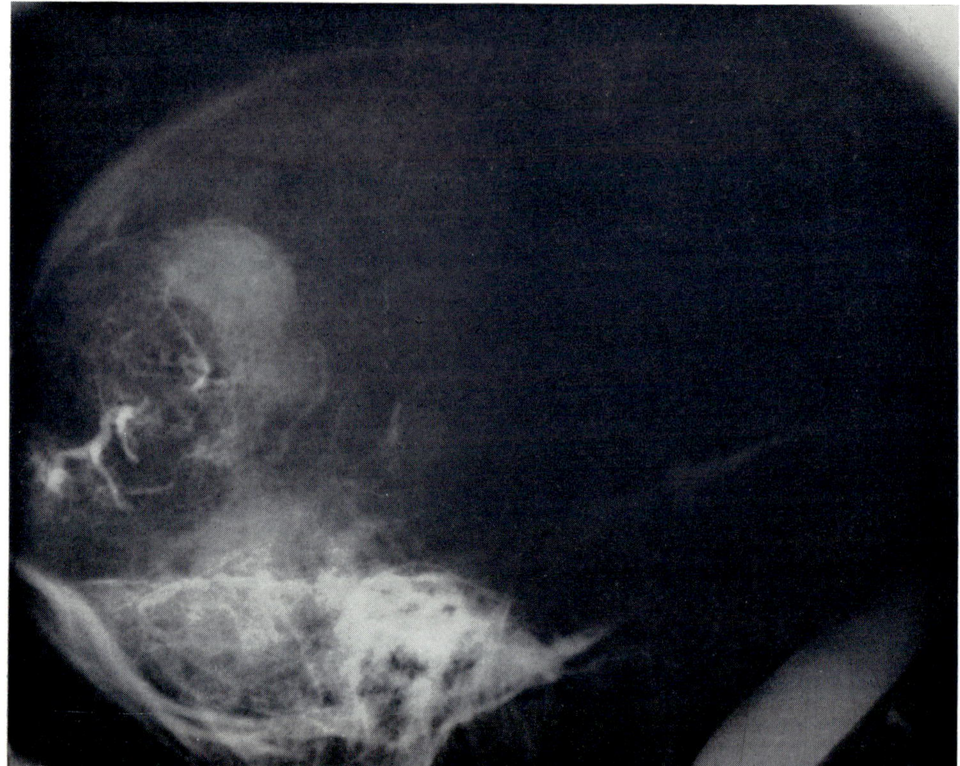

Figure 42 D.

Deficits of the Caudal Cerebral Syndrome

There are three basic deficits produced by caudal cerebral lesions: central hemianopia, complex disorders of recognition (including receptive aphasia) and visual seizures.

A. Central hemianopia

Homonymous hemianopia, in which visual half-fields of the same side (right or left) are lost, is always due to a lesion of the visual pathways posterior to the optic chiasm. At the level of the chiasm, hemianopia is usually bitemporal. The most common form of homonymous visual field deficit is central hemianopia. This results from a lesion of the opposite optic radiation or calcarine cortex. It is a geniculocalcarine or thalamocortical sign. In contrast, the less common homonymous defect is tract hemianopia, due to a lesion of the opposite optic tract. This

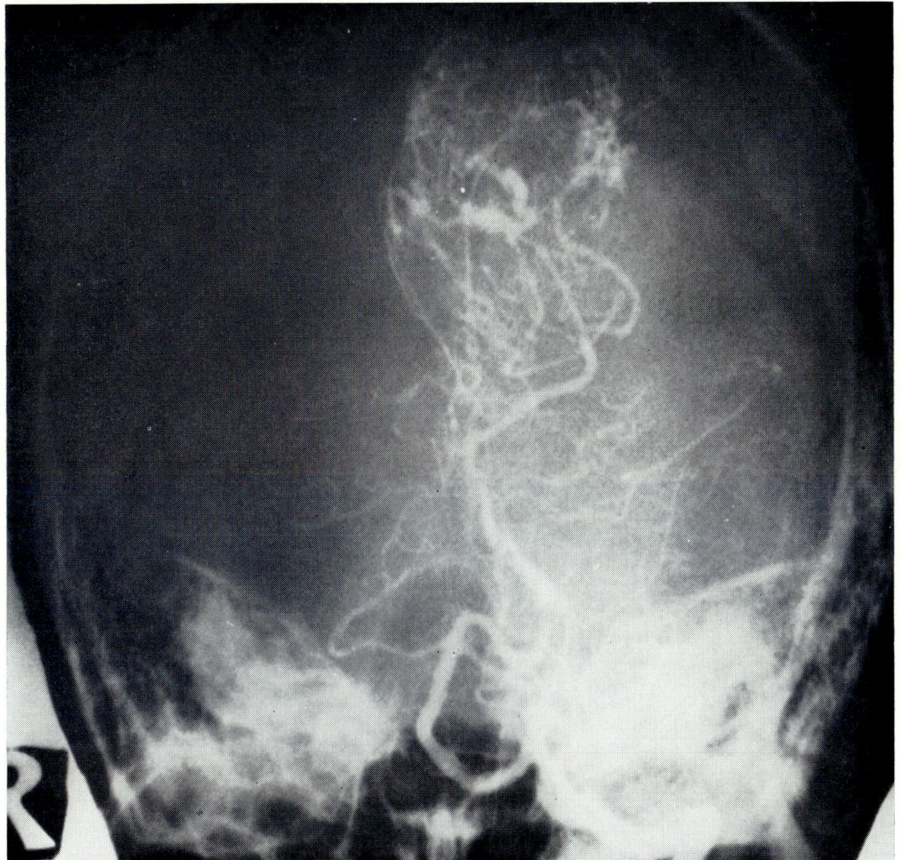

Figure 42 E.

is a pregeniculate (prethalamic) basal rather than caudal sign. The differentiation between central and tract hemianopia depends primarily upon the character of the visual field cut itself. Secondarily, the presence or absence of ocular signs is helpful in differentiation. Finally, associated regional signs may point to either hemispheral or subhemispheral disease.

1. Visual field signs.
   a. Lack of awareness of visual deficit—this is most often due to central hemianopia and indicates a caudal lesion; this impaired awareness may take a number of forms.
      (1) Striking objects and groping are more common with caudal lesions.
      (2) The patient may be partially aware of visual deficit, consider-

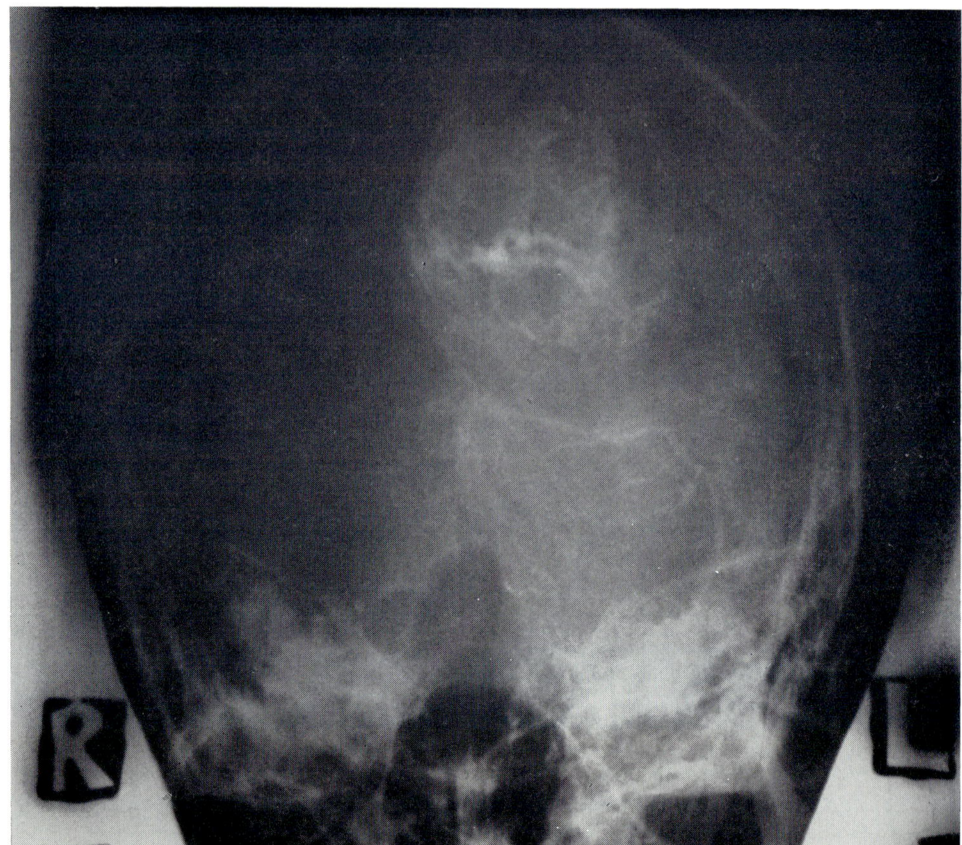

Figure 42 F.

ing the symptoms to be monocular or due to inadequate lighting.

(3) Negative hemianopia—the patient is merely aware of "something missing" on the hemianopic side.

(4) White hemianopia—the patient is only aware of visual deficit when placed in the dark, the half-fields opposite the caudal lesion appearing bright white.

(5) Black hemianopia—the patient is fully aware of black bisection of objects; this is more common with rostral than with caudal lesions of the visual pathway.

(6) Hemichromatopsia—the patient with a caudal cerebral lesion on either side may be hemianopic for colored objects in the opposite visual field, while black-white perception is intact.

This differs from innate color blindness and also from acquired color agnosia. In the latter, a dominant caudal cerebral lesion results in inability to recognize colors which the patient sees (i.e. it may occur without any visual field defect). It also differs from aphasic disturbances in which the patient has an anomia for colors along with other language defects.

(7) Riddoch's sign—the patient is unaware of stationary objects opposite a caudal cerebral lesion, while perception of small moving objects is intact. There may be associated loss of depth perception.

(8) Unilateral visual neglect—double simultaneous visual stimulation reveals a loss of awareness (inattention) for the test object opposite the lesion, even when visual fields are otherwise normal.

b. Central vision—this is usually preserved in central hemianopia.

(1) Macular sparing—this indicates a caudal cerebral lesion, occurring especially with lesions of the occipital pole. Parietotemporal lesions either split or spare the macula. Macular sparing is absent in tract hemianopia. It is possibly an artifact of ocular fixation with the establishment of a pseudofovea. Sparing of the temporal crescent, like macular sparing, indicates an occipital lesion. The temporal crescent or most peripheral retina is represented most deeply and rostrally in the calcarine region.

(2) Macular splitting—this results from rostral lesions of the visual pathway. It does not occur if the optic fixation reflexes (i.e. occipital oculomotor field) are impaired. If the patient is able to fixate, the macula may be split, as it is in hemianopias of tract and rostral parietotemporal radiation lesions. Partial hemianopias may not bisect the fixation point.

(3) Conventional visual acuity remains unimpaired whether the macula is spared or split. Cerebral lesions, even when associated with papilledema and homonymous hemianopia often present normal acuity. Visual acuity also remains normal in lesions confined to the optic tract. However, most optic tract lesions are the result of tumors (craniopharyngioma, pituitary adenoma, optic-hypothalamic glioma) which to some extent also involve the optic chiasm. Such chiasmatic involvement impairs visual acuity. The combination of homonymous hemianopia with primary optic atrophy makes the diagnosis of an optic tract lesion certain.

c. Congruity—central hemianopic field cuts tend to be "congruous" or symmetrical.
   (1) The greater the symmetry, the more caudal the lesion.
   (2) Incongruous or asymmetrical hemianopias indicate a lesion of the opposite optic tract or temporal radiation.

d. Quadrantanopia—while the visual field cut of radiation or calcarine origin is usually hemianopic, it may be quadrantic.
   (1) Superior quadrantanopia—this is the most common homonymous quadrant defect; it is almost always due to a lesion of the temporal radiation including "Meyer's loop" (most rostral of the optic radiations curving around the temporal horn). While lesions of the occipital pole almost uniformly produce hemianopia, infracalcarine lesions may produce superior quadrant defects. Temporal lobe field cuts usually result from a mass lesion such as a glioma or abscess. Occipital lobe field cuts are usually of vascular origin.
   (2) Inferior quadrantanopia—this is a less common homonymous deficit; it is due to a lesion of the superior optic radiations at parietotemporal border; it is less often the result of a supracalcarine occipital lesion. If the inferior quadrant defect gradually becomes a hemianopia, a parietal glioma with caudal cerebral extension is the most likely diagnosis.
   (3) Since the optic tract is small and compact, tract lesions produce hemianopia rather than quadrantanopia.

e. Development of homonymous hemianopia.
   (1) Slowly developing central hemianopia indicates a caudal cerebral tumor; rapid development most commonly is vascular in origin.
   (2) A caudal cerebral glioma is usually parietotemporal rather than occipital. The typical course is a gradually progressive central hemianopia with initial involvement of the periphery of the visual field and ultimate central field defect. The field defect may be preceded by visual inattention on the side opposite the tumor. Hemichromatopsia for colored objects typically precedes black-white hemianopia.
   (3) A temporal pole glioma may initially spare the visual pathways. Glioblastoma of the temporal pole causes relatively rapid uncal herniation. Temporal gliomas proceeding caudally produce an incongruous superior quadrantanopia. Hemianopia develops as the posterior temporal and temporoparietal

region is involved. The defect becomes increasingly congruous as it extends caudally.

(4) Sudden, completely congruous central hemianopia followed by improvement in the central field is virtually always vascular.

2. Ocular signs associated with homonymous hemianopia.
   a. The fundi, pupils and ocular motility are often normal in caudal cerebral lesions producing central hemianopia.
   b. Diminished or absent optokinetic nystagmus (OKN), readily demonstrated with a tape measure, on the side opposite a caudal cerebral lesion may be the sole abnormality.
      (1) The OKN response must be clearly asymmetrical to be a valid sign.
      (2) The deficit is on the hemianopic side; it may precede hemianopia.
      (3) The OKN response remains symmetrical in optic tract lesions.
      (4) Thalamic and brain stem lesions also produce a decreased OKN response.
   c. Papilledema with homonymous hemianopia.
      (1) Choked discs and central hemianopia point to a caudal cerebral tumor, either intracerebral (e.g. temporoparietal glioma) or extracerebral (e.g. tentorial meningioma).
      (2) Choked discs with tract hemianopia indicate a mass lesion involving the optic tract with third ventricular extension and foraminal block (e.g. craniopharyngioma).
      (3) The visual field defects associated with papilledema (enlargement of the blind spot and peripheral construction) are superimposed upon the hemianopia.
      (4) If the fundi are normal, artifactual enlargement of the blind spot may accompany the use of small test objects or poor illumination. An abnormal blind spot is an early sign of glaucoma. In glaucoma, ring scotomas and nasal visual field defects rather than homonymous hemianopia occur. The normal blind spot is always temporal to the fixation point, since the optic disc is nasal to the fovea. Pseudopapilledema may be indicated by a blind spot which is not enlarged. Apparent peripheral field constriction may result from visual inattention. "Tubular vision" may occur in cortical blindness, double hemianopia and hysteria. In hysteria, the peripheral constriction may remain the same despite distance from the tangent screen.
   d. Primary optic atrophy with homonymous hemianopia.

(1) Primary atrophy of the optic disc is never the result of a caudal cerebral lesion.

(2) Primary optic atrophy with homonymous hemianopia is a sign of an optic tract lesion.

(a) When present, the atrophy is usually greater in the disc opposite the lesion.

(b) The atrophy is less marked than that of optic nerve or chiasm lesions.

e. Secondary optic atrophy-disc atrophy consequent to papilledema has no localizing value; it indicates long-standing intracranial hypertension. The disc is not only pale, but its margins are blurred or irregular, the optic cup has lost its definition, and there is often evidence of previous retinal hemorrhage.

f. Behr's sign—tract hemianopia is often accompanied by a larger pupil opposite the lesion. This does not occur in central hemianopia.

g. Horner's syndrome—miosis and ptosis occasionally occur ipsilateral to a temporal tumor. Involvement of the sympathetic plexus around the carotid as it emerges from the cavernous sinus medial to the temporal lobe may be responsible. If ptosis is absent, the small pupil on the side of the tumor may give the erroneous impression that the opposite pupil is dilated ("pseudo-Behr's sign"). The presence of superior quadrantanopia (or central hemianopia) indicates a temporal (or temporoparietal) mass on the side of the small pupil. With uncal or hippocampal herniation, the ipsilateral pupil becomes dilated, and the field cut escapes detection due to progressive stupor and coma.

h. Cogan's sign—parietal lesions produce conjugate contralateral eye deviation when the patient forcibly closes his lids while the examiner tries to open them. This occurs also in brain stem lesions and in some normal persons.

i. Wernicke's hemianopic pupillary sign—there is loss of the light reflex in optic tract lesions if the light source can be confined to the nonfunctioning portion of the retina. This does not occur in central hemianopia. However, it is difficult to demonstrate due to intraocular scatter of light.

3. Regional signs associated with homonymous hemianopia—the presence of regional deficits clarifies the localization in central and tract hemianopia. Cerebral dominance plays a very significant role in caudal (central) lesions; it does not in basal (tract) lesions.

a. Right homonymous central hemianopia—this field cut is associated with the regional signs of a left (major) caudal cerebral syndrome.
   (1) Receptive aphasia.
   (2) Alexia.
   (3) Agraphia.
   (4) Acalculia.
   (5) Visual agnosias.
   (6) Bilateral body-image agnosias.
   (7) Ideomotor apraxia.

b. Left homonymous central hemianopia—this field cut is associated with the regional deficits of a right (minor) caudal cerebral syndrome.
   (1) Spatial agnosias.
   (2) Unilateral body-image agnosias.
   (3) Constructional apraxia.
   (4) Apraxia for dressing.

c. Geniculate hemianopia—lesions involving the lateral geniculate body usually include the adjacent thalamus and corticospinal tract. The signs are contralateral to the lesion.
   (1) Central homonymous hemianopia.
   (2) Hemisensory deficit.
   (3) Thalamic pain (vascular lesions).
   (4) Hemiplegia.

d. Homonymous tract hemianopia—signs resulting from involvement of regional structures may accompany this field defect.
   (1) Hypothalamic and pituitary disorders.
   (2) Optic chiasm—associated bitemporal hemianopia with increased optic atrophy and decreased visual acuity.
   (3) Third ventricular extension or cisternal block-signs of intracranial hypertension and hydrocephalus.
   (4) Sphenoid ridge signs.
   (5) Uncinate seizures.

4. Double hemianopia—this results from bilateral involvement of the optic radiations ("cerebral blindness"). Like "cortical blindness," vascular disease with basilar thrombosis and bilateral posterior cerebral occlusion is the most common cause. Hypoxia, vertebral angiography, encephalopathy, Schilder's disease and various toxins also produce the syndrome. Responsible lesions of neurosurgical interest are occipital trauma and certain tumors.

   The patient with double hemianopia typically gropes about, but does not complain of his virtually complete blindness. He may even deny his severe visual loss or admit to only "poor lighting." Markedly constricted visual fields with bilateral tubular vision may be present. Apathy, euphoria, confabulation and spatial disorientation are common. The pupils are usually dilated and reactive. Extraocular movements may be impaired especially in convergence. Optokinetic nystagmus is bilaterally lost. Sudden onset, tendency for improvement and normal optic discs indicate a vascular etiology. Consecutive onset of unilateral hemianopia, papilledema and ultimate double hemianopia indicates a caudally situated tumor. A tentorial meningioma or a caudal cerebral glioma with extension through the splenium of the corpus callosum ("caudal butterfly") may be responsible. Bilateral posterior cerebral arterial compression during transtentorial herniation may result in bioccipital calcarine ischemia; any supratentorial mass may be responsible. However, the presence of coma in these cases masks the presence of visual loss.

B. Complex disorders of recognition

These disturbances result from caudal cerebral lesions involving the parietotemporal or parieto-occipital cortex or underlying white matter. They are "complex" because the elemental forms of sensation are relatively or entirely intact. They are complex in another sense, in that "cerebral dominance" is critical in these disorders. The sidedness of the cerebral lesion determines the character of the recognition deficit. It is clinically useful to define two distinct syndromes depending on whether the major or minor hemisphere is involved. The signs as listed apply to right-handed patients.

1. Left (major) caudal cerebral syndrome—the basic triad of aphasia, agnosia and apraxia is involved.
   a. Disorders of recognition of language and number.
      (1) Receptive aphasia.
      (2) Alexia.
      (3) Agraphia.
      (4) Acalculia.
   b. Disorders of perceptual recognition (agnosia).
      (1) Visual agnosias.
      (2) Bilateral spatial agnosia.
      (3) Bilateral body-image agnosias.
   c. Disorders of perceptually related movement (apractognosia).
      (1) Ideomotor apraxia.
      (2) Ideational apraxia.
2. Right (minor) caudal cerebral syndrome—the basic components are the dual deficits of agnosia and apraxia in the absence of aphasia. The

agnostic and apraxic difficulties differ from those of the dominant hemisphere.

a. Disorders of perceptual recognition (agnosia).
   (1) Left hemispatial agnosia.
   (2) Left body-image agnosias.
b. Disorders of perceptually related movement (apractognosia).
   (1) Constructional apraxia.
   (2) Apraxia for dressing.

These complex disorders of recognition usually occur in various combinations rather than in isolated fashion. They may or may not be associated with central hemianopia opposite the lesion. The signs are often partial (e.g. dysphasia, dyscalculia) rather than complete. The lateralizing value of these deficits is diminished in the left-handed patient. The presence of "sinistral signs" (Ch. 5) renders the detection of hemianopia particularly important, since the field cut definitely lateralizes the lesion to the opposite side.

1. Major (left) caudal cerebral signs.
   a. Receptive aphasia—the basic defect in sensory aphasia is an inability to understand speech. While expressive difficulties are often present, the major deficiency is in recognition. Receptive aphasia indicates a left parietotemporal lesion in virtually all right-handed (and two-thirds of left-handed) patients.
      (1) Conversation exceeds comprehension—the patient tends to be garrulous; this is the reverse of expressive aphasia in which there is a general reduction in the quantity of speech.
      (2) Jargon aphasia—speech is confused in words, grammar and meaning.
      (3) Paraphasia—in speaking, the patient employs the wrong words and is typically unaware of his errors.
      (4) Clang associations—the words which the patient selects often reveal some connection with the proper words.
      (5) Parietal dysnomia—the patient usually has great difficulty in naming common objects. He is often unconcerned by his inability to name them. The words he employs to describe the object reveal jargon. Paraphasia is present in his writing when asked to write the name of the object. This dysnomia can be differentiated from the following:
         (a) Temporal dysnomia—the patient has great difficulty finding words in both spoken and written language. Comprehension may be relatively intact, as may be reading, read-

ing aloud, and writing from dictation (i.e. nominal aphasia).

(b) Frontal dysnomia—the patient mispronounces the correct name, or if unable to supply the correct name due to severe speech reduction, he makes negative gestures or says No when the examiner supplies false names. He writes the name correctly.

(6) Verbal perseveration—the patient's words are repeated by him in a stereotyped manner.

(7) Repetition sign—the patient is unable to correctly repeat words spoken to him.

(8) Automatic speech—conventional phrases may be properly employed.

(9) Articulation is normal; the patient's difficulties in verbal expression stem from impaired recognition.

(10) Alexia and agraphia are associated with receptive aphasia; the patient is unable to comprehend written material and is unable to write correctly.

(11) Receptive aphasia should be carefully differentiated from general confusion or disorientation. The aphasic speech deficit has both lateralizing and localizing value, while the other disturbances are nonspecific.

(a) Special object-naming ("pin"—"pen"—"penny") and sequence-naming (months of the year, forward and reverse) will often uncover subtle dysnomia and perseveration.

(b) Generalized confusion which is increasing and associated with restlessness is a common sign of intracranial hypertension; it may be a prelude to stupor, coma and transtentorial herniation.

(c) Disorientation to time, place and person also has diffuse cerebral implications. Disorientation in time is the most sensitive and persistent abnormality of the three spheres in organic cerebral disease. Disorientation in place and person without disorientation in time suggests hysteria.

(12) Global aphasia—this is a virtually total loss of communication resulting from severe combined receptive and expressive deficits.

(a) The total amount of speech is markedly reduced and may be totally absent (the patient remaining alert enough to test).

(b) The patient's comprehension of speech is also markedly reduced and may be totally absent.

(c) Acute lesions of the deep temporoparietal white matter, thalamus and basal ganglia ("lenticular zone") of the dominant hemisphere characteristically produce this major deficit.

(d) Acute cortical lesions (contusion, laceration) of presylvian, intrasylvian, suprasylvian, retrosylvian, and infrasylvian regions of the dominant hemisphere (sectors 2, 3, 4, 5, 6, and 7) may also produce a global aphasia. With recovery, the deficit is chiefly expressive if rostral (sectors, 2, 3, 4), and chiefly receptive if caudal (sectors 5, 6, 7).

b. Alexia—an inability to understand written or printed letters or words as a result of a dominant caudal cerebral lesion.

(1) Aphasic alexia—receptive aphasia is usually associated with severe reading difficulties resulting from poor comprehension, often compounded by right homonymous hemianopia. This is accompanied by agraphia. The combination of aphasia, alexia and agraphia is the most common form. It is usually vascular, but may result from trauma or neoplasm of the dominant parietotemporal region.

(2) Agraphic alexia—a less common reading-writing disorder without significant aphasia. This is frequently associated with Gerstmann's syndrome (finger agnosia, right-left disorientation, acalculia and agraphia). It is due to vascular, traumatic or neoplastic lesions of the dominant parieto-occipital region.

(3) Pure alexia—this is a rare reading disorder occurring without significant aphasia and agraphia. Right homonymous hemianopia and color agnosia are associated. The onset is sudden and almost exclusively due to thrombosis of the dominant posterior cerebral artery. The infarct involves the major occipital lobe and splenium of the corpus callosum.

(4) Pseudoalexia—this is a common false-localizing sign. "Dyslexia" is a term most often used to denote an inability to learn to read ("developmental dyslexia"). It has also been employed to indicate a partial deficit. A third usage suggests that the reading disability represents a pseudoalexia.

(a) Frontal dyslexia—dominant fronto-opercular lesions with expressive aphasia reveal a defect in reading aloud. The patient understands what he reads, but has some difficulty in remembering series of words. He looks back to the beginning of a sentence frequently. What he does read aloud is poorly pronounced and accompanied by buccofacial apraxia.

(b) Parietal dyslexia—dominant parieto-opercular lesions with conduction aphasia also reveal a defect in reading aloud. The patient reads hesitantly and understands most of what he reads. He is relatively unconcerned by this disability.

(c) Caudal pseudoalexia—in true alexia the patient is unable to interpret the words that he sees. In pseudoalexia due to a dominant caudal lesion, the reading difficulty is a result of right homonymous hemianopia, the right halves of words or sentences escaping visual detection. In pseudoalexia due to a nondominant caudal lesion, reading disturbance results from unilateral left-sided spatial neglect or from left homonymous hemianopia. These patients have difficulty finding the beginnings of lines and skip lines as a result. True alexia almost always indicates a dominant left-sided lesion. Pseudoalexia occurs with left- or right-sided lesions. A reading disturbance may also be an early sign of an occipital lesion, resulting from impaired ocular fixation reflexes (i.e. occipital oculomotor field) which precede the onset of other visual deficits.

c. Agraphia—defective writing in the absence of paralysis has clinical use as an adjunctive sign.

(1) Aphasic agraphia—all forms of aphasia are associated with writing disturbances. The demonstration of agraphia is important in the differentiation of an aphasia from general confusion, since written and spoken language are affected together. Agraphia is most common in the presence of aphasia, but does occur without it. Agraphia is generally associated with left cerebral lesions.

(2) Frontal dysgraphia—this accompanies expressive aphasia. The patient can copy correctly but cannot write well to dictation. Spontaneous writing is limited to common words and is otherwise defective. Spelling errors are present. Kinetic (motor) apraxia of the right hand severely impairs writing.

(3) Parieto-occipital dysgraphia—this is the writing disorder associated with Gerstmann's syndrome. Like the frontal form, the patient can copy well but cannot write to dictation. There are also defects in spontaneous writing with irregular script, graphic perseveration and paragraphia including erroneous letters or words. Finger agnosia, right-left disorientation, and acalculia complete Gerstmann's syndrome. Alexia may be associated, without significant aphasia.

(4) Parietotemporal dysgraphia—the writing disorder of receptive

aphasia is typically severely disturbed. Writing is often unintelligible and includes the jargon which confuses speech. Spontaneous writing, writing to dictation and copying are all defective. Alexia is associated.

(5) Spatial dysgraphia—while the dysgraphias listed above are all associated with dominant cerebral lesions, spatial dysgraphia occurs as a result of nondominant caudal cerebral involvement. The patient tends to leave a large margin on the left. His writing on the right side of the page may suddenly shift in direction. Copying may reveal gross neglect of the left-sided portions of words or lines. Gross abnormalities in copying accompany associated constructional apraxia.

(6) Micrographia—writing is reduced in size and is often barely legible. It is most commonly seen in Parkinson's disease, but may occur with deep cerebral tumors involving the basal ganglia. It also occurs with macropsia secondary to retinal disease.

(7) Macrographia—writing is enlarged in size and is usually due to cerebellar lesions resulting in dysmetria. It may result from the visuospatial disorders of left or right caudal cerebral lesions. It also occurs with micropsia due to retinopathy.

d. Acalculia—inability to calculate may occur in diffuse cerebral dementias. It may also accompany frontal, parietal, temporal or occipital lesions of a focal nature. Calculation defects accompany both left and right cerebral lesions. Disturbances in the recognition and manipulation of numbers which have some localizing value are as follow:

(1) Aphasias are usually associated with calculation difficulty; counting and simple sums may be correct, but beyond this some degree of dyscalculia occurs with the dominant cerebral language disorder.

(2) Acalculia of Gerstmann's syndrome—results from a dominant parieto-occipital lesion. It is associated with bilateral finger agnosia. It is most marked for computations made on paper or "motor arithmetic." Defects of "mental arithmetic" are present, but less severe. The patient may be unable to add on paper, while able to mentally multiply.

(3) Alexia for numerals—associated with alexia for words. Inability to comprehend written and spoken numerals, letters and words occurs in dominant parietotemporal lesions producing receptive aphasia. Dysnomia for numbers may also be present.

(4) Spatial dyscalculia—incorrect alignment of numbers on paper

with associated left-sided spatial neglect occurs in nondominant caudal cerebral lesions. Finger counting is disturbed in the left hand. Abnormalities in copying numbers occur due to the presence of constructional apraxia.

(5) Frontal dyscalculia—there is a general deterioration in calculation appropriate to the general level of torpor. The patient may add and subtract but not multiply or divide. Significant amnesia is usually accompanied by calculation disorders most marked for division and least for addition. The patient may exhibit perseverate calculation as in the subtraction of 7's from 100: 93, 83, 73. Dominant frontal lesions are associated with improper pronunciation of numbers along with other expressive difficulties.

e. Visual agnosias—these are disorders of the perceptual recognition of objects, pictures or colors which occur with dominant parieto-occipital lesions.

(1) Visual object agnosia—an inability to identify common objects which are seen, though they can be named when presented to the other senses. The patient is unconcerned or unaware of the deficit. Right homonymous hemianopia is often associated.

(2) Picture agnosia—an inability to interpret the content of pictures; often accompanied by alexia.

(3) Color agnosia—an acquired deficit in naming colors which may occur without visual field defect.

(4) Frontal visual agnosia—patients with frontal lesions may have difficulty identifying objects as a result of visual inattention. This is associated with gaze inertia, easy distractability and apparent concentric contraction of visual fields due to failure of attention.

f. Bilateral spatial agnosia.

Dominant or bilateral caudal cerebral lesions may result in an impaired recognition of the relative position of body parts or objects in space. This is associated with "right-left disorientation" (e.g. the patient may be requested to touch his left ear with his right hand). These patients cannot find their way about. They walk in the wrong direction, walk into objects and present "near-far disorientation." They are spatially disoriented for length and width of objects. Given the direction of the north, they cannot determine the south. They may demonstrate "spatial ataxia." Bilateral spatial agnosia is usually accompanied by ocular signs including a tendency to stare with impaired blinking, ocular fixation and convergence palsy. Right homonymous hemianopia, or double hemianopia, may be associated. This form of spatial agnosia produces bilateral deficits; it differs from the unilateral left spatial neglect of minor hemisphere lesions.

g. Bilateral body-image agnosias.

These are disorders of the perceptual recognition of fingers (finger agnosia) or body parts (asomatognosia) resulting from dominant parieto-occipital lesions. These defects are always bilateral and therefore differ from the unilateral body-image agnosias (hemiasomatognosia and anosognosia) of the minor hemisphere.

(1) Finger agnosia—the patient is unable to recognize or name the fingers, including his fingers and those of the examiner. The defect applies to the fingers of both hands and is most marked for the index, middle and ring fingers. The patient can correctly identify other body parts. The fingers are not paralyzed or apraxic. This is the chief component of Gerstmann's syndrome (also includes right-left disorientation, agraphia and acalculia). The syndrome may be partial. It may be associated with other deficits (e.g. alexia, right homonymous hemianopia).

(2) Asomatognosia—this is a bilateral agnosia involving a lack of recognition for all body parts. The patient cannot identify his own anatomy, nor that of the examiner. Right-left disorientation is commonly associated.

(3) Right-left disorientation—the inability to determine the sidedness of body parts occurs with Gerstmann's finger agnosia and with asomatognosia. There may also be an inability to determine the sidedness of objects in external space. Right-left disorientation with near-far disorientation is a common feature of bilateral spatial agnosia.

h. Ideomotor apraxia—perceptually related movement is impaired. This form of apractognosia results from a dominant parietal, parietotemporal or parieto-occipital lesion.

(1) The motor disability is bilateral.

(2) The motor impairment is marked in the absence of paralysis.

(3) The patient is unable to imitate movements which are demonstrated to him; he is also unable to perform movements to command.

(4) Spontaneous movements are relatively intact.

(5) The apraxia involves all four extremities.

(6) The patient employs hesitant, roundabout movements to accomplish the motor task.

(7) The patient usually does not notice his disability.

i. Ideational apraxia—this is also an apractognosia. The disturbance in perceptually related movement in this instance is more severe. This apraxia may result from either dominant caudal cerebral or diffuse cerebral disease.

(1) The patient appears quite absentminded.

(2) He has little or no concept of the required motor task.

(3) He performs an unrelated or only tangentially related movement, if at all, upon request.

(4) This apraxia also involves all four extremities.

Note: These apraxias should be differentiated from "kinetic (motor) apraxia" which is an excessively clumsy hand due to a premotor frontal lesion on the opposite side. All fine hand movements are impossible, although the arm may be used for gross movement.

2. Minor (right) caudal cerebral signs.

The right frontal pole and the right temporal pole are particularly "silent" regions of the brain. An early lesion of either of these poles may present little more than flattening of the left nasolabial fold. The right caudal pole, however, is not silent. Deficits produced by a lesion of the subordinate hemisphere are not burdened by the communication blockade of aphasia. The patient who can understand and produce speech is more readily tested for agnosia. Agnosias are disorders in which the patient does not recognize the significance of sensory stimulation, the elemental sensations being intact. It is Jacksonian "imperception." It is interesting that this silent, non-talking hemisphere is revealed by the Freudian term "agnosia." The personal and extrapersonal agnosias of the subordinate hemisphere apply to the left body-half and left side of space. Any associated hemiplegia involves the left extremities, the normally less useful left hand escaping awareness in Babinskian "anosognosia." The master right hand remains free from paralysis, rendering its perceptually deficient drawing and constructive capacities most vivid. Such personal, spatial and constructive defects are combined in the production of the curious, perceptually dependent "apraxia for dressing" typical of right-sided lesions. The subordinate parietotemporal or parieto-occipital lesion is thus characterized by unilaterally predominant left-sided agnosias and right-sided apractognosias in the absence of an aphasic barrier. This stands in marked contrast to the bilateral agnosias, bilateral apraxias and communication deficiencies of the speech hemisphere.

Complex perceptual deficits of the minor (right) caudal cerebral syndrome include hemispatial agnosia, hemiasomatognosia, anosognosia, constructional apraxia and apraxia for dressing.

a. Hemispatial agnosia.

This is a unilateral neglect of space to the left characteristic of a right caudal cerebral lesion. The patient directs his visual attention to the right. Spontaneous turning of his head to the right may be intermittent. He may not turn his head or his gaze to the left at all, even when conversing with an examiner standing on his left side. It is well for an examiner to routinely stand at a patient's left so that this sign is not overlooked. The patient bumps into objects on the left despite intact vision. Other features include the following:

(1) Spatial dysnomia—the patient fails to name objects visually presented to his left side, but names them as they are moved to his right. Aphasia is not present.

(2) Spatial dysgraphia—the patient leaves an excessive margin on the left side of his writing paper. The patient may be unable to spontaneously write or to copy. Writing reveals hemispatial and constructional deficits.

(3) Spatial dyslexia—the patient may read single lines well, but be unable to locate the following line. If there is serious difficulty with reading a line from left to right, the same line printed vertically may be read correctly.

(4) Pseudoaphasia—these spatial language disorders of dysnomia, dysgraphia and dyslexia due to a minor hemisphere lesion may simulate a mild aphasia in which verbal comprehension and expression are otherwise intact. They may erroneously suggest that the patient has right-sided dominance for speech.

(5) Spatial dyscalculia—the patient may be unable to count objects correctly. Finger counting is especially disturbed in the left hand. The patient has difficulty in copying numbers and in aligning them correctly on paper.

(6) Unilateral disorientation—while right-left disorientation occurs with dominant (e.g. Gerstmann's syndrome) or bilateral caudal lesions, a unilateral inability to determine the position of left-sided objects or body parts may occur with caudal lesions of the minor hemisphere. The patient recognizes right-sidedness but fails on left-sided identification. When requested to raise his right arm, the patient does so. When requested to raise an unparalyzed left arm, the patient either does nothing or again elevates the right. This may be difficult to separate from the left-sided poverty of movement due to neglect which frequently accompanies a right caudal lesion.

b. Hemiasomatognosia—this uncommon deficit is an agnosia for the left body-half, a "hemidepersonalization." The patient is unaware of his left body-half and often is unaware of the left side of space. He looks to the right.

c. Anosognosia.

This is a more common deficit in which the patient is not aware of coexistent left hemiplegia. The most common cause is a right parietotemporal or right posterior capsule infarction. The anosognosia is typically transient in vascular hemiplegia, lasting only several days, while the hemiplegia is dense and persistent. A right caudal tumor is much less common, but should be suspected if the anosognosia accompanies a more gradually progressive left-sided motor paralysis. If the patient is confronted by his paralyzed left extremities, he is typically unconcerned and may deny the disability. The normally less useful left hand, following the paralysis, is now totally ignored by the patient. This deficit is commonly associated with left central hemianopia, left hemisensory deficit and constructional apraxia of the right hand.

d. Constructional apraxia.

This perceptually dependent movement disorder (apractognosia) consists of an inability to draw, to assemble and to arrange objects. This disability can be detected in both hands, but the normal capacity of the left hand is limited, especially in drawing. Abnormalities are thus most vividly demonstrated in the right master hand. Significant paralysis of a hand obviously prevents detection of its skilled or praxic ability. Significant aphasia also interferes in that the patient may not understand the requirements of the test. Thus, while constructional apraxia occurs with both left and right parietotemporal or parieto-occipital lesions, it is a more dramatic deficit when it results from a lesion of the nondominant hemisphere. If a dominant caudal lesion occurs without aphasia and paralysis, the presence of bilateral visual or spatial agnosias or ideomotor apraxia will interfere in constructional performance. In contrast, a lesion of the right parietal, parietotemporal, or parieto-occipital region leaves the ipsilateral master hand free to draw and build. The patient is required to copy, to draw from memory, or to construct simple objects with match sticks or blocks. Typical constructional deficits include the following:

(1) The copy is smaller than the sample.
(2) The copy is crowded to the right, revealing left-sided spatial neglect.
(3) "Closing-in" occurs with close approximation to the sample or overlapping of the copy upon the sample.

(4) Details are omitted, often those on the left.

(5) Perspective is omitted, the patient drawing a square when instructed to copy a cube.

(6) Lines are tilted, wavy or interrupted.

(7) Constructional perseveration—lines shown in the sample are repeated many times in the copy.

(8) The patient is often pleased with his efforts despite poor performance.

e. Apraxia for dressing.

The inability to properly dress obviously may accompany any diffusely dementing process. The patient with a dominant cerebral lesion with bilateral ideomotor apraxia of all four extremities may have difficulties in dressing himself as a part of the more generalized loss of skilled movement. The localizing value of apraxia for dressing only exists when it occurs in relative isolation. Under these circumstances, this deficit points to a right parietotemporal or right parieto-occipital lesion. The patient may put his arm in the wrong sleeve of his jacket, although his general mentation, vision and skilled movement appear normal. A left-sided unilateral clothing disarray may point to an underlying hemispatial neglect. Constructional apraxia is commonly associated.

3. Localizing principles in complex disorders of recognition.

Diffuse cerebral disease may present multiple disorders of recognition along with general disturbances in memory, orientation in time and place, mood and motor behavior. In neurosurgery, such diffuse cerebral involvement is commonly seen in head trauma, brain swelling and cerebral hypoxia.

In focal cerebral disease, the maximal localizing value from the complex recognition deficits may be obtained by application of the following principles:

a. The patient should be alert enough to allow a fair test.

b. Handedness should be determined.

c. Specific speech tests should be employed even if the patient's conversation appears normal. Dysphasia, even if subtle, implicates the left hemisphere in virtually all right-handed and in two-thirds of left-handed patients. Thus a cerebral speech disorder lateralizes the responsible lesion.

d. If conversation is markedly reduced and comprehension is relatively intact, the lesion is rostral (left frontal). If comprehension is reduced and conversation is excessive and erroneous, the lesion is caudal or deep cerebral (left parietotemporal). The character of the dysphasia localizes the lesion.

e. The visual fields should be carefully tested. The visual pathways constitute the major horizontal system of the brain with clearly definable deficits. The character of the field cut both lateralizes and localizes. In contrast, the major motor and sensory systems take a vertical course. As a consequence, the Babinski sign lateralizes but does not localize. It may be of cerebral, brain stem or spinal cord origin.

f. To define an agnosia, the primary sensory system involved must be relatively intact. To define an apraxia, the primary motor system involved must be relatively intact.

g. The combination of aphasia, agnosia and apraxia (the aphasia being receptive and the agnosia and apraxia being bilateral) indicates a caudal dominant lesion: left parietotemporal.

h. The combination of agnosia and apraxia (the agnosia and apraxia being bilateral) in the absence of aphasia also indicates a caudal dominant lesion: left parieto-occipital.

i. The combination of agnosia and apraxia (the agnosia being unilateral to the left and the apraxia being constructional in the right hand) in the absence of aphasia indicates a caudal nondominant lesion: right parietotemporal or right parieto-occipital.

j. The combination of aphasia and apraxia (the aphasia being expressive and the apraxia being kinetic in the right hand) indicates a rostral dominant lesion: left frontal.

C. Visual seizures

Caudal cerebral parietotemporal or parieto-occipital lesions result in three basic neurological deficiencies. Destructive lesions produce central hemianopia and complex disorders of recognition. Irritative lesions produce visual seizures. Temporal lobe epilepsy also may produce a visual ictal experience. These visual seizure disorders can usually be differentiated from visual hallucinations of a nonepileptic nature occurring in migraine, drug intoxication, oculo-optic and psychogenic disturbances.

1. The epileptic visual aura.

As described by Penfield (1954), this includes: ". . . darkness before the eyes going on to blindness, lights, stars, whirling and moving lights, and colored lights. These things may be seen in the visual field opposite the involved hemisphere, which the patient may explain as being seen with the eye on that side. More often, however, the phenomena appear straight ahead. As a rule such sensations increase rapidly in intensity, the light becomes so bright that the patient can see nothing, or the darkness advances to complete blindness, which may be followed by unconsciousness and some form of generalized convulsion."

2. The basic characteristics of the visual seizure due to focal cerebral disease are as follow:
   a. Stereotyped aura—the visual aura is relatively constant in the individual patient. Nonepileptic visual hallucination is usually more variable in content.
   b. Rapid evolution—the visual aura proceeds more rapidly and is of shorter duration than the visual phenomena occurring with migraine. Scotomas, hemianopias, headaches and episodic attacks may occur in both focal cerebral epilepsy and migraine.
   c. Relation to immediate environment—focal cerebral seizures are relatively unrelated to the immediate surroundings. Visual hallucinations of psychogenic origin often relate to environmental events.
   d. Oculocephalic turning—head and eyes turn toward the opposite side at the onset of the seizure, especially if the visual phenomena are projected to that side. Oculocephalic turning without a visual aura occurs in frontal adversive seizures.
   e. While the visual aura is usually followed by generalized convulsion and loss of consciousness, the seizure may be limited to the visual events. In the latter case, the aura may be vividly described by the patient.
3. Visual phenomena of localizing significance.
   a. Photopsias—these are subjective flashes of white or colored lights of an unformed type; these often indicate an occipital, parieto-occipital or temporo-occipital lesion.
   b. Formed visual seizures—subjective visualization of familiar objects, figures, faces or events usually indicate a temporal or temporoparietal lesion. Associated features favoring a temporal lesion include sensations of unpleasant odor, of sound, of unusual familiarity (déjà vu) or strangeness accompanied by automatic behavior during the attack.
   c. Metamorphopsias—these are visual distortions of the form of objects occurring on an episodic basis. They have relatively little localizing value. The structural characteristics become irregular, tilted, enlarged (macropsia), small (micropsia), inverted, flattened, or distorted as to color and movement. They are associated with vertigo. These visual aberrations may accompany drug intoxication or hysteria, but may also be seen in oculo-optic or cerebral epileptic lesions. Temporal lobe epilepsy or parieto-occipital visuospatial agnosia should be considered.
   d. Paliopsia (visual perseveration)—this is the subjective impression of an after-image of a removed object. While it may indicate a parieto-occipital lesion, it is a relatively nonspecific, rather than

epileptic, visual sign. It occurs with hemianopia, the persistent image transiently projected in the blind half of the visual field.

e. In the final analysis, the diagnosis of visual seizures due to a focal cerebral lesion must rest on the demonstration of other clinical, radiological or electroencephalographic signs.

Deformities (Angiographic and Pneumographic) of the Caudal Cerebral Syndromes

A. Angiographic deformities

1. Caudal intracerebral mass (e.g. posterior parieto-temporo-occipital glioma) —the majority of retrosylvian tumors are intracerebral rather than extracerebral; however, they are still less common than rostral cerebral gliomas.

a. Rostral displacement (lateral view) .

(1) Angiographic sylvian point—forward displacement of the last middle cerebral vessels at the posterior end of the sylvian fissure is the most prominent single sign of a retrosylvian mass.

(2) "Telescoping" of the sylvian triangle in the rostral direction.

(3) "Onion-peeling" of the middle cerebral arteries and superficial sylvian veins in curved layers convex forward.

(4) Forward displacement and separation of middle cerebral cortical branches on the lateral convexity.

(5) Forward displacement and separation of posterior cerebral cortical branches on the mesial cerebral surface on the lateral vertebral angiogram.

b. Midline shift (AP view) .

(1) The internal cerebral vein is shifted to a greater degree than the anterior cerebral vessels.

(2) There may be minimal contralateral deep venous shift with no anterior cerebral shift.

(3) A great shift of the internal cerebral vein suggests deep central cerebral extension of the tumor to the region of the basal ganglia.

(4) Medial shift of the basal vein and posterior cerebral artery occurs with transtentorial herniation.

(5) Deep cerebral venous compression in the region of the vein of Galen may produce evidence of marked intracranial hypertension due to generalized cerebral edema (i.e. delayed circulation time, generalized narrowing and straightening of vessels, brain herniations distant from the tumor site) .

c. Paradoxical depression of the angiographic sylvian point—on the lateral view, in addition to a rostral displacement of the angiographic sylvian point, the retrosylvian mass will also frequently elevate this point since the greater bulk of these tumors is often temporo-occipital. However, on the frontal view, rostral displacement of the angiographic sylvian point takes the form of apparent depression of the point (when compared to the opposite normal side). On the frontal view, this paradoxical depression of the point may mimic the appearance of a superior parietal mass.

d. Angiographic glioma signs—early and deep draining veins, tumor blush which does not persist due to multiple arteriovenous shunts, and failure to define an extracerebral supply to the tumor favors the diagnosis of glioma. Avascularity of the mass is also compatible with the diagnosis.

2. Caudal extracerebral mass (e.g. tentorial meningioma)—meningiomas may arise from the posterior third of the sagittal sinus, posterior falx or tentorium. Tentorial meningiomas may be mesial, incisural or lateral; they may be supra- or infratentorial or both. This entire group of caudal meningiomas is much less common than the parasagittal meningiomas of the central third of the longitudinal sinus. They are also less common than the basal meningiomas of the floor of the anterior fossa, tuberculum and sphenoid ridge. The caudal meningioma, however, is more common than the unusual intraventricular meningioma. Characteristics of the caudal meningioma include the following:

a. Rostral displacement (lateral view)—angiographic sylvian point, sylvian telescoping and onion-peeling on the carotid study.

b. Elevation of all the cortical branches (rather than separation of the branches) of the posterior cerebral artery on the lateral vertebral angiogram in medial tentorial meningiomas.

c. Elevation of all the posterior cortical branches of the middle cerebral artery (in addition to rostral displacement) on the lateral carotid angiogram in lateral tentorial meningiomas.

d. Midline shift (AP view)

(1) Medial tentorial meningioma—the carotid angiogram may reveal no midline shift. The vertebral angiogram may show deflection of the mesial cortical posterior cerebral arteries in a lateral direction, away from the posterior falx as they approach the medial tumor.

(2) Lateral tentorial meningioma—the carotid angiogram may show internal cerebral venous shift across the midline, without anterior cerebral shift. On the vertebral study the lateral tumor does not deflect the posterior cerebral arteries laterally.

(3) Medial shift of the posterior cerebral artery on the vertebral angiogram, or basal vein on the carotid study as they course around the brain stem, indicates transtentorial herniation.

e. Partial or complete obstruction of the superior sagittal or transverse sinus with reversal of flow and collateral venous filling may occur. Transverse sinus asymmetry is not abnormal. The right transverse sinus may be much larger and the left sinus may at times be difficult to demonstrate normally.

f. In addition to the usual sources of meningeal arterial supply to the tumor, there may be evidence of the following:

(1) Tentorial artery—the internal carotid normally supplies a branch to the cavernous sinus and tentorium which is usually not seen on the normal angiogram. It may be visible in the presence of a tentorial meningioma, extending from the intracavernous carotid caudally.

(2) Meningeal branches of the occipital scalp artery which are a prominent source of supply to the tumor.

(3) Meningeal branches from the ascending pharyngeal artery enlarging foramina at the cranial base other than foramen spinosum (e.g. foramen lacerum; hypoglossal and jugular foramina).

g. Angiographic meningioma signs—arterial sunburst and a prolonged tumor cloud may be noted.

h. If the posterior cerebral arteries do not fill from the carotid system, the carotid angiograms may not clearly reveal the tentorial location of the meningioma, although the angiographic sylvian point will be displaced forward.

3. Caudal arteriovenous malformation—small arteriovenous malformations (AVM) capable of producing subarachnoid, intracerebral and intraventricular hemorrhage may be missed on angiography. The typical AVM is supratentorial and most often within middle cerebral territory. It takes a wedge-shape with the apex pointing at the ventricle. The angiographically visible arteriovenous malformations usually have the following characteristics:

a. Extremely rapid circulation time.

b. Appearance of enlarged, tortuous draining veins during the early arterial phase, often with direct A-V shunting.

c. Enlarged and multiple arterial vessels of supply.

d. Enlarged draining veins may empty directly into the major venous sinuses (e.g. straight or transverse sinus in the case of caudal AVM).

e. Contralateral filling may be present and the caudal AVM may also be supplied by the vertebrobasilar system.
f. Evidence of hematoma or cyst (encephalomalacic, due to ischemia or previous bleeding) in the vicinity of the AVM may be present in the form of an adjacent avascular mass.
g. Both true and false aneurysms are occasionally associated. The false aneurysm looks like a dye-filled sac because of rupture of the AVM into an adjacent cyst.
h. Evidence of ventricular enlargement with stretching of pericallosal arteries (lateral) and flattening of the thalamostriate vein as it passes to the midline (AP) as a result of previous subarachnoid hemorrhage (communicating hydrocephalus) may be present.
i. Aneurysm of the great vein of Galen—usually presents in infancy or early childhood with obstructive hydrocephalus. Occasionally it can be seen with an associated arteriovenous malformation of the brain either in childhood or later.
j. Extracerebral external carotid arteriovenous malformation may be present (e.g. cirsoid aneurysm of the scalp) .
k. Angiograms in Sturge-Weber's disease may be negative despite extensive cerebral and meningeal angiomatosis of small pial vessels. The circulation time is normal. Occasionally there is a diffuse density in the caudal cerebral region on angiography corresponding to the malformation. Other abnormalities may include abnormal veins and arterial occlusions. Less often, Sturge-Weber's angiomatosis is frontal rather than caudal. The plain skull x-ray with characteristic "railroad track calcifications" is often more helpful than angiography in this disorder.

B. Pneumographic deformities
1. Caudal cerebral tumors produce generally similar pneumographic deformities whether they are intra- or extracerebral.
2. The lateral brow-down film is usually most significant.
3. Caudal (retrosylvian) tumors are "periatrial," the atrium being the junction of the body and temporal and occipital horns of the lateral ventricle.
4. The occipital horns are the most normally variable part of the ventricular system. They are commonly quite asymmetrical. The larger of the two occipital horns is usually the left. The occipital horn may appear amputated when it is merely absent as a normal variant.
5. The most significant single finding is forward dislocation of the atrium (when compared to the opposite side) .
6. The atrium, even though dislocated, is rarely obliterated as commonly

occurs in more rostral tumors adjacent to other parts of the ventricular system.

7. The atrium, and the occipital horn, in addition to rostral dislocation are commonly shifted superiorly (e.g. temporo-occipital glioma or tentorial meningioma).
8. The closer the tumor to the ventricular system, the greater the incidence of local irregularities of the atrial walls.
9. Marked dilatation (i.e. hydrocephalus) of the ventricular system is uncommon in caudal cerebral tumors despite their frequently large size.
10. In contrast, cerebral edema due to translated pressure upon deep cerebral draining veins by the caudal mass commonly occurs. This may produce diminution of general ventricular size, distant (i.e. rostral) ventricular shifts and herniations.
11. On the PA view the involved atrium may appear locally widened due to its foreshortening. Midline caudal tumors may separate the two atria.
12. Enlargement of the ventricular system due to a caudal mass occurs with tumors within, rather than external to, the atrium. In the adult, the relatively smooth globular intra-atrial tumor is most likely a meningioma (intraventricular). An irregular mass within the atrium may be an epidermoid (cholesteatoma) or a glioma with intraventricular extension (glioblastoma, oligodendroglioma). In childhood and adult life a cerebral ependymoma may extend into the atrial region. In infancy, the choroid plexus papilloma most often involves the region of the atrium.

Additional Diagnostic Clues in Caudal Cerebral Syndromes

A. Plain skull x-rays

1. Rostral displacement of a calcified pineal—this is an uncommon finding in supratentorial mass lesions and indicates a caudal mass. The pineal may be undisplaced. There may be pineal shift across the midline opposite a caudal mass.
2. Calcification of the glomus of the choroid plexus within the atria of the ventricles occurs normally. However, it may occur only unilaterally or one may be calcified in a higher position than the other. Gross rostral displacement of a calcified glomus suggests a caudal cerebral mass.
3. Calcification of the tentorium may occur normally and may simulate the hyperostosis of a caudal meningioma. Calcification at the tentorial union with the falx may mimic pineal calcification on the frontal view.

4. The presence of a caudal meningioma may be indicated by occipital hyperostosis or erosion and increased vascular markings. Calcification within the tumor itself may be visible as in meningiomas at the other sites. Supratentorial-subtentorial plain x-ray changes of these types point to the peritorcular location of the tumor.
5. Tumor calcification may also be present in oligodendrogliomas and astrocytomas.
6. A significant minority of arteriovenous malformations contain calcifications visible on plain x-ray.
7. "Railroad-track" calcification of parallel linear type characterize the caudal cerebral atrophy occurring in Sturge-Weber's disease. The parallel calcifications occur at sulci.
8. Pressure atrophy of the sella—indicates intracranial hypertension of at least one month's duration but does not indicate the tumor site. The tentorial meningioma is particularly apt to be exceedingly large at the time of diagnosis, with chronic papilledema and marked erosion of the dorsum sella as evidence of prolonged intracranial hypertension. Middle sphenoid ridge and olfactory meningiomas provide other examples of large tumors often detected late.

B. EEG

1. Slow wave (delta) abnormalities from occipital leads suggest a focally destructive caudal cerebral lesion. This may be the result of intracerebral or extracerebral tumor, but can also be due to vascular infarction.
2. Reduction of alpha rhythm on the side of the neoplastic or vascular lesion is common.
3. Like other parasagittal meningiomas, those of the posterior third of the longitudinal sinus are occasionally missed as a result of their slow growth and midline location. However, some focal abnormality is usually detected related to the large size of the caudal meningioma at the time of its clinical presentation. If the tumor is entirely subtentorial the EEG may be normal.
4. Advanced intracranial hypertension due to any intracranial mass may result in generalized slowing and increased amplitudes. This effect of generalized bilateral slowing and increased amplitude may be most marked at the occipital leads, but does not necessarily indicate a caudal tumor. Since brain tumors are more common rostrally, this EEG change more often indicates a rostral mass (i.e. frontal, frontotemporal, frontoparietal) with increased intracranial pressure. The same effect can be produced by posterior fossa tumors. Marked bifrontal delta activity with generalized slowing commonly occurs with upper brain stem compression. The responsible supratentorial mass

may be variously located and may be intra-or extracerebral. A posterior fossa mass with obstructive high pressure hydrocephalus may produce the same result.

5. Irregular delta activity from occipital leads without more general electrographic disturbance may indicate a caudal tumor, but parasagittal tumors near the cranial vertex and third ventricular tumors may produce the same abnormalities.
6. An atrial intraventricular meningioma commonly results in lateralized slow waves projected to the temporal or posterior temporal region.
7. Irritative foci with spikes and sharp waves may be recorded with gliomas, meningiomas or malformations resulting in cerebral seizures. They may be recorded between attacks.

C. Brain scan

1. The brain scan is most valuable in the caudal cerebral region in the diagnosis of tentorial meningiomas, glioblastomas, metastatic carcinomas and caudal arteriovenous malformations.
2. The caudal cerebral region is much more commonly involved by vascular infarction than by neoplasm or malformation. A negative scan immediately following an acute neurological caudal deficit increases the likelihood of vascular ischemia (the scan becoming positive later). A positive scan at the outset of the caudal deficit may indicate a tumor or malformation.
3. A negative scan does not rule out an intracerebral glioma.
4. The normal increased density at the site of the torcular is greatly exaggerated in tentorial meningiomas. A positive posterior fossa scan may be due to subtentorial meningioma or cerebellar hemangioblastoma in the adult.

CHAPTER 8

TEMPORAL LOBE SYNDROMES

Anatomical and Physiological Correlates

Sector: 7 and 8; the temporal lobe and middle fossa
Angiogram: Infrasylvian
Pneumogram: Temporal

Neuroanatomy of the Temporal Region

A. Intratemporal

The caudal cerebral syndromes (Ch. 7) included the posterior temporal region where it becomes continuous with the posterior parietal and occipital lobes (sector 6). That caudal region surrounds the atrium of the lateral ventricle. Proceeding outward from the atrium, the optic radiation (both upper and lower portions of the geniculocalcarine tract) are encountered. At the cortical level, Wernicke's area and visual association areas are notable in that posterior temporoparietal and temporo-occipital region.

Proceeding rostrally into the midtemporal lobe (sector 7), the temporal horn and hippocampus are the central structures. The digitations of the pes hippocampi can be seen protruding into the floor of the temporal horn. Medially, the hippocampal gyrus borders the tentorial incisura (Fig. 43). Meyer's loop (lower portion of the geniculocalcarine tract) courses around the lateral border of the temporal horn, its anterior fibers proceeding as far rostrally as the tip of the horn, before turning caudally to join the upper optic radiation fibers in the caudal cerebral white matter.

The temporal pole (sector 8) lies rostral to the tip of the temporal horn (Fig. 44). The optic radiation does not enter the temporal pole. The uncus is the medial surface of the temporal pole. It overhangs the tentorial incisura medially. The amygdala lies within the temporal pole, bulging into the rostromedial rostrodorsal tip of the temporal horn.

The connections of the temporal lobe are widespread and are based on the following three fundamental facts:

1. The neocortex of the temporal lobe is widely connected with the neocortex of the frontal, parietal and occipital regions.

2. The paleocortex and primitive ganglia of the temporal lobe (hippocampus and amygdala) have wide cerebral connections, most notably with the ancient midline and basal "limbic structures."

3. The temporal lobe is essentially a bilateral structure with both rostral (anterior commissure) and caudal (hippocampal commissure) interconnections.

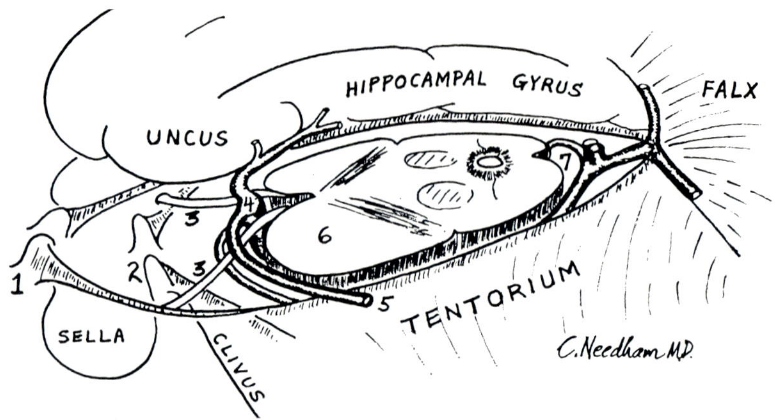

Figure 43. The uncus, hippocampal gyrus and tentorial door. The uncus and hippocampal gyrus constitute the medial surface of the temporal lobe. They lie along the tentorial edge. The "door of the tent" contains the midbrain caudally and the perichiasmatic-hypothalamic region rostrally. (1) The free edge of the tentorium inserts into the anterior clinoid process. (2) The fixed edge of the tentorium inserts as the "petroclinoid ligament" into the posterior clinoid process. (3) The oculomotor nerve passes medial to the uncus, and over the petroclinoid ligament, to enter the cavernous sinus. (4) The basilar artery bifurcates into the posterior cerebral arteries. The oculomotor nerve passes forward between posterior cerebral and superior cerebellar arteries. (5) The posterior cerebral artery runs along the tentorial edge, to supply the medial temporal and occipital regions. (6) The position of the pyramidal tract within the cerebral peduncle of the midbrain. (7) The basal veins of Rosenthal are shown at their juncture with the amputated internal cerebral veins, to form the great vein of Galen adjacent to the tectum of the midbrain.

Afferent and efferent projections

1. Afferent.
   a. Medial geniculate nucleus of the dorsal thalamus—to the primary auditory cortex (Heschl's transverse gyri of the temporal operculum) via the sublenticular part of the posterior capsule.
   b. Transcallosal projections from the opposite auditory cortex to the auditory association cortex (first temporal gyrus, adjacent to Heschl's gyri).
   c. Ipsilateral association projections to the general temporal cortex including the auditory association area—from frontal, parietal, occipital and insular cortex.
   d. Uncinate fasciculus—from the frontopolar and frontobasal regions to the temporal pole.
   e. Cingulum bundle—from the limbic lobe and paralimbic cortex at the medial surface of the hemisphere to the hippocampal gyrus (with which the cingulate gyrus is continuous caudally; rostrally,

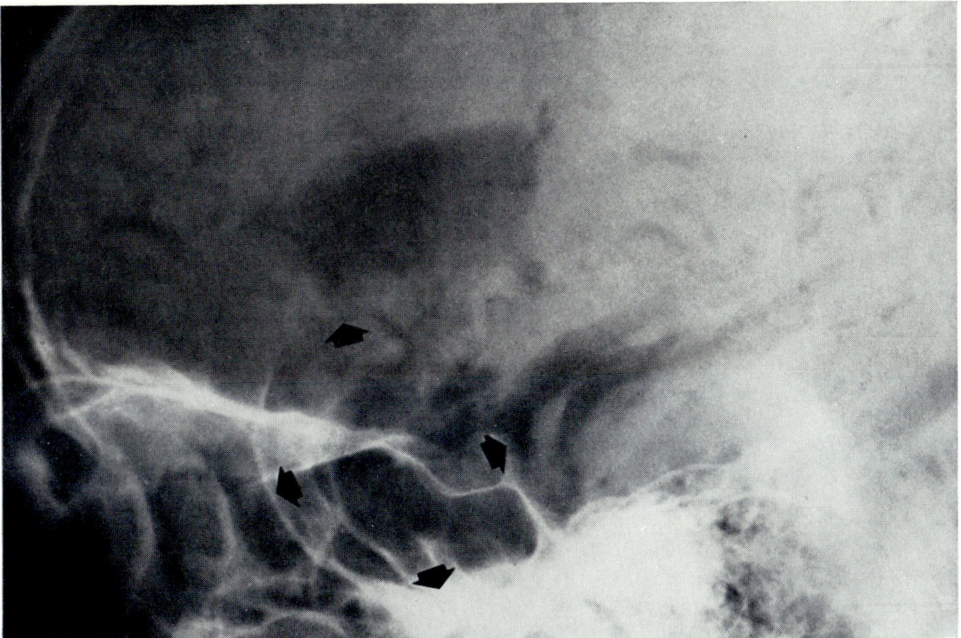

Figure 44. The temporal pole. The temporal pole is indicated by arrows. The pole lies rostral to the tip of the temporal horn. The pole contains the amygdala deeply and the uncus medially. The rostral and basal arrows point to the bony margins of the middle fossa.

the cingulum, through the paraolfactory area of Broca, transverse gyrus of the insula and gyrus ambiens of the uncus, becomes continuous with the uncus and hippocampal gyrus). The rostral cingulum interdigitates with the uncinate fasciculus.

f. Hypothalamic, preoptic, septal and frontobasal projections to the amygdala; includes the diagonal band of Broca, lateral olfactory stria and direct hypothalamo-amygdalary tracts.

g. Anterior commissure—from the opposite temporal pole and septum to the amygdala, including fibers from the stria terminalis.

h. Hippocampal commissure—from the fornix of the opposite hippocampus.

i. Limbic nuclei of the dorsal thalamus (e.g. anterior nuclei)—indirectly via the cingulum to the hippocampal gyrus.

j. Medial dorsal nucleus of the dorsal thalamus—periventricular system to the amygdala.

k. Reticular formation of the brain stem—indirectly via the septum (from intralaminar nuclei of the dorsal thalamus and from tegmentum of the midbrain via tegmentohypothalamic fibers of the medial forebrain bundle).

2. Efferent.
   a. Corticogeniculate and corticotectal tracts—from the auditory cortical areas to the medial geniculate nucleus and inferior colliculus.
   b. Short and long association bundles and transcallosal projections from the temporal cortex to frontal, parietal, occipital and insular cortex of the ipsilateral hemisphere and opposite temporal cortex.
   c. Uncinate fasciculus—from the temporal pole to frontopolar and frontobasal cortex.
   d. Cingulum bundle—from the hippocampus to the limbic lobe and paralimbic cortex of the medial surface of the hemisphere.
   e. Preoptic, hypothalamic and septal direct connections from the amygdala.
   f. Commissural projections to the opposite temporal lobe via the anterior and hippocampal commissures.
   g. Stria terminalis—from the amygdala to the septum and anterior commissure.
   h. Stria medullaris—from the septum to the lateral dorsal nucleus of the thalamus and habenula; contains projections from the amygdala.
   i. Periventricular system—from the amygdala to the medial dorsal nucleus of the dorsal thalamus.
   j. Fornix—from the hippocampus via the fimbria to the mammillary bodies, septum and midbrain tegmentum (to the "limbic midbrain region of Nauta" and reticular core of the brain stem).
   k. Hippocampal rudiment—continuous with the supracallosal gyrus and paraterminal body.

B. Extratemporal (middle fossa)—for clinical and radiological analysis of mass syndromes of the temporal region, the regional anatomy of the middle fossa (including the tentorial edge) bordering the temporal lobe is critical.
   1. The medial surface of the temporal lobe (anterior-uncus, posterior-hippocampal gyrus) lies at the tentorial edge (incisura) of the opening ("door") of the tentorium (Fig. 43).
      a. The free margin of the tentorium inserts on the anterior clinoid of the sella. The anterior clinoid is the medial tip of the sphenoid ridge. It is immediately above the optic foramen (optic nerve and ophthalmic artery) at the orbital apex.
      b. The fixed margin of the tentorium inserts on the posterior clinoid. This margin passes forward beneath the free margin as the "petroclinoid ligament." This ligament runs from the petrous

ridge to the posterior clinoid; it may be calcified on x-ray. The oculomotor nerve runs over this ligament as it passes through the interpeduncular cistern on its way to the cavernous sinus. The posterior communicating artery lies close to the oculomotor nerve as it courses back from the internal carotid to the posterior cerebral artery.

c. The uncus overhangs the medial edge of the tentorium anteriorly. The oculomotor nerve lies just medial to it. Also medial to the uncus is the cerebral peduncle, connecting the cerebral hemisphere with the base of the midbrain. The corticospinal tract descends in the cerebral peduncle. The midbrain occupies the posterior two-thirds of the tentorial door. The anterior third of the tentorial door contains the subhemispheric optic system (optic nerves, chiasm and optic tracts), the circle of Willis and hypothalamus. The anterior choroidal artery and the optic tract are also adjacent to the medial surface of the uncus.

d. The oculomotor nerve emerges from the midbrain between the posterior cerebral artery and the superior cerebellar artery just above the basilar bifurcation (at the superior border of the belly of the pons). As the oculomotor nerve passes forward in the interpeduncular cistern, the posterior cerebral artery turns backward and ascends around the cerebral peduncle in the crural cistern to reach the tentorial edge adjacent to the hippocampal gyrus. The posterior cerebral artery follows the tentorial edge and medial surface of the temporal and occipital lobes. The proximal portion of the posterior cerebral artery between the basilar bifurcation and the juncture of the posterior communicating artery is the "mesencephalic artery." It constitutes the posterior part of the circle of Willis. The medial relations of the hippocampal gyrus are the posterior cerebral artery, tentorial incisura, basal vein of Rosenthal, and the lateral and dorsal surfaces of the midbrain.

e. The basal vein of Rosenthal arises from the deep middle cerebral vein (insular cortex), the anterior cerebral vein (anteromedial frontal lobe and anterior corpus callosum), and the lenticulostriate veins (central cerebral region). These veins join at the anterior perforated region and the basal vein passes horizontally backwards, medial to the uncus and above the anterior choroidal artery to lie medial to the hippocampal gyrus. It ascends with the posterior cerebral artery around the brain stem near the tentorial edge. Above the colliculi and below the splenium it joins with the internal cerebral veins and the opposite basal vein to form the great vein of Galen; this in turn is joined by the posterior vein of the corpus callosum, internal occipital veins and the superior cerebellar veins. The vein of Galen joins the inferior longitudinal sinus to form the straight sinus. The origin of the straight sinus marks the apex of the tentorial door. It is the highest, most posterior and midline peak of the tentorium. The apex of the tentorial door is a critical point.

(1) The pineal, tectum of the midbrain overlying the aqueduct, superior cerebellar vermis and splenium of the corpus callosum, internal cerebral veins joining the vein of Galen—these are all structures which can be identified in the cerebral midline at the apex of the tentorial door.

(2) The hippocampal gyri of the temporal lobe course mediosuperiorly at the tentorial edge. They become continuous with the cingulate gyrus posteriorly in the region of the isthmus, just adjacent to the midline and behind the splenium.

f. Critical pathways to CSF circulation at the tentorial opening include the cisterns of the tentorial door which surround the upper brain stem as it joins the hemisphere, and the aqueduct within the midbrain. The quadrigeminal cistern (dorsal to the colliculi) is continuous with the ambient cistern (around the lateral surface of the midbrain). The wings of the ambient cistern encircle the pulvinar of the dorsal thalamus. The ambient cistern itself is continuous with the crural cistern which is the lateral extension of the interpeduncular cistern. The latter is continuous with the prepontine cistern below and with the suprasellar cistern rostrally. The sylvian cistern is continuous with this and runs along the sphenoid ridge between the temporal and frontal lobes.

g. The sphenoid ridge begins laterally at the pterion and extends medially to the anterior clinoid. The sphenoparietal sinus runs along the edge of the ridge to join the cavernous sinus medially at the orbital apex. The middle cerebral veins in the sylvian fissure empty into these sinuses. The cavernous sinus forms the lateral border of the sella. It lies just medial to the temporal lobe. The cavernous sinus contains the carotid artery with its sympathetic plexus, the venous drainage of the orbit (ophthalmic veins), the ophthalmic division of the trigeminal nerve, the oculomotor, trochlear and abducens nerves. These nerves pass into the orbit through the superior orbital fissure. With the optic nerve and ophthalmic artery passing through the optic foramen, they constitute the neurovascular stem of the eye. The orbital apex thus forms the rostromedial edge of the middle fossa, at its juncture with the anterior fossa and pituitary fossa. The cranio-orbital junction can be involved by a mass of the temporal pole, frontal base, sella, cavernous sinus and posterior orbit.

h. Meckel's cave, lateral to the cavernous sinus and beneath the temporal lobe, contains the trigeminal gasserian ganglion underneath a dural cover. The ophthalmic division passes forward into the cavernous sinus. The maxillary division leaves the middle fossa through the foramen rotundum. The mandibular division, with the motor root of the trigeminal, leaves through the foramen ovale. The retrogasserian root of the trigeminal passes posteriorly from the medial middle fossa through the porus trigemini, into the posterior fossa where it enters the lateral pons.

i. The foramina of the middle fossa form a curved line across the medial floor of the fossa. This "crescent" begins rostromedially and ends caudolaterally. The superior orbital fissure is most rostromedial; the foramen rotundum is next, followed by foramen ovale; the foramen spinosum (middle meningeal artery) is most caudolateral of these foramina. The foramen lacerum (carotid artery and sympathetic plexus) lies just caudomedially to the crescent; it is immediately in front of the petrous ridge. Between the caudal end of the foramen lacerum and the caudal end of the crescent (foramen spinosum) is the innominate canal (lesser superficial petrosal nerve).

j. The foramina of the middle fossa and their contents form the rostromedial and medioinferior extradural boundaries of the temporal lobe. The petrous ridge forms the boundary between the middle and posterior fossae. It runs diagonally backward and laterally beneath the temporal lobe. The fixed edge of the tentorium is attached to the petrous ridge along the margin of the superior petrosal sinus, forming the caudal margin of the middle fossa and superior-rostral margin of the posterior fossa. The superior petrosal sinus connects the cavernous sinus with the transverse sinus caudally, at the point where the transverse sinus turns downward to become the sigmoid sinus.

k. The gasserian ganglion in Meckel's cave of the medial middle fossa passes backward beneath the fixed margin of the tentorium (under the medial end of the superior petrosal sinus) as the retrogasserian root of the trigeminal which then crosses the posterior fossa. In contrast, just medially, the oculomotor nerve passes forward and over the fixed margin of the tentorium (over the petroclinoid ligament) to enter the cavernous sinus. The abducens nerve passes rostral to the belly of the pons, upon the clivus, to enter the cavernous sinus below the level of the petroclinoid ligament. The trochlear nerve, after dorsal decussation in the region of the colliculi, passes forward beneath the tentorial edge to enter the cavernous sinus.

l. The greater superficial petrosal nerve lies on the anterior surface of the petrous bone. It enters the middle fossa through the hiatus of the facial nerve and runs rostromedially to a point beneath the gasserian ganglion.

m. The middle meningeal artery enters the middle fossa through the foramen spinosum. The accessory middle meningeal artery usually enters through the foramen ovale. The middle meningeal artery runs across the floor of the middle fossa in a rostrolateral direction to the lateral wall of the fossa where it divides into an anterior and posterior branch. The artery may groove the inner table or may run within the temporal bone in the squamosal region (*Note:* Fracture of the temporal bone leads to tearing of the middle meningeal artery with acute epidural hematoma. Fracture of the base of the middle fossa will also tear the middle meningeal trunk closer to its origin from the foramen spinosum; such a basal fracture may not be evident on lateral views of the skull). The middle meningeal artery at the foramen spinosum is just lateral to Meckel's cave.

n. The middle meningeal artery (rostrally) and the greater superficial petrosal nerve (caudally) form a "V" across the floor of the middle fossa. The artery and nerve are widely separated laterally but converge medially. The point of convergence lies immediately lateral to the gasserian ganglion.

o. The middle cerebral artery forms the "angiographic sylvian triangle" upon the surface of the insula of Reil. The insula and the "trifurcation" of the middle cerebral artery lie deeply between the temporal and frontal lobes. The insula forms the mediodorsal relation of the temporal lobe. The insular cortex overlies the basal ganglia. The lateromedial sequence is temporal lobe, insula, extreme capsule, claustrum, external capsule, putamen, globus pallidus, internal capsule, thalamus, and third ventricle.

p. The frontal and parietal opercula are the dorsal relations of the temporal lobe. The opercula (frontal, parietal and temporal) form the "cover" of the insula. The middle cerebral arteries emerge from the sylvian fissure after passing outward upon the opercula. The major portion of the opercula is frontal. The opercula and their adjacent convexity walls are formed by the following:

(1) Frontal-pars orbitalis and frontolateral cortex (Broca's area and precentral facial-motor region).

(2) Parietal-postcentral facial-sensory and supramarginal gyri.

(3) Temporal—the transverse gyri of Heschl form the deep temporal operculum in the middle region of the temporal lobe. The auditory association areas surround this region in the first temporal convolution. The rostral temporal operculum is the roof of the temporal pole. Wernicke's area is located on the convexity of the posterior part of the superior temporal gyrus. It becomes continuous with the auditory association area rostrally and with posterior parietal cortex caudally.

Blood Supply of the Temporal Region

A. Arterial

1. Anterior choroidal artery.
   a. Uncus and amygdala of the temporal pole.
   b. Hippocampus and the choroid plexus of the temporal horn; Meyer's loop of the geniculocalcarine tract.
2. Middle cerebral artery, cortical branches.
   a. Anterior temporal branch—to the temporal pole, lateral surface.
   b. Middle temporal branch—to the midtemporal lobe, lateral surface.
   c. Posterior temporal branch—to the caudal cerebral portion of the temporal lobe.
3. Posterior cerebral artery.
   a. Anterior temporal branch—to the uncus, hippocampal and fusiform gyri in their rostral portions on the medial surface of the temporal lobe.
   b. Posterior temporal branch—to the posterior part of the hippocampal gyrus and medioinferior part of the temporal lobe.

B. Venous

1. Superficial middle cerebral (sylvian) vein—to the sphenoparietal and cavernous sinuses.
2. Anterior temporal cerebral vein—to the sphenoparietal sinus.
3. Lesser anastomotic vein of Labbé—to the superficial middle cerebral and greater anastomotic veins; to the transverse sinus.
4. Inferior temporo-occipital veins—to the transverse sinus.

Infarction Syndromes of Arterial Occlusion in the Temporal Region

1. Occlusion of the anterior choroidal artery—despite the fact that the anterior choroidal artery may supply the globus pallidus, optic tract, Meyer's loop and the temporal pole, no clearly defined, characteristic syndrome results.
2. Occlusion of the cortical temporal branches of the middle cerebral

artery usually is clinically associated with more proximal middle cerebral occlusion.

a. Contralateral hemiplegia.
b. Contralateral hemisensory deficit.
c. Contralateral hemianopia.
d. Aphasia—major hemisphere.
e. Stupor or coma—especially in acute and deeply situated occlusion.

3. Occlusion of the cortical temporal branches of the posterior cerebral artery—usually clinically associated with posterior cerebral occlusion also involving the occipital lobe.
   a. Homonymous hemianopia—contralateral.
   b. Alexia and visual agnosia--dominant side.

   Posterior cerebral occlusion may occur with hippocampal herniation as a result of a temporal or other supratentorial mass. Progressive coma due to midbrain compression obscures the clinical evidence of occipital infarction.

Neurophysiology of the Temporal Region

A. Middle fossa mass—experimental production of a middle fossa mass has been shown in animals to result in ipsilateral oculomotor palsy beginning with pupillary dilatation and ending in coma. Midbrain compression secondary to unco-hippocampal herniation occurs.

B. Temporal lobe
   1. Stimulation.
      a. Representation of tone is present in the auditory cortex according to sound frequency.
      b. Temporal and parietal cortical stimulation may produce vertigo. Vestibular sensation may have a cortical representation in this region.
      c. Stimulation of the posterior superior temporal and temporoparietal region may produce speech arrest.
      d. Stimulation of temporal cortex may produce motor responses with head and eye turning to the opposite side and extremity movement. It is considered an accessory motor field.
      e. Stimulation of temporal lobe cortex or the amygdalohippocampal complex (in temporal lobe epilepsy) may result in a typical experiential seizure with automatism.
      f. A variety of epileptogenic agents (e.g. alumina cream, cobalt, penicillin) have been employed to produce seizures in animals. The general cortex is quite epileptogenic and the hippocampus is extremely so under these experimental conditions. The thalamus and brain stem appear to be rather less epileptogenic, although

convulsive activity can be produced. Seizures occur with application of the particular agent to temporal cortex, hippocampus or amygdala.

2. Ablation.
   a. Unilateral ablation of auditory cortex does not result in readily detectable deafness. However, clinical lesions in the region of the auditory cortex of the human dominant hemisphere may produce "word deafness," a variant of Wernicke's sensory aphasia in which the patient can hear sounds but cannot interpret words; extreme jargon is characteristic.
   b. Temporal lobectomy in man (i.e. in temporal lobe epilepsy).
      (1) Temporal lobectomy in the nondominant side does not impair the verbal reception or expression of speech. Some impairment in nonverbal communication may be detected on neuropsychological testing.
      (2) Anterior temporal lobectomy (5 cm) on the dominant side does not impair the reception or expression of speech. Transient postoperative dysphasia, especially with dysnomic predominance, indicates reactive edema in the remaining posterior temporal lobe.
      (3) Posterior temporal lobectomy on the dominant side results in permanent and severe receptive dysphasia due to involvement of Wernicke's area.
      (4) Temporal lobectomy anterior to the temporal horn spares the visual radiation. Temporal lobectomy through the temporal horn (pes hippocampus level) results in contralateral superior homonymous quadrantanopia due to excision of Meyer's loop. This visual field defect is ordinarily asymptomatic. Posterior temporal lobectomy near the junction of the temporal horn with the atrium, like occipital lobectomy, will result in contralateral homonymous hemianopia. Destruction of the dominant periatrial temporo-occipital region can be expected to result in visual agnosia in addition to aphasic and hemianopic disturbances.
      (5) Bihippocampal destruction results in severe memory disorder. Unilateral hippocampal excision spares memory if the opposite temporal lobe is normal. Unilateral temporal lobectomy in patients with bitemporal epilepsy is apt to result in severe memory disturbance. Testing of recent memory with the use of pictures, objects and sentences during the carotid amytal speech test (see Ch. 5, "Frontolateral Syndromes") is helpful in the detection of bitemporal disturbance. Demonstration of

memory impairment (pretest memory being normal) during the test is taken as evidence of bitemporal disorder.

(6) Temporal lobectomy for temporal tumors may produce more variable results in terms of speech, memory and visual field involvement. This results from the combination of preoperative deficit, temporal lobe edema or distortion, or deep tumor extension.

c. Klüver-Bucy syndrome—various combinations of bitemporal lesions, especially of the amygdala or amygdala and hippocampi, in experimental animals may produce the following:

(1) "Psychic blindness"—the animal may no longer recognize its natural enemies and exhibits generally placid responses.

(2) Hyperphagia.

(3) Hypersexual activity.

Note: In contrast, electrostimulation of the amygdala may produce arousal responses similar to reticular activation and rage attacks similar to hypothalamic stimulation.

NEUROSURGICAL SYNDROMES OF THE TEMPORAL REGION

Development

A. Acute middle fossa epidural hematoma syndrome

The typical epidural hemorrhage results from fracture across the lateral wall or base of the middle fossa with tearing of the middle meningeal artery. A "lucid interval" is less common than progressive obtundation without restoration of consciousness. The usual course is rapidly downhill with dilatation of the ipsilateral pupil, hemiparesis usually contralateral to the clot and deepening coma. A classical temporal lobe uncal herniation syndrome occurs, with midbrain compression and intracranial hypertension of rapid onset. A bounding tachycardia often precedes the more usual bradycardia with arterial hypertension; ultimately, arterial hypotension with thready tachycardia appear in the late phase of brain stem decompensation. Vital sign changes may be particularly variable in the childhood epidural (e.g. systemic hypertension may not occur; bradycardia alone may appear at the outset). Venous epidurals are more common in childhood and may result in slower progression. Slower progression may result from eccentric epidural bleeding due to tearing of the distal branches of the meningeal artery tree (e.g. anterior fossa epidural with contralateral facial weakness preceding evidence of hemiparesis). The supratentorial epidural at any site ultimately (within two or three hours to several days even if eccentric in location or venous in origin) leads to uncal or hippocampal temporal lobe herniation with ipsilateral oculomotor palsy; contralateral hemiparesis (ipsilateral cerebral peduncle); occasionally ipsilateral hemiparesis (Kernohan's notch of the opposite peduncle against the tentorial edge); and decerebration with noisy hyperventilation (often Cheyne-Stokes). The posterior fossa epidural is much less common than the supratentorial epidural. Persistent vomiting, stupor progressing to coma, various ocular palsies, nystagmus, hemiparesis, quadriparesis and decerebration may occur. Bradycardia and arterial hypertension with early hypoventilation (preceding cardiovascular collapse) are typical. Occipital fracture may be associated with such posterior extradural hematomas.

B. Bitemporopolar syndrome

Confusion, disorientation, stupor and coma may follow contrecoup contusion of the temporal poles against the rostral boundary of the middle fossae. Subfrontal contusion is commonly associated. Temporal lobe contusion with edema or traumatic intratemporal hematoma may result in uncal herniation. Tearing of bridging veins from the temporal pole to the sphenoparietal and cavernous sinuses may lead to subtemporal-middle fossa acute subdural bleeding. The acute middle fossa epidural syndrome may be exactly simulated by traumatic edema or intracerebral or subdural hematoma either within the middle fossa or more generally within the supratentorial compartment. The occurrence of focal or generalized convulsions is common in cerebral contusion, but does not rule out the presence of an associated expanding clot.

C. Middle fossa basal skull fracture syndrome

Cerebrospinal fluid otorrhea, bleeding from the middle ear, blood behind the tympanic membrane and ecchymosis over the mastoid (Battle's sign) indicate fracture of the petrous temporal bone of the middle (or posterior) fossa. Naso-oral hemorrhage and CSF rhinorrhea may also occur (commonly the result of anterior fossa fracture). Peripheral facial palsy and unilateral deafness on the side of the fracture are common. Brain stem contusion, traumatic diabetes insipidis and optic nerve trauma at the cranio-orbital junction are occasionally associated. Meningitis may result from continuity of CSF pathways with the middle ear, mastoid, nasopharynx, or sphenoid sinus. Traumatic carotid-cavernous fistula with progressive exophthalmos and cranial bruit may result. Traumatic occlusion of the carotid artery within the carotid canal may result in contralateral hemiplegia, ipsilateral retinal pallor and progressive stupor. The acute epidural, subdural or intracerebral hematoma may of course be associated with signs of basal skull fracture, in which case progressive coma, hemiplegia and oculomotor palsy dominate the clinical picture.

D. Ruptured middle cerebral aneurysm (Fig. 45)

The aneurysm is commonly located at the "trifurcation" of the middle cerebral artery within the sylvian fissure. Acute subarachnoid hemorrhage occurs with sudden severe headache, occipital and neck pain and stiffness, photophobia and retinal hemorrhage as nonlocalizing signs. Focal cerebral seizures or hemiparesis on the opposite side favor middle cerebral aneurysm rupture over aneurysm at another site. Intratemporal hematoma is common (Fig. 46). Hematoma may be intrainsular. The latter produces a dense flaccid complete hemiplegia. The intratemporal or sylvian hematoma produces progressively worsening hemiparesis and an uncal herniation syndrome. Coma may result from herniation, arterial spasm, brain edema or deep intracerebral hematoma. Barring this, the patient may remain quite alert, typically complaining of headache and neck pain. Examination may reveal only a mild drift of contralateral extremities and may be otherwise negative.

E. Temporal lobe abscess (Fig. 47) —may present acutely after otitis media or mastoiditis. Transverse sinus occlusion may be associated with cortical thrombophlebitis (the same circumstances may lead to cerebellar ab-

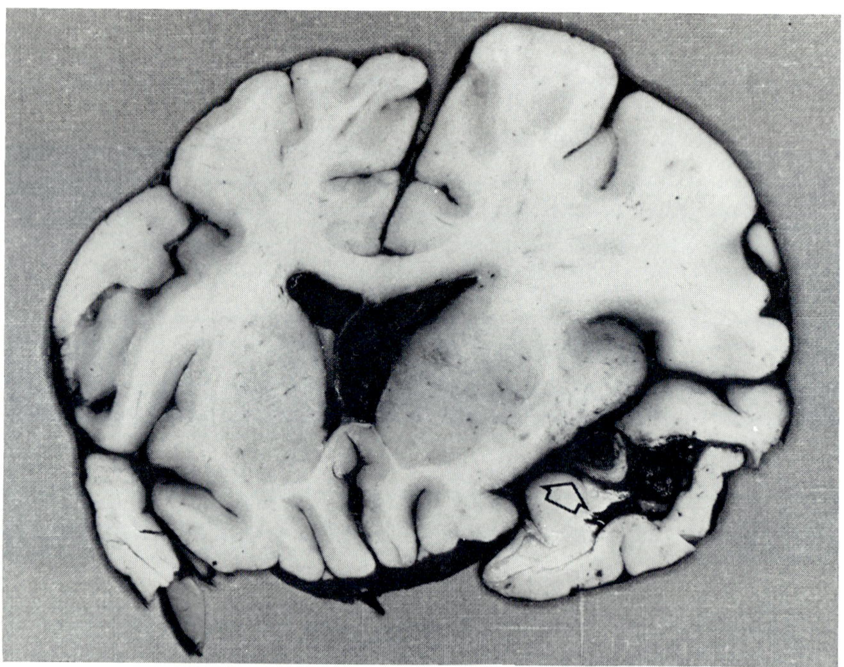

Figure 45. Middle cerebral aneurysm with temporal hematoma-cerebral section. The arrow indicates the aneurysm between the insula and expanded temporal pole. Hematoma in the temporal pole is present. The hemorrhage extends into the ventricular system.

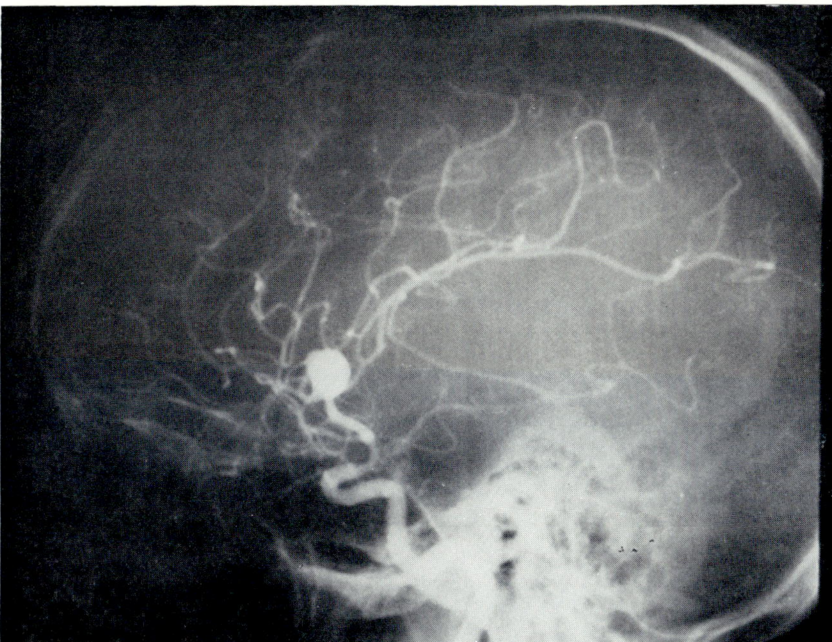

Figure 46. Aneurysm with temporal hematoma. There is elevation of the posterior part of the sylvian triangle with evidence of an avascular temporal mass. Rupture of the aneurysm resulted in the temporal hematoma.

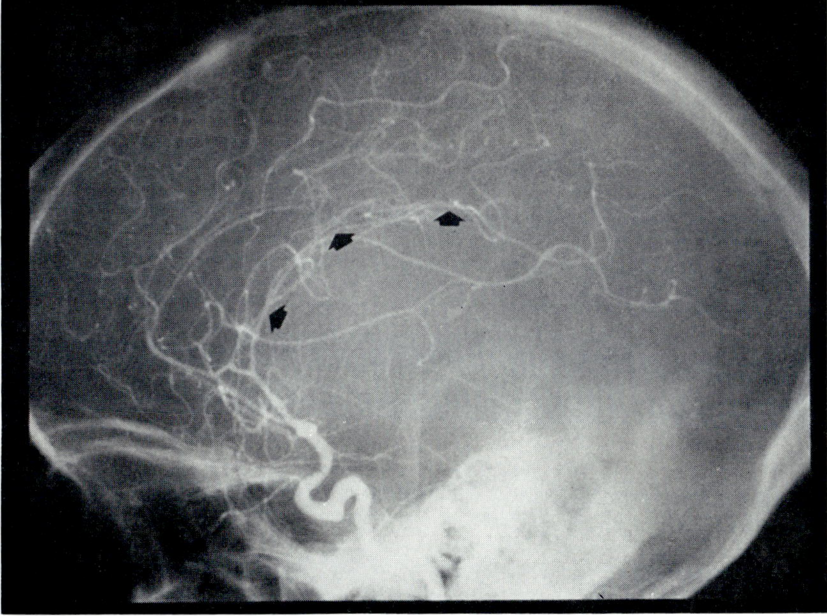

Figure 47. Temporal abscess. Marked elevation of sylvian arteries by a hypovascular temporal mass proved to be due to a temporal lobe abscess.

scess). Associated cerebritis with temporal abscess may rapidly lead to an uncal herniation syndrome, with septic signs and obtundation followed by deepening coma, oculomotor palsy and contralateral hemiparesis. The abscess may be occult and present as a brain tumor syndrome with papilledema and without septic signs.

F. Petrositis—infection extending to the region of the apex of the petrous bone commonly results in trigeminal facial pain which may be combined with various deficits or followed by serious complications as a result of otitis.
   1. Gradenigo's syndrome—petrositis with ipsilateral trigeminal pain and ipsilateral abducens palsy (sparing of the oculomotor nerve makes a superior orbital fissure—cavernous sinus syndrome unlikely).
   2. Ipsilateral Horner's syndrome with ptosis and miosis.
   3. Carotid artery thrombosis.
   4. Cavernous sinus thrombosis

G. Temporal lobe glioma—glioblastomas of the temporal lobe (Fig. 48) characteristically have a more rapid course than glioblastomas situated elsewhere. The tumor is in a relatively silent region, relatively close to

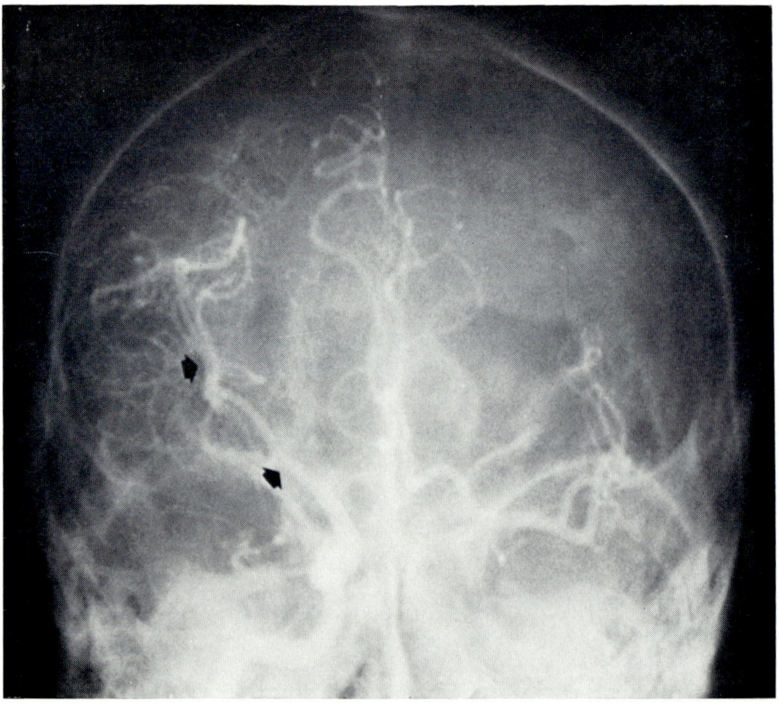

Figure 48. Temporal glioblastoma. The tumor is indicated by the marked elevation of the middle cerebral artery and hypervascularity in the temporal region.

the uncus. Temporal lobe astrocytomas may present with a seizure disorder months before development of symptoms of intracranial hypertension. Such seizures may be focal motor beginning in the opposite face or hand, generalized or of psychomotor type. The latter are most commonly nonneoplastic in etiology. Deep extension of the tumor is common.

H. Tumor of the base of the middle fossa—nasopharyngeal carcinoma, lymphoepithelioma, metastatic carcinoma, chordoma and tumors of the glomus jugulare may invade the cranial base and invade the nerves (and vessels) passing through the various foramina. Foramina of the posterior fossa and their contents similarly may be involved. Craniofacial pain and multiple cranial nerve palsies are characteristic. The facial pain is commonly due to trigeminal involvement. Sensory loss does not occur in trigeminal neuralgia and indicates the presence of tumor. Sudden onset of facial pain suggests aneurysm. Middle fossa invasion by tumor may secondarily compress the temporal lobe. Multiple cranial nerve palsies also may follow locally invasive chromophobe adenoma, aneurysm at the orbital apex, mucocele of the sphenoid sinus, basal meningioma, cerebellopontine angle tumors, brain stem glioma, vertebrobasilar aneurysm and hydrocephalic attacks.

I. Peritemporal meningioma syndromes

Various meningiomas can involve the temporal lobe by gradual compression of its lateral, rostral, medial or caudal margins.

1. Sylvian meningioma (Fig. 49)—a large convexity tumor typically producing focal motor seizures and eventual hemiparesis on the contralateral side and chronic papilledema. Focal sensory seizures may occur with temporoparietal convexity meningiomas.
2. Globular meningioma of the pterion (Fig. 50)—outer sphenoid ridge large meningioma with focal contralateral motor seizures, eventual hemiparesis and chronic papilledema is typical.
3. Alar meningioma of the middle sphenoid ridge (Fig. 51)—may be quite silent and attain huge size; unilateral anosmia, compression of the optic tract, seizures and chronic papilledema occur.
4. Clinoidal meningioma of the inner sphenoid ridge—may be detected relatively early due to central blindness, optic atrophy and oculomotor palsy while the tumor is still of small size.
5. Meningioma of Meckel's cave—gassero-petrosal syndrome—the tumor lies at the medial margin of the middle fossa and extends into the posterior fossa. Unilateral trigeminal pain and sensory loss, oculomotor palsy, facial palsy, tinnitus, deafness, nystagmus, ataxia and chronic papilledema occur. The tumor is usually large and grows

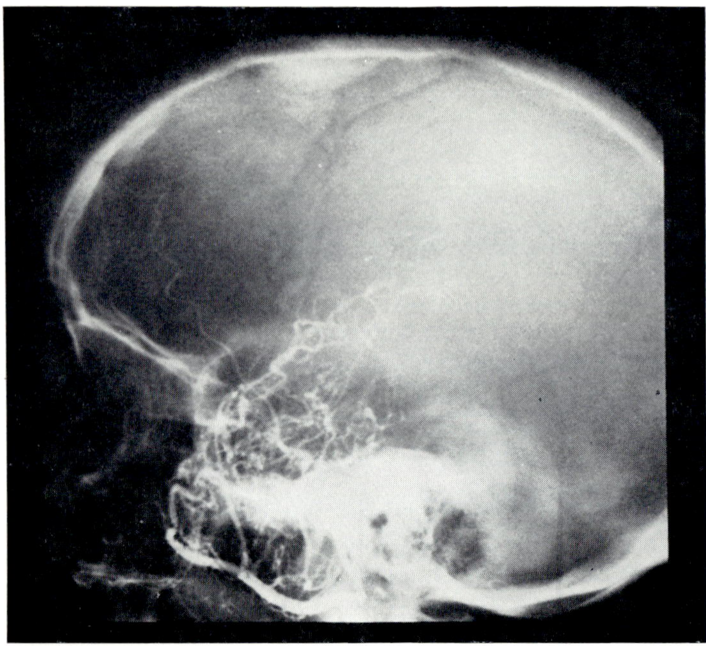

Figure 49. Sylvian meningioma. There is extensive external carotid supply to this extracerebral tumor.

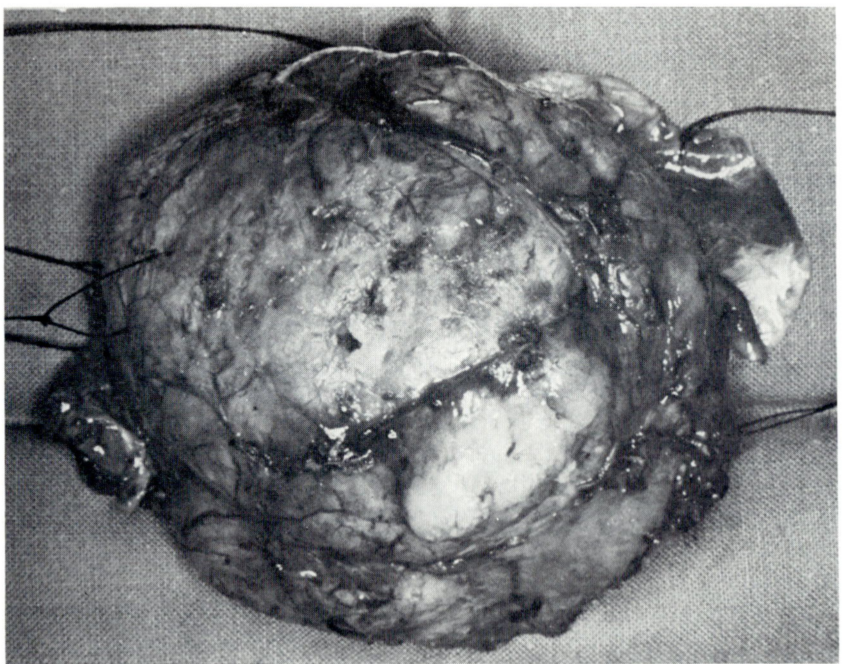

Figure 50. Globular meningioma of the pterion. The tumor and its dural attachment are shown. This tumor of the outer sphenoid ridge exerted its mass effect on the temporal pole and adjacent frontal lobe. It differs from the flat pterional meningioma en plaque associated with marked temporal-orbital hyperostosis.

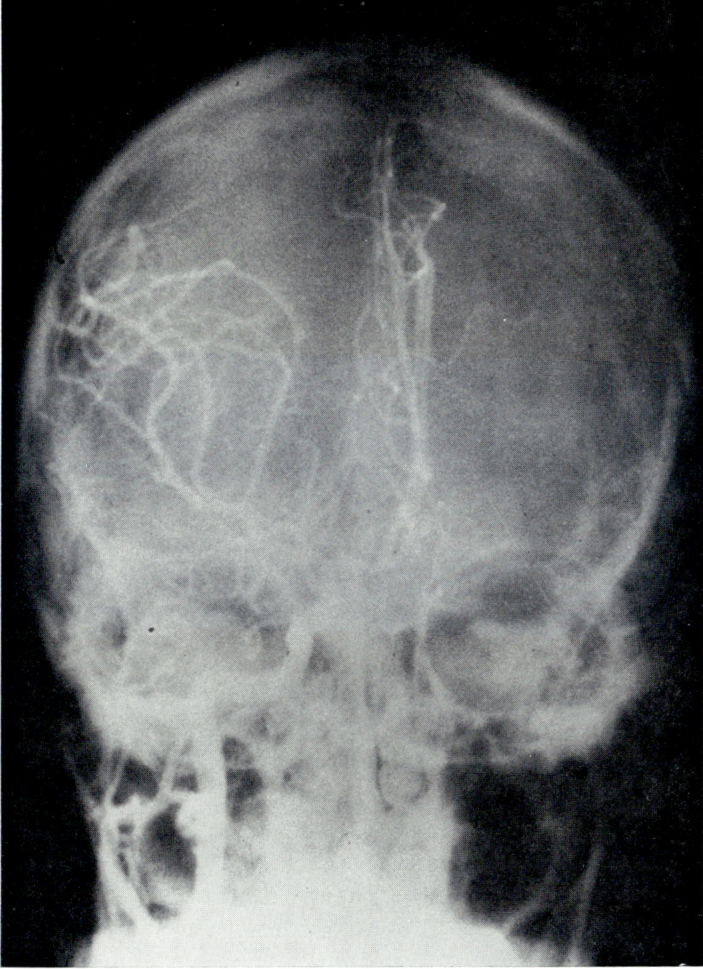

Figure 51. Sphenoid meningioma. A large meningioma arose from the middle (alar) ridge, producing marked elevation of the middle cerebral artery and subfalcial herniation of the pericallosal arteries. There had been apparent clinical silence for many years, a feature characteristic of middle ridge tumors.

over the petrous ridge. It slowly compresses the cerebral peduncle and brain stem.

6. Lateral tentorial meningioma—may compress the undersurface of the posterior temporo-occipital region adjacent to the transverse sinus. These are usually quite large tumors with hemianopia and chronic papilledema. Ataxia, nystagmus and hypotonia due to extension below the tentorium may be associated. The meningioma may occlude the transverse sinus.

Deficits of the Temporal Syndromes

The signs of localizing value indicating a temporal lobe lesion are of two basic types: ictal and nonictal. The seizure disorder of temporal lobe epilepsy is rather characteristic and is ordinarily separable from other forms of focal cerebral attack. Its interest to the neurosurgeon consists not only in the surgical therapy of medically intractable focal cerebral seizures, but also in the diagnostic significance of the syndrome.

A. Temporal lobe epilepsy

Temporal lobe epilepsy is basically an ictal disorder of memory. The temporal fit is a "time" fit. Nonictal disorders of time and memory are common in cerebral disease. Memory may be regarded as remote, recent and current; it is time-based. Any disturbance in consciousness may distort the sense of time and recall. Diffuse cerebral injury commonly affects time orientation. While disorientation to place and person also occurs, time disorientation appears first in the clouding of consciousness and persists longest in the process of return to normalcy. Retrograde amnesia for events preceding cerebral injury is commonly associated with time disorientation. The length of post-traumatic amnesia is the single best indicator of the duration of unconsciousness in unwitnessed coma, the two being directly proportional. Continuous anterograde amnesia (i.e. an impairment in "current" memory) as a result of bihippocampal destruction is a well-recognized, although fortunately rare entity. This does not necessarily localize so complex a function as memory, just as division of the optic chiasm producing total blindness does not localize the complex function of vision. It should be recalled that localization of a lesion and its deficit or dysfunction is fundamentally different from localization of normal function in the normal brain. The only valid conclusion is that both hippocampi form a vital link in memory mechanisms and that both medial temporal lobes must be damaged to produce this specific form of nonictal memory disorder.

Temporal seizures are a relatively common form of epilepsy. The temporal lobe attack is an instance in which a time-memory disorder has localizing clinical value. The ictal experience recalled by the patient may possess the intangible quality of the present, occurring "now," or of some past time, remote memories detailed with the vitality of present occurrence. Time may seem to stop or to accelerate. Oculomotor automatism accompanies the visual and auditory ictus, the patient staring about as though witnessing a familiar scene. There may be a sense of undue familiarity (déjà vu) as though the event was previously experienced. Unfamiliarity, a sense of environmental strangeness (derealization), a sense of detachment from self (depersonalization), a sense of witnessing oneself (autoscopy), anxiety and fear may occur. These feelings of dread may be heightened by visual distortions (metamorphopsia), apparent enlargement (macropsia), or smallness (micropsia) of seen objects, faces, persons or events. Auditory sensations of tinnitus, noise, the sound of bells, musical notes, songs and symphony may occur.

While there may be total recall of the ictal experience, with the patient describing it in detail, description is often limited. The patient may report a dreamlike quality (dreamy state seizures). He may be unwilling to discuss the attack because of its unpleasant nature. Recall may be possible only in the immediate postictal period. While ictal events may be partially obscured, total loss of memory for the attack also may occur. Complete amnesia, like postictal paralysis, is most common when the temporal attack is followed by generalized convulsion with total loss of consciousness and prolonged postictal stupor. The entire episode may have occurred during the night, the patient awakening in the morning with headache, sore tongue and neck, and urinary incontinence as lonely witnesses of the nocturnal ictus. Episodic amnesias may occur and should always suggest temporal epilepsy.

If all this is forgotten, and the clinician is confronted with merely a history of some obscure behavioral disorder, perhaps with aggressive overtones, some memory defect or variation in consciousness of an episodic nature, a leading consideration should be temporal lobe epilepsy, even if convulsion is not reported. The localizing features of greatest value occur at the very beginning of the attack. This is true of all the focal cerebral epilepsies (e.g. deviation of gaze away from an irritative cerebral lesion witnessed at the very outset of a seizure has greater lateralizing value than eye deviation occurring in the midst of generalized convulsion). The best localizing signs which label any complex hallucinatory experience as both epileptic and temporal in origin are as follow:

1. Epigastric aura.

   This peculiar sensation beginning in the pit of the stomach and rising in the chest to the throat, occurring at the very beginning of the attack, is most characteristic of temporal lobe epilepsy. The feeling is variously described, but begins in the abdomen and may be confined to the epigastrium. The patient frequently does not volunteer this information. The amnesia of generalized convulsion may obliterate any recall of any warning to the seizure. However, the epigastric aura is part of the ictus itself, and as such may occur in some attacks as an isolated phenomenon. More commonly it occurs with other temporal features such as automatism, not followed by generalized convulsion. Such partial seizures are frequently seen in patients already on anticonvulsants. The carefully constructed questions: Have you ever had an attack in which you did not lose consciousness? or Have you ever thought you were about to have an attack and then you did not? Why did you think an attack was coming? will often be rewarded with the spontaneous answer: Yes, I remember an odd feeling in my stomach. This is particularly valuable when the patient has previously denied any type of warning.

2. Olfactory aura.

   The unpleasant odor (parosmia) classically described with temporal epilepsy (uncinate attack) is much less common than the epigastric aura. An unpleasant taste (gustatory aura) is even less common. At times an unpleasant mixture of odor and taste is described. The odor of rotten eggs should always raise the possibility of temporal lobe astrocytoma, especially if it represents a change in the attack pattern.

3. Speech arrest.

   The patient may have sudden difficulty with speech at the outset of an attack. He may be unable to speak at all, although retaining the semiawareness characteristic of temporal epilepsy. Anomia is particularly characteristic of dominant temporal lobe epilepsy. This cerebral language disorder may be the sole clinical sign of left-sided origin. It should be separated from the nonlocalizing dysarthria of "slurred speech." The latter is common in many types of convulsive disorder and is prominent postictally. It is a disorder of articulation rather than of language. The form of words and their position in sentences remains intact in dysarthria. Anomia is not a feature of dysarthria. Anarthria, a complete speechless paralysis of the muscles of articulation, is much less common in the context of epilepsy.

4. Automatism and other motor features.

   Lip-smacking and masticatory movements are commonly seen during the temporal attack. They differ from the less complex chewing and biting movements occurring in brain stem trauma. Temporal epilepsy is associated with a variety of semipurposeful movements of a stereotyped nature. While picking at clothing is common, picking at the nose and mouth is most suggestive of temporal automatism. More elaborate automatisms including walking or more complex activities with an external appearance of normality sometimes occur. Automatized aggressive activity is not unusual. Focal motor activity of a nonpurposeful nature also occurs in temporal lobe epilepsy. Focal motor convulsions usually involve the opposite face or hand and arm. The attack may become generalized with or without this focal motor component. Todd's paralysis of parts convulsed is common postictally and should be detected in the early postictal phase when it is most marked. It points to a contralateral lesion.

In summary, visual and auditory hallucinations commonly occur in a variety of conditions, most notably in drug intoxication, toxic states, hysteria and epilepsy. Drug intoxication should always be ruled out first. The drug induced, toxic, or metabolic encephalopathy can each result in generalized convulsion. Pseudoseizures occur in hysteria. In addition, certain epileptics have occasional hysterical attacks. The episodic nature of the visuo-auditory hallucinations is an important epileptic characteristic, but also occurs in drug ingestion and hysteria. Certain features of the attack (e.g. déjà vu) suggest temporal lobe epilepsy. Epigastric aura with automatism indicates involvement of one or both temporal lobes. Focal motor seizures and postictal Todd's paralysis place the lesion on the opposite side. Ictal or postictal dysphasia indicates the dominant hemisphere. Parosmia raises the possibility of temporal astrocytoma. Most temporal lobe seizure disorders are not the result of a space-occupying process. Atrophy of the lobe is common. Occasionally, hemispheral atrophy from childhood may coexist, with a smaller contralateral hemiface, hand and foot. Subarachnoid cyst, subdural hygroma, juvenile subdural hematoma or arteriovenous hamartoma may be associated with the atrophic lobe. The temporal lobe may also appear grossly normal. Birth trauma, anoxia and chronic viral encephalopathy have been implicated.

B. Temporal lobe epilepsy and brain tumor

When temporal lobe epilepsy results from a tumor, it is most often an astrocytoma. The clinical points indicating a temporal astrocytoma syndrome are as follows:

1. At the time of diagnosis, the glioma, regardless of grade, has usually spread beyond the confines of the temporal lobe.
2. A temporal lobe astrocytoma may or may not be associated with seizures; if seizures occur they may be focal motor, generalized, or compatible with the syndrome of temporal lobe epilepsy; the latter does not necessarily indicate a low grade at the time of tumor diagnosis.
3. The features of temporal lobe epilepsy which should arouse suspicion of the temporal astrocytoma include the following:
   a. Aura—if an unpleasant odor is noted, astrocytoma should be suspected.
   b. Ictus—a basic change in the character of a previously stereotyped attack pattern.

(1) Increasing frequency of attacks despite previously adequate anticonvulsant control.
(2) Development of focal motor seizures which vary as to site of onset.

c. Postictal phase—unusually prolonged Todd's paralysis.
d. Interictal period.
(1) Development of a visual field cut not previously noted.
(2) Conversion of superior quadrantanopia to hemianopia.
(3) Development of any symptoms or signs of increased intracranial pressure.

4. Extracerebral regional tumors associated with seizures are the globular outer-ridge sphenoid and sylvian meningiomas; the characteristic syndrome includes the following:
a. Chronic papilledema is very common in these meningiomas (temporal astrocytoma may occur with or without swollen discs).
b. Focal motor seizures commonly occur with these meningiomas. They may produce spikes and sharp waves from the temporal leads. However, the clinical syndrome of temporal lobe (psychomotor) epilepsy virtually never occurs with meningiomas. Focal motor seizures also occur with frontal, parietal or temporal gliomas.
c. Contralateral facial weakness—this also occurs with frontal, frontoparietal or temporal astrocytoma.
d. Absence of a visual field cut—this negative sign is important, the presence of superior quadrantanopia or hemianopia favoring a temporal glioma over an extracerebral tumor.

5. Temporal lobe abscess—this may also produce focal motor or generalized convulsions; temporal lobe epilepsy does not occur; the characteristic features are as follow:
a. History or evidence of otitis media or mastoiditis.
b. Systemic signs—fever, leukocytosis, elevated sedimentation rate; may be entirely absent.
c. Coexistent meningeal signs—these may be present or absent in brain abscess cases.
(1) Nuchal rigidity—may indicate meningitis, or transtentorial herniation as a result of the temporal mass.
(2) Spinal rigidity.
(3) Kernig's sign—with the patient supine and the hip flexed perpendicular to the trunk, an attempt to extend the knee results in intense pain.
(4) Brudzinski's neck sign—passive flexion of the neck results in reflex flexion of the hips and knees.

(5) Brudzinski's leg sign—passive extension of the leg results in reflex flexion of the opposite hip and knee.

(6) Photophobia—a common symptom of meningeal irritation, especially when combined with pain and stiffness of the neck.

d. Acute papilledema, contralateral facial weakness and hemianopia are often present.

e. May present as a relatively silent temporal lobe mass, much as a frontal abscess consequent to frontoethmoidal sinus infection may be silent until elevated pressure occurs.

f. An intracranial inflammatory mass associated with visual field cut indicates temporal lobe abscess related to middle ear infection. Hemianopia may also occur with cerebral abscesses resulting from hematogenous sources. The absence of hemianopia when focal suppuration is suspected should suggest frontal or cerebellar abscess, epidural or subdural empyema.

C. Nonictal signs of temporal lobe lesions

Deficits which specifically indicate a lesion confined to the temporal lobe are few. Many clinical signs which help to substantiate the presence of a temporal lesion are due to compression of, or extension to, neighboring structures (e.g. contralateral central facial weakness). Infrasylvian lesions which spare speech may be readily missed until the signs of increased intracranial pressure and brain shift occur. Even at this point, the expanding temporal lesion may still be confused with a frontal mass. Sign silence in the presence of symptoms of intracranial hypertension should in itself raise the possibilities of tumor of either temporal pole, tumor of the nondominant temporal lobe, frontopolar tumor, intraventricular tumor, hydrocephalus and venous sinus thrombosis. The nonictal temporal lobe and temporal satellite signs include the following:

1. Visual field signs.
2. Ocular signs.
3. Auditory and vestibular signs.
4. Motor signs.
5. Speech signs.
6. Bitemporal signs.

The localizing diagnostic value of these signs is greatest when they occur in combination.

1. Visual field signs.

a. Character of the field cut.

The single nonictal temporal lobe sign of greatest localizing value is superior homonymous quadrantanopia opposite the lesion. In unusual circumstances the responsible lesion will be occipital, beneath the calcarine sulcus. Incongruity favors a temporal lesion, but a symmetrical field cut may also result from a temporal lesion, especially if situated more posteriorly. Posterior temporoparietal or temporo-occipital (i.e. a caudal retrosylvian cerebral lesion) visual field deficit is indicated by central hemianopia opposite the lesion. While macular sparing is suggestive of hemianopia of occipital origin, hemianopia due to posterior temporal lesions may spare or split the macula.

b. Character of the lesion.

(1) Intracerebral.

The responsible intracerebral masses of neurosurgical interest, glioma and abscess, are more commonly temporal than occipital. Gradual conversion of a quadrantanopia to hemianopia is usually due to temporal lobe glioma. Intratemporal hematoma resulting from trauma, from the "slit hemorrhage" of hypertension, from ruptured middle cerebral aneurysm or arteriovenous malformation, or from intragliomatous bleeding may result in hemianopia most marked in the superior quadrants. The visual field defect usually accompanying trauma to the occipital pole is either hemianopia or total blindness, and often hemianopia following total blindness. Superior quadrantanopia, then, almost always indicates a temporal lobe lesion. The lesion responsible for superior quadrantanopia is often space-occupying and of a surgical nature rather than the result of infarction. The field cut produced by most vascular infarctions is hemianopic rather than quadrantic. More posterior or deeply situated tumors (e.g. caudal or central cerebral gliomas) commonly produce hemianopia and are less readily differentiated from infarction on the basis of visual field study.

(2) Extracerebral (Fig. 52).

Superior quadrantanopia favors a temporal intracerebral rather than extracerebral lesion. Hemianopia is also more likely due to an intracerebral rather than an extracerebral mass. Hemianopia as a result of extracerebral lesions in the temporal region can occur under certain conditions.

(a) Acute middle fossa extradural (or subdural) hematomas associated with progressive coma do not permit visual field examination.

(b) Chronic subdural hematoma with visual field abnormality usually consists of peripheral constriction due to chronic papilledema. The finding of a hemianopia suggests an intracerebral lesion. In the elderly patient, cerebral infarc-

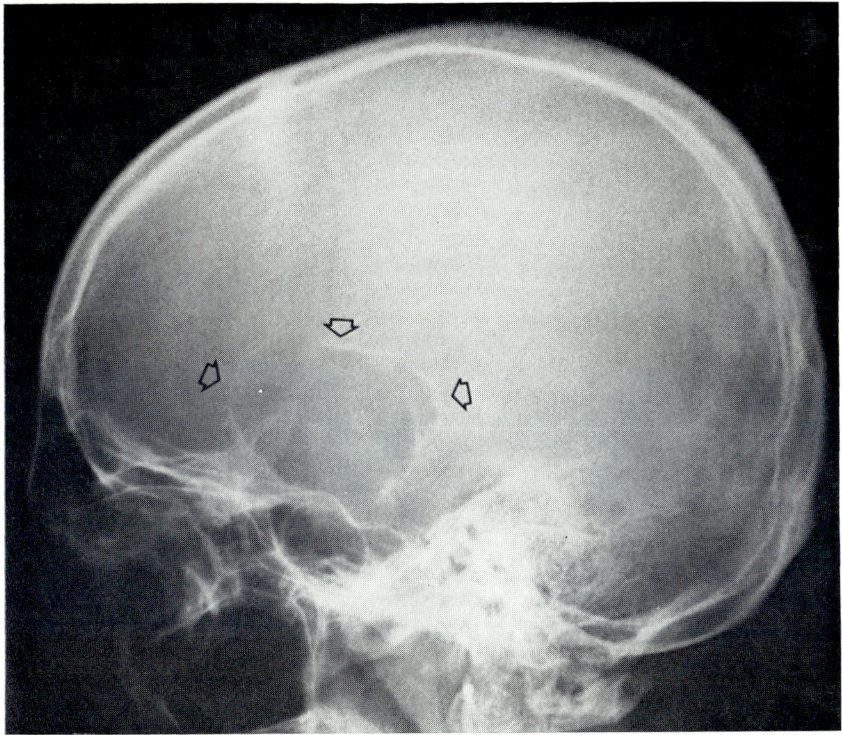

Figure 52. Epidermoid tumor of the pterion. This epidermoid calvarial tumor was extradural in the region of the pterion. Epidermoid tumors also occur in intradural locations.

tion may occasionally coexist with the chronic subdural, producing a hemianopia.

(c) Alar meningioma of the middle sphenoid ridge may produce tract hemianopia, acting as a mass which both compresses the temporal pole and medially adjacent optic tract.

(d) Clinoidal meningioma of the inner sphenoid ridge produces unilateral blindness, optic atrophy and oculomotor palsy rather than hemianopia.

(e) Globular pterion meningioma of the outer sphenoid ridge or intrasylvian meningioma compress the temporal pole but produce peripheral constriction of the fields due to papilledema, rather than hemianopia.

(f) Meningioma en plaque of the pterion results in gross hyperostosis of the temporal bone and orbit with exophthalmos, but without hemianopia, in women of middle age. Intracranial pressure remains normal.

(g) Nontemporal meningiomas resulting in hemianopia—these are caudal cerebral tumors of the posterior third of the sagittal sinus, falx or tentorium. They are characteristically also associated with peripheral field constriction due to chronic papilledema.

2. Ocular signs.
   a. Pupillary signs—in most temporal lobe lesions the pupils are normal in size and in reaction to light. Abnormal pupils suggest the presence of a mass.
      (1) Most cases of temporal lobe epilepsy are not associated with mass lesions. During an attack the pupils may be abnormal. Between attacks the pupils are normal. If the seizure is one involving a sense of unreality, anxiety or fear, the pupils are often dilated and brisk. If the attack continues into generalized convulsion with total loss of consciousness, the pupils may be widely dilated and sluggish. They remain equal. If, in the interictal period between attacks, pupillary inequality is noted, a temporal lobe astrocytoma should be suspected.
      (2) Partial Horner's syndrome—a small pupil with partial ptosis may occur ipsilateral to a temporal tumor. This may give the false impression of a dilated pupil on the opposite side, especially if ptosis is minimal.
      (3) Behr's sign—involvement of the optic tract (medial to the uncus) produces a large pupil on the opposite side. Tract hemianopia and eventual optic atrophy are associated.
      (4) Oculomotor palsy—temporal lobe masses (e.g. glioblastoma, acute abscess) tend to produce relatively rapid transtentorial herniation in contrast to tumors of similar growth rate in other parts of the hemisphere. Low-grade astrocytoma may present as a seizure disorder long before signs of transtentorial herniation occur. Despite the grade, the glioma has usually extended beyond the confines of the temporal lobe at the time of diagnosis. The most common sign (apart from obtundation) of transtentorial herniation is pupillary inequality, with the dilated pupil on the side of the mass, followed by sluggishness of the light reflex, extraocular oculomotor palsy and eventual loss of pupillary reaction. The other signs of uncal-hippocampal herniation occur, with progressive coma, contralateral or occasionally ipsilateral hemiplegia, noisy respiration, hypertension and bradycardia, generalized rigidity especially prominent in the neck and legs, decerebrate extensor rigidity of all extremities, loss of oculocephalic reflexes, and ultimate hypo-

tension, tachycardia and hypoventilation. While this rapid transtentorial syndrome may occur with any supratentorial expanding mass, it is a particularly prominent feature in the acute extradural and intracerebral middle fossa hematomas. The acute subdural produces the same signs, the hematoma extending over the convexity of a swollen, usually contused brain.

b. Extraocular motor signs.
   (1) Oculomotor palsy—the eye on the side of the mass looks outward and downward with ptosis and associated pupillary enlargement. This occurs with uncal herniation of any supratentorial source. It may occur without uncal or hippocampal herniation due to "central transtentorial herniation." In this instance, the brain stem is shifted downward by a supratentorial mass, stretching the oculomotor nerve (s) over the petroclinoid ligament (s). The signs of brain stem compromise noted above ensue. Oculomotor palsy also may occur without either form of transtentorial herniation in "clinoidal" inner ridge sphenoid meningiomas. These tumors compress the optic nerve and medial aspect of the temporal pole.
   (2) Abducens palsy—lateral rectus weakness indicates elevated intracranial pressure. It is either unilateral or bilateral. It does not safely lateralize the lesion. It may occur well before transtentorial herniation. Its occurrence in temporal lobe epilepsy suggests astrocytoma.
   (3) Spontaneous nystagmus—fairly frequent in temporal lobe tumor. Its direction does not safely lateralize the temporal mass. Gross nystagmus of coarse type is even more common in cerebellar tumors. It is coarser in the direction of the tumor. Nystagmus in the presence of field cut indicates a temporal tumor. Occasionally, large cerebellar tumors compress the occipital poles sufficiently to produce hemianopia. This falsely localizing sign must be weighed against the prominent ataxia, hypotonia and hyporeflexia in these cerebellar cases.

c. Funduscopic signs—temporal lobe lesions including mass lesions often have normal fundi.
   (1) Most cases of temporal lobe epilepsy have normal optic discs.
   (2) Temporal lobe seizures complicated by development of papilledema indicate an astrocytoma, possibly glioblastoma.
   (3) Temporal tumors may also present with normal fundi and no seizures.
   (4) Evidence of chronic papilledema and focal motor seizures be-

ginning in the opposite face, hand or arm is quite compatible with an outer sphenoidal or sylvian meningioma, or with temporal glioma or abscess, or with chronic subdural hematoma. Frontal or frontoparietal tumors may produce the same clinical picture.

3. Auditory and vestibular signs.
   a. For practical clinical purposes, deafness does not result from a unilateral temporal lesion.
   b. Bitemporal destruction of Heschl's gyri is virtually unknown as a clinical source of central deafness. Bitemporal polar contusion is common, but Heschl's gyri are relatively protected in the operculum of the midtemporal region. The opercular syndrome results from bilateral opercular infarctions (usually sequential vascular occlusions due to carotid or middle cerebral thrombosis or embolism). This produces pseudobulbar palsy rather than central deafness.
   c. Auditory signs of a temporal lesion are either ictal (auditory hallucinations) or aphasic (impaired recognition of language sounds).
   d. Vestibular signs include the following:
      (1) Sense of imbalance or vertigo occurring in temporal lobe epilepsy.
      (2) Spontaneous nystagmus in temporal lobe tumors.
      (3) Asymmetries in optokinetic and caloric nystagmus in temporal lesions.
      (4) While both vertigo and nystagmus may have ocular, cerebral, brain stem, cerebellar or peripheral etiologies, particular attention should be directed to the posterior fossa.
4. Motor signs.
   a. A non-mass lesion of the temporal lobe (e.g. most cases of temporal lobe epilepsy) characteristically presents no motor deficit and no Babinski sign.
   b. A mass lesion of the temporal lobe commonly produces a motor deficit by transsylvian compression of the lower motor region. The motor signs include the following:
      (1) Contralateral central facial weakness.
      (2) Contralateral faciobrachial weakness.
      (3) Contralateral hemiparesis including the face with relative sparing of the leg.
      (4) Contralateral Babinski sign and hyperreflexia are commonly present. The facial paralysis and Babinski sign may appear in isolation opposite a temporal (or frontal) mass.

(5) Motor dysphasia (major hemisphere)—simulating a lesion within Broca's region.

c. A mass lesion of the temporal lobe can thus closely simulate a frontal mass. The differential diagnosis is clinically established by the following:

(1) Demonstration of a homonymous field cut—heavily favors a temporal mass over a frontal mass. A temporal polar mass rostral to the temporal horn (and Meyer's loop) may spare the visual radiation but compress the optic tract. Frontal pseudohemianopia may occasionally cause difficulty. Large frontobasal tumors or small inner ridge sphenoidal meningiomas may compress the optic nerve, but the visual loss is central and monocular rather than homonymous. Tuberculum meningiomas may produce binocular visual loss due to compression of both optic nerves and the anterior chiasm, but the visual impairment is usually worse on one side and is not homonymous.

(2) Unilateral anosmia—heavily favors a frontobasal lesion (olfactory meningioma or frontal glioma). It may be produced by middle ridge sphenoid meningiomas which also compress the temporal pole. It does not result from an intratemporal mass.

(3) Rothfield's sign.

(a) Passive straight leg raising ipsilateral to a temporal (or temporoparietal) lesion results in flexion of the hip, knee and ankle on the side opposite the tumor.

(b) Passive straight leg raising contralateral to a frontal lesion lesion produces flexion of the hip, knee and ankle on the side of the tumor.

(4) Demonstration of nominal or receptive dysphasia—favors a dominant temporal or temporoparietal lesion. A predominantly expressive dysphasia can result from either a dominant frontal or temporal mass, although most often indicating a frontal lesion.

(5) Optokinetic nystagmus—there may be an asymmetry produced in the absence of hemianopia, favoring a temporal rather than frontal mass.

d. A temporal mass may also produce motor deficit by uncal-transtentorial herniation. This differs from the transsylvian motor deficit (described above in 4b.) which commonly exists before uncal herniation. Both motor deficits are associated with pyramidal signs. The two forms of motor deficit are differentiated as follow:

(1) Distribution of the paralysis.

(a) Transsylvian compression always includes contralateral facial weakness as part of the paralysis; the paralysis may be limited to the face; if hemiparesis occurs there may be relative sparing of the leg; the hemiparesis is always contralateral; the progression of hemiparesis tends to be gradual (compared to uncal herniation).

(b) Cerebral peduncle compression (by uncal herniation) always includes the leg ("leg" fibers are outermost in the peduncle and "face" fibers are most medial); the hemiparesis usually is equally distributed in the contralateral arm and leg; the face is usually included in the paralysis, but may be spared; the leg is never spared. The progression of the hemiparesis is rapid. The hemiparesis may be a prelude to decerebration. While the hemiparesis is usually contralateral, it is at times ipsilateral due to compression of the opposite peduncle by the tentorial edge (Kernohan's notch).

(2) Presence of associated signs.

(a) Progressive obtundation—occurs rapidly in uncal herniation with the production of coma.

(b) Oculomotor palsy—a reliable sign of transtentorial herniation with ipsilateral pupillary dilatation.

(c) Other components of the transtentorial syndrome—vital sign changes, etc.

5. Speech signs—nominal dysphasia (i.e. temporal anomia).

Temporal lobe lesions on either side may be associated with normally expressive and receptive speech. In the dominant hemisphere a temporopolar mass may compress Broca's region and thereby produce a predominantly expressive dysphasia. In the caudal portion of the dominant temporal lobe, where the posterior superior temporal gyrus (Wernicke's region) becomes continuous with the parietal supramarginal gyrus above, a lesion results in predominantly receptive dysphasia. In the intermediate portion of the midtemporal lobe, a lesion may result in nominal dysphasia or anomia. This is a variant of dysphasia in which there is a particular inability to name words. There is often a variable mixture with other speech deficits, but a midtemporal lesion will at times produce a relatively pure form. Under these circumstances, anomia has a localizing value to the major temporal lobe. A temporal tumor may present an anomia before a more generalized receptive speech disorder occurs. The patient is usually aware of his inability to name a word correctly. Although he "word-hunts," he cannot recall the correct term. This lack of recall is sometimes referred to as "amnestic aphasia." Memory for the correct term is impaired. The patient understands the meaning of the word, if the word is spoken to him. The correct word, however, is quickly forgotten. In this relatively pure temporal anomia, there is no lack of recognition (of the word), impaired recognition characterizing caudal cerebral (parieto temporal) lesions. In temporal anomia, the patient not only understands the meaning of the word, but instantly recognizes the correct word when it is presented to him. The patient is not garrulous and does not use jargon as in receptive dysphasia. When questioned as to the proper word for an object, the anomic patient is apt to stop his speech if he cannot name it, rather than to continue a flow of speech, misnaming the object in the process. There is no general speech reduction or mispronounciation of words as in Broca's expressive dysphasia. Anomia or nominal dysphasia is a fragment on a spectrum of interrelated speech disorders. The basic impairment appears to be one of memory, rather than one of perception or articulation. In its relatively pure form, anomia may be regarded as a nonictal memory disturbance of the temporal lobe devoted to language.

6. Bitemporal signs.
   a. Signs of bitemporopolar contusion.
      (1) The patient is confused and disoriented. Time disorientation is most prominent and persistent.
      (2) Intermittent aggressive behavior is common.
      (3) Focal cerebral or generalized seizures commonly occur.
      (4) Marked temporal contusion with a swollen temporal lobe may result in hemiparesis with relative sparing of the leg. The hemiparesis is on the side opposite the greater contusion.
      (5) Associated brain edema, subfrontal contusion, or extracerebral or intracerebral hematoma result in progressive coma. Continuous and spontaneous restless motor activity suggests contusion of the orbital cortex. Restlessness may also result from progressive intracranial hypertension preceding transtentorial herniation. Traumatic subarachnoid hemorrhage is another source of restlessness.
      (6) When hemiparesis is progressive and does not spare the leg, transtentorial herniation should be suspected. Increasing generalized rigidity ("Gegenhalten"), increasing nuchal rigidity, oculomotor palsy, systemic hypertension, bradycardia and deepening coma indicate herniation through the incisura, and hematoma is the likely source. Extradural, subdural or intracerebral hematoma may be responsible. A markedly contused

temporal lobe may produce the same picture. Subtemporal subdural hematoma consequent to tearing of the bridging veins at the temporal pole occasionally produces a temporal hernia without a large hemispheral convexity accumulation of subdural clot.

b. Psychomotor seizures.
   (1) Typical temporal lobe epilepsy in a significant minority of cases represents bitemporal rather than unitemporal damage.
   (2) Bilaterality can be demonstrated electrographically and with the use of memory testing during the carotid amytal test.
   (3) Bitemporal anoxia may accompany various forms of craniocerebral trauma, including birth trauma.

c. Tentorial packing.
   (1) Bihippocampal herniation results in compression of the tectum and tegmentum of the midbrain. The brain stem is dislocated downward. The oculomotor nerves may be stretched over the petroclinoid ligaments. Deep cerebral venous drainage and incisural circulation of CSF around the brain stem is impaired. Brain stem ischemia and central stem hemorrhages occur.
   (2) Tentorial packing occurs as a result of generalized supratentorial mass effect as in diffuse cerebral edema.
   (3) Signs are similar to those of uncal herniation. Forward flexion of the head may result in pupillary dilatation and loss of reflex upward gaze. The patient is invariably obtunded and coma is progressive. Tentorial packing may be responsible for terminal deterioration with complete bilateral ophthalmoplegia. Upward herniation of the superior cerebellar vermis due to cerebellar tumor may produce a similar picture.

d. Anterograde amnesia—an impairment in "current memory" resulting in a continuous forgetting. This is a rare clinical entity resulting from bitemporal damage to both hippocampi. The impairment is nonepisodic, in contrast to the more common "ictal amnesias" of temporal lobe epilepsy. It is readily separated from the common nonictal amnesias of retrograde type. In "retrograde amnesia" memory is impaired for events occurring before the time of cerebral trauma; it is not impaired specifically for continuously acquired new information occurring after cerebral trauma; it is reflected into the past rather than into the future. In "post-traumatic amnesia," which is also common, memory is impaired for events immediately following cerebral trauma; it is not permanently continuous. Duration of post-traumatic amnesia correlates with duration of coma. Retrograde and post-traumatic amnesias do not necessarily implicate the temporal lobe. Anterograde amnesia does not occur unless both hippocampi are damaged.

Acute Middle Fossa Epidural Syndrome (and Its Differentiation from Other Traumatic Comas)

The combined clinical-radiological nature of this acute middle fossa mass syndrome requires its special consideration at this point. The combination of clinical signs, plain x-rays and echo-encephalography often permit accurate clinical diagnosis without angiography. This is helpful due to the urgent necessity for operative intervention. The acute epidural hematoma most commonly results from traumatic laceration of the middle meningeal artery within the lateral wall or floor of the middle fossa. The arterial hemorrhage produces rapid uncal herniation. The hematoma, temporal lobe and midbrain lie in a direct horizontal plane. The force is directly translated to the upper brain stem. The temporal lobe is literally pushed toward the midline. The brain stem reticular formation is progressively impaired by compression, ischemia and ultimately by central stem hemorrhages. The level of coma rapidly deepens during this process with eventual cardiorespiratory collapse. Central stem hemorrhages may extend to the lower level of the pons. Early hematoma evacuation, before serious brain stem compromise, can result in excellent recovery. A number of features, both clinical and radiological, characterize the acute middle fossa epidural syndrome.

1. A history or evidence of head injury; a history of "lucid interval" between initial unconsciousness and the progressive coma phase is relatively uncommon. Some evidence of bruising about the face or scalp may be present; in particular, a bruise with swelling in the temporal region may be noted.
2. Progressive stupor and coma—this is the most common form of sensorial impairment.
3. Pupillary inequality—the larger pupil is almost always on the side of the clot. There is progressive sluggishness and ultimate loss of its light reflex and extraoculomotor palsy.
4. Hemiparesis—the motor deficit is usually on the opposite side; the paralysis may be mild or severe. A Babinski sign and hyperreflexia on the side opposite the clot are common.
5. Temporal skull fracture—this is quite common on the side of the clot; the middle meningeal artery is torn as it passes through a groove on the inner table of the temporal bone or as it passes within the bone; the fracture may be lateral or in the floor of the middle fossa; such

basal fracturing can be missed on plain films. Even a lateral temporal fracture can be missed on plain x-rays in early childhood.

6. Pineal (or echo) shift of the midline to the side opposite the clot is characteristic.

While the above features may be compatible with any unilateral supratentorial expanding mass, the presence of all six makes an acute middle fossa epidural hematoma the leading diagnosis. Pineal (or echo) shift away from a temporal skull fracture in the middle meningeal region is particularly significant. The temporal fracture is usually best seen on the lateral view, while the midline shift is noted on the PA (or AP) film. In the absence of satisfactory pineal calcification, ultrasonic echo-encephalography gives a rapid and highly accurate assessment of the deep midline. The probe should be placed in the temporal region of each side of the head and each midline trace compared. In the presence of marked temporal scalp contusion, the midline echo may be erroneous.

An acute epidural hematoma may be present lacking some of these features. This is especially true if the epidural is eccentric, if it compresses a major venous sinus, or if it lies in the posterior fossa. These epidurals are less common than the classical acute middle fossa epidural clot. Bleeding from diploic venous channels leads to a slower rate of epidural clot formation and a slower deterioration. An intermediate rate of deterioration can be seen if peripheral branches of the middle meningeal artery are torn. An anterior fossa epidural may be limited by the attachment of the dura to the undersurface of the coronal suture. Such a frontopolar (eccentric) epidural, whether of venous or peripheral arterial origin, may not shift the midline. An epidural hematoma may lie immediately beneath a depressed skull fracture; this is also true of the subdural and intracortical hematomas. An epidural hematoma over the vertex, which compresses the longitudinal sinus, typically leads to bilateral brain swelling without significant midline shift. The posterior fossa epidural, often associated with an occipital skull fracture, may lead to rapid deterioration due to brain stem compression combined with obstructive hydrocephalus. The fracture line may cross the transverse sinus and Towne's (AP) view is valuable. The pineal (and echo) are characteristically in the midline in subtentorial epidural hematomas.

The acute subdural or intracerebral hematoma, and acute traumatic brain swelling with unilateral hemispheral predominance, can produce a similar syndrome. The middle fossa and temporal lobe need not be involved. The subdural usually covers most of the cerebral convexity and may or may not enter the middle fossa. Either uncal or central transtentorial herniation can occur. As in epidurals, various sorts of cranial fracturing may also be present. However, these masses are somewhat less likely to be associated with temporal fracturing (through meningeal vessel grooves) on the side of a dilated pupil. An acute subdural is occasionally present on the side opposite a cranial fracture as a result of contrecoup tearing of bridging veins. In the majority of cases, the acute subdural or intracerebral clot or unihemispheral brain swelling will shift the midline to the opposite side. However, the acute subdural is more apt to be bilateral than the epidural hematoma. This results in a midline pineal which is shifted downwards on the lateral view. The intracerebral hematoma is most commonly frontopolar, central cerebral or in the temporal lobe. The frontopolar intracerebral hematoma may not displace the pineal from the midline until it reaches large size. It may displace the pineal backward (on lateral view) without producing midline shift. The central cerebral and temporal lobe hematomas characteristically displace the midline to the opposite side. Traumatic brain swelling is commonly bilateral and does not shift the midline. Swelling may be marked in one temporal lobe, and in these cases the midline is often shifted to the opposite side.

In summary, the following is true with regard to the midline shift of the pineal (or echo) in the traumatically comatose patient.

1. Shift across the midline makes a unilateral supratentorial hematoma most likely.
2. The responsible hematoma may be epidural, subdural or intracerebral.
3. Certain forms of unilaterally predominant brain swelling may be responsible for the midline shift.
4. When the midline pineal (or echo) is *not* shifted in the traumatically comatose patient an acute middle fossa epidural hematoma is unlikely.

When the midline pineal (or echo) is *not* shifted in the traumatically comatose patient, the following diagnoses must be ruled out:

1. Bilateral subdural hematomas.
2. Traumatic brain swelling—cerebral or brain stem contusion may be associated.
3. Frontopolar (or occipitopolar) lobar hematoma.
4. Eccentric epidural or subdural hematomas.
5. Traumatic occlusion (or epidural compression) of a major venous sinus with secondary brain swelling.
6. Posterior fossa epidural or subdural hematomas (intracerebellar hematoma due to trauma is still less likely).
7. Coma due to acute traumatic anterior pituitary infarction—resistant hypotension or shock without evidence of blood loss; resistant coma without evidence of intracranial hypertension.

In addition, a second major group of traumatic comas results from various forms of associated extracranial injury. This group must also be differentiated from the head-injured comatose patient without shift of the pineal (or echo).

1. Coma due to blood loss shock.
   a. Hemothorax—commonly with rib fractures.
   b. Hemoperitoneum—commonly with rib fractures or blunt abdominal trauma leading to ruptured spleen or liver.
   c. Fractured pelvis and femoral head fractures.
   d. Retroperitoneal hematoma—often with renal contusion and hematuria and fractured transverse processes.
   e. Acute gastrointestinal hemorrhage—may be the result of stress ulceration.
   f. Extremely severe fracturing of the cranial base or very extensive scalp laceration with laceration of major scalp arteries may result in blood loss shock and resultant coma.
2. Coma due to anoxia without shock.
   a. Aspiration.
   b. Pulmonary contusion—commonly with rib fractures.
   c. Pneumothorax—rib fractures usually present.
   d. Compression injury of the thorax with reduced cerebral venous return.
   e. Primary cerebral anoxia secondary to uncontrolled status epilepticus.
3. Coma due to anoxic—hypotensive high spinal injury—cervical x-rays should be routinely taken in head injury cases.
4. Coma due to cerebral fat embolism—usually associated with extremity long bone fracture. Petechiae on upper thorax, axillae, conjunctiva and retina are characteristic. Tachypnea with tachycardia is common, with multiple cotton-wool densities on chest x-ray. Progressive stupor and coma, sometimes with decerebration are noted. Retinal hemorrhage may be prominent.

Another important group of head-injured patients are those in whom head trauma is secondary to some other pathological process. Convulsive disorders commonly result in craniocerebral injury as a result of ictal falling. Similarly, a ruptured aneurysm, arteriovenous malformation, or hypertensive intracranial hemorrhage may at times present with the combination of coma and signs of cephalic trauma. Examination of the fundi in the acutely head-injured case revealing chronic papilledema should suggest underlying brain tumor or chronic subdural hematoma with secondary trauma. A history or evidence of chronic alcoholism should be accepted as suggestive of cranial trauma even if history and examination for trauma signs are negative. There may be acute bleeding into a chronic subdural in these cases.

Neurological examination in the acutely head-injured, comatose patient should emphasize the following points:

1. Level of consciousness to noxious stimulation.
   a. Stupor—obtunded but arousable.
   b. Semicoma—not arousable, but purposeful movement present.
   c. Coma—not arousable; no purposeful movement apart from reflex withdrawal.
   d. Decorticate—not arousable; rigid flexion of upper extremities and extension of lower extremities.
   e. Decerebrate—not arousable; rigid extension and hyperpronation of all extremities.
   f. "Coma de passe"—not arousable; total flaccidity and arreflexia; cardiorespiratory collapse.

   Note: Level of consciousness can be followed with cotton-wisp testing of corneal responsiveness (brisk, sluggish or absent corneal response from light to deeper stages of obtundation); asymmetry may indicate either cranial nerve five or seven involvement.
2. Vital signs—blood pressure, pulse, respiration and temperature.
3. Signs of craniofacial injury—compound scalp injury, palpable depressed fracture, basal skull fracture ecchymoses, CSF rhinorrhea or otorrhea, and so forth.
4. Signs of associated trauma—cervical, carotid, chest, abdomen, spine, pelvis, extremities.
5. Pupillary equality, reactivity and size.
6. Oculocephalic reflexes—conjugate or disconjugate gaze on head turning.
7. Retromandibular or supraorbital noxious stimulation may induce facial grimace with facial asymmetry not previously detected.
8. Suprasternal noxious stimulation—may induce previously undetected extremity movement or purposeful movement. Undetected hemiparesis may become obvious.
9. Posture of extremities may indicate hemiparesis; degree of spontaneous movement on each side should be compared; degree of withdrawal response on each side should be compared. Slight inward rotation of the arm with persistent tendency toward hyperpronation on painful stimulation indicates decerebrate coma even if gross decerebration is absent.
10. Tone.
    a. Nuchal rigidity.
    b. Generalized mild increase in tone ("Gegenhalten").
    c. Nuchocrural rigidity—increased tone in the neck and legs.
    d. Hypertonia of decortication, decerebration and opisthotonus.

e. Unilateral hypotonia (flaccidity) of hemiplegic limbs.
f. Unilateral hypertonia (spasticity) of hemiparetic limbs.

11. Deep tendon reflexes—noted particularly for symmetry; unilateral hyperreflexia in hemispasticity; unilateral hyporeflexia in hemiflaccidity; generalized arreflexia in medullary failure, profound anoxia, drug intoxication and spinal injury.
12. Babinski sign (and other pyramidal signs)—commonly present in cerebral or brain stem contusion either unilaterally or bilaterally. A unilateral Babinski sign opposite a dilated pupil indicates hematoma until proven otherwise. The Babinski sign may become bilateral with sufficient compression due to a unilateral hematoma.

Deformities (Angiographic and Pneumographic) of Syndromes of the Temporal Region

A. Angiographic

1. Angiographic findings in acute middle fossa epidural hematoma. (Angiograms are commonly not required; pneumograms are contraindicated; angiography may be required in cases of eccentric epidurals not in the middle fossa and in equivocal cases).
   a. Lateral distribution of an avascular mass (i.e. clot), devoid of all vessels, lying between the middle cerebral cortical vessels and the inner table of the temporal bone (AP view) is characteristic. The avascular mass is relatively segmental in contrast to the more widely distributed convexity subdural hematoma. Temporal fracture overlying the avascular region is common; the fracture may be linear or depressed.
   b. A slightly irregular cortical margin at the site of an epidural clot is common (AP view); local irregularity is less common in subdural hematoma.
   c. Shift of the internal cerebral vein (AP view) to the opposite side is typical; it may exceed the degree of anterior cerebral shift. Medial shift of the anterior choroidal artery indicates uncal herniation. Subdural or intracerebral hematomas may result in similar midline shifts. Displacement of the anterior cerebral artery is usually less obvious in epidurals than in subdurals.
   d. Elevation of the horizontal part of the middle cerebral artery (AP view) may be seen in epidural hematoma of the floor of the middle fossa.
   e. Lateral view—may be normal while the AP view is markedly abnormal; may reveal elevation of the sylvian triangle either anteriorly, posteriorly or diffusely.
   f. Traumatic aneurysm of the middle meningeal artery is a rare

event but can be seen in association with the epidural hematoma; seen only with common carotid injection (i.e. the middle meningeal is a branch of the external carotid system).

2. Angiographic findings in epidural hematoma at other sites (not the typical middle fossa clot).
   a. Displacement of the superior longitudinal sinus away from the inner table by an avascular mass—due to an epidural rather than subdural collection; the sinus may become occluded; adjacent fracture (vertex) is common.
   b. Displacement of the transverse sinus away from the inner table by an avascular mass—either a caudal epidural or a subtentorial epidural; the latter typically extend upward over the occipital pole in contrast to posterior fossa subdural hematomas.
   c. Posterior fossa epidural—hydrocephalus on carotid angiograms (pericallosal artery stretching on lateral view; thalamostriate vein depression on AP view). Separation of the torcular or transverse sinus away from the inner table may be seen on carotid angiograms; occipital skull fracture is often present; vertebral angiograms may be negative. Posterior inferior cerebellar artery depression through the foramen magnum (e.g. as in tonsillar herniation) into the cervical canal does not necessarily indicate a posterior fossa mass.
   d. Eccentric epidurals (frontopolar or caudal cerebral) these may not shift the midline until large; normal AP and lateral carotid angiograms may result, the clot being seen only on oblique view. Marked round shift (AP view) of the anterior cerebral artery (in excess of internal cerebral vein shift) favors a frontal mass. "Rolling out" of the angle between the anterior cerebral and pericallosal arteries (lateral view) favors a frontal intracerebral rather than an extracerebral mass; a normal angle with a frontal round shift favors a frontal epidural. Oblique views indicate eccentric epidurals when the following occur:
      (1) A large avascular mass under the frontal boss can be seen when the head is rotated toward the side of the clot and side of carotid injection.
      (2) A large avascular mass under the region of the lambdoid suture can be seen when the head is rotated toward the side opposite the clot and carotid injection.
3. Angiographic findings in transtentorial temporal herniation (these mesial temporal herniations are anterior, posterior or complete).
   a. Uncal (anterior) herniation.
      (1) AP view, medial displacement.

(a) Anterior choroidal artery.
(b) Basal vein.
(c) Posterior communicating and posterior cerebral arteries.

(2) Lateral view.
(a) Stretching of the anterior choroidal artery.
(b) Downward displacement of the posterior communicating and posterior cerebral arteries.
(c) Downward displacement of the basilar bifurcation on vertebral angiogram.

b. Hippocampal (posterior) herniation.
(1) AP view, medial displacement.
(a) Posterior cerebral artery—vertebral or carotid angiogram.
(b) Basilar artery, upper portion—vertebral angiogram.
(2) Lateral view—"step" in distal segment of the posterior cerebral artery from its depressed position to the tentorial edge; vertebral or carotid angiogram (the posterior cerebral artery retains its "embryonic state" in one of three carotid angiograms, demonstrating filling from the carotid system).

c. Unco-hippocampal (complete) herniation—marked displacement of the anterior choroidal, posterior communicating and posterior cerebral arteries and the basal vein toward the midline (AP); marked downward displacement of the entire posterior communicating-posterior cerebral complex with a distal step (lateral), plus downward shift of the basilar bifurcation (lateral vertebral).

4. Angiographic findings in supra-alar temporal pole herniation—the middle cerebral artery and superficial middle cerebral (sylvian) vein are displaced superiorly (with the temporal lobe) across the sphenoid wing and into the base of the anterior fossa (lateral view). This unusual herniation suggests a slowly enlarging subtemporal mass. More rapidly enlarging temporal and middle fossa masses result in uncal or hippocampal herniation.
5. Angiographic findings in infra-alar frontobasal herniation into the middle fossa—the middle cerebral artery and sylvian vein are displaced backward from the sphenoid ridge by a frontobasal hernia. This indicates a frontopolar tumor.
6. Angiographic findings in extratemporal masses of the middle fossa.

a. Sphenoid ridge meningiomas.
(1) Elevation.
(a) Middle cerebral artery, horizontal portion—the "knee" may be elevated or even reversed (AP).
(b) Sylvian triangle, anterior portion (lateral).
(c) Carotid bifurcation—may be elevated.

(d) Anterior cerebral artery—may be elevated near its origin in medial ridge masses extending into the anterior fossa.

(2) Medial displacement.

(a) Supraclinoid carotid siphon.

(b) Anterior choroidal artery—indicating uncal herniation (more common with middle or outer ridge globose meningiomas which grow to large size than with clinoidal tumors of the inner ridge).

(3) Angiographic meningioma signs—extracerebral supply from the maxillary artery, middle and accessory meningeal arteries are prominent. Recurrent supply from the ophthalmic artery may be noted. Persistent tumor cloud and "sunburst sign" are typical.

b. Less common meningiomas of the middle fossa.

(1) Intrasylvian meningioma.

(a) "Splitting" of the middle cerebral arterial branches—some lie above and some below the sylvian mass.

(b) Usually lateral and intrasylvian, with medial displacement of middle cerebral arteries away from the temporal squama.

(c) Typical angiographic meningioma signs.

(2) Subtemporal meningioma of the middle fossa floor.

(a) Upward displacement of all the middle cerebral arterial branches.

(b) Upward displacement of the anterior choroidal artery —can differentiate an extratemporal from an intratemporal mass.

(c) Typical angiographic meningioma signs.

(3) Meningioma of Meckel's cave ("gassero-petrosal" or "saddle tumor").

(a) Upward displacement of the middle cerebral artery.

(b) Marked upward displacement of the anterior choroidal artery.

(c) Medial displacement and localized kinking of the basal vein.

(d) Medial displacement of the posterior cerebral artery.

(e) Typical angiographic meningioma signs including extracerebral supply from meningeal vessels in both the middle and posterior fossae.

c. Nonmeningiomatous extratemporal tumors—another group of tumors of the floor of the middle fossa may elevate the temporal lobe, the sylvian vessels and anterior choroidal artery. The displacement is similar to that of the subtemporal or saddle meningioma, but angiographic meningioma signs are absent.

(1) Metastatic carcinoma of the cranial base.

(2) Trigeminal neuroma.

(3) Epidermoid tumor.

(4) Chordoma of the clivus with extension to the middle fossa.

(5) Subtemporal invasive chromophobe adenoma—may also extend into the posterior fossa.

(6) Chronic subtemporal subdural hematoma—may be present as a "juvenile subdural hematoma" with unilateral enlargement of the middle fossa seen best on basal views.

7. Angiographic findings in intratemporal tumors.

a. Elevation.

(1) Middle cerebral artery, horizontal part—anterior temporal tumor.

(2) Angiographic sylvian point—posterior temporal tumor.

(3) Superficial middle cerebral (sylvian) vein.

(4) Carotid bifurcation.

b. Medial displacement.

(1) Anterior choroidal artery.

(2) Posterior communicating and posterior cerebral arteries.

(3) Carotid bifurcation.

(4) Basilar vein.

(5) Internal cerebral vein.

(6) Angiographic sylvian point.

c. "Draping sign"—usually due to an intratemporal tumor which elevates the sylvian vessels above the tumor, with draping of the temporal cortical arteries over the caudal pole of the mass. Upward deviation of the anterior choroidal artery or any meningioma signs indicate pseudodraping of temporal vessels about an extratemporal mass.

d. Angiographic glioma signs—early draining veins, prominent A-V shunts, brief tumor cloud or avascular temporal mass are all compatible with temporal glioma.

B. Pneumographic features of the temporal region

1. Tumors.

Intracerebral and extracerebral temporal tumors are not absolutely differentiated by pneumography; however, the following points are helpful:

a. Lateral view.

(1) Intratemporal tumors commonly produce failure to fill (i.e. occlusion) the uppermost temporal horn.

(2) Narrowing of the temporal horn occurs in both intratemporal and extratemporal tumors; occlusion is less common in extratemporal tumors.
(3) The involved temporal horn is not usually dilated, but the opposite lateral ventricle is often enlarged.
(4) Intratemporal polar tumors may amputate or truncate the tip of the temporal horn.
(5) Globular sphenoid meningiomas (outer and middle ridge) produce upward deviation of the temporal horn; narrowing without occlusion is common. The normal temporal horn deviates downward at its tip.
(6) Extracerebral tumors of the middle fossa floor also produce upward deviation of the temporal horn without occlusion.

b. Frontal view.
(1) The temporal horns on each side should be compared.
(2) Slight asymmetry of the temporal horns may be due to a temporopolar tumor with unilateral occlusion of the tip of the horn.
(3) Sharp medial deviation of a temporal horn may be due to globular sphenoid meningioma.
(4) The temporal horn on the tumor side may be small (or absent) while the temporal horn on the opposite side may be normal or enlarged.
(5) The lateral ventricle and its septum are commonly involved on the tumor side.
(a) The lateral angle is elevated.
(b) The floor is elevated, but less so than the lateral angle.
(c) The lower portion of the septum (and upper third ventricle) are commonly shifted to the opposite side.

2. Temporal lobe epilepsy.

In most cases, temporal lobe epilepsy is not related to temporal tumor, and evidence of an atrophic process is common.

a. Enlargement of the temporal horn on the atrophic side is characteristic; the enlargement is usually slight to moderate.
b. Smallness of the middle fossa on the atrophic side (best seen in basal views of the skull) suggests an early onset.
c. Smallness of the hemicalvarium on the side of cerebral atrophy may be present. Thickened calvarial bone with reduced brain markings and large air sinuses may be present on the atrophic side. The entire ventricular system on this side may be enlarged.
d. The skull may be entirely normal with an abnormal pneumogram.

e. Local narrowing of the temporal horn should suggest astrocytoma.
f. Failure to fill the uppermost temporal horn in a case of temporal lobe epilepsy indicates temporal astrocytoma.

Additional Diagnostic Studies in Temporal Syndromes

A. Plain skull x-rays

1. Temporal fracture through the middle meningeal artery region—common in acute epidural hematoma of the middle fossa.
2. Fracture through the floor of the middle fossa—may also result in an epidural hematoma and the fracture may be missed on lateral view and even on basal view.
3. Middle fossa basal fracture—may show an air-fluid level in the sphenoid sinus (brow-up lateral) ; the fracture may extend into a large lateral wing of the sphenoid sinus in the middle fossa floor; it may extend into the cavernous sinus, sella or petrous ridge; CSF rhinorrhea or otorrhea may result. Pneumocephalus may be seen on plain skull x-ray (typically a suprasellar gas bubble) .
4. Depressed skull fracture—may be associated with underlying cerebral contusion, epidural, subdural or intracortical hematoma and cortical laceration.
5. Erosion or absence of one anterior clinoid—parasellar tumor, inner sphenoidal meningioma or aneurysm.
6. Hyperostosis of the clinoid—meningioma.
7. Sphenoid ridge erosion or hyperostosis—meningioma.
8. Pterional erosion or hyperostosis—meningioma; excessive hyperostosis extending into the orbit suggests "meningioma en plaque" of the pterion.
9. Pressure atrophy of the sella may be so prominent that erosion of the pterion (lateral view) due to a globose outer ridge meningioma may be overlooked if attention is directed to the sella alone.
10. Excessive and tortuous vascular markings of middle meningeal and accessory meningeal arteries—meningioma.
11. Enlargement of basal foramina—spinosum and ovale—suggests meningioma.
12. Erosion of the cranial base—suggests metastatic carcinoma.
13. Enlargement of the middle fossa (basal view) —suggests juvenile subdural hematoma.
14. Smallness of the middle fossa or hemicalvarium—suggests temporal or hemispheral atrophy, respectively.
15. Erosion of the petrous apex with evidence of mastoiditis—petrositis (e.g. Gradenigo's syndrome) .

16. Neoplastic erosion of the petrous apex—acoustic neuroma, meningioma, epidermoid, chordoma, invasive chromophobe adenoma, or metastatic carcinoma to the cranial base.

B. EEG

1. Random spike discharge in one or both temporal regions is commonly noted in temporal lobe epilepsy. Serial EEG's are necessary to lateralize the focus. The routine EEG may be normal, especially if the patient is on anticonvulsants at the time of the study. Specialized pharyngeal or sphenoidal electrodes which record activity from the medial and inferior temporal surfaces may reveal spikes and sharp waves when routine EEG studies are negative. Sleep EEG's may be helpful. Specialized EEG tests involving convulsive threshold to Metrazol® or chronic depth electrode studies may assist in lateralization of the focus and identify cases of bitemporal epilepsy. Careful EEG analysis is also required to identify those cases in which the psychomotor attack is the result of an irritative focus elsewhere in the limbic system (i.e. cingulate gyrus).
2. Slow waves recorded from temporal leads should suggest the possibility of temporal tumor, with or without a history of epilepsy of any type. This is particularly true of delta activity which may indicate temporal intracerebral or extracerebral tumor. Such activity may reflect the presence of a frontal tumor as well. Slow activity in the theta range from temporal leads is commonly normal.

C. Brain scan

1. The brain scan is usually unremarkable in cases of temporal lobe epilepsy.
2. A positive scan in the temporal region may indicate sphenoidal or sylvian meningioma, temporal glioblastoma or metastatic tumor, or arteriovenous malformation. Lower-grade gliomas of the temporal lobe often produce negative scans.
3. The chief value of the scan in head-injury cases lies in the identification of the chronic subdural hematoma. The usual subdural pattern over the hemispheral convexity may be present. A subdural pattern limited to the middle fossa may be noted in cases of juvenile subdural hematoma resulting from tearing of bridging veins from the temporal lobe to the sphenoparietal sinus.

CHAPTER 9

CENTRAL CEREBRAL SYNDROMES

Neuroanatomy of the Central Cerebral Region

THE CENTRAL SENSORY and motor nuclei of the thalamus and basal ganglia, pierced by the internal capsule, comprise the central cerebral region. The term "basal ganglia" actually includes the corpus striatum and amygdala. The term "central motor ganglia" eliminates the amygdala and refers to the corpus striatum and its motor satellites in the deep central regions of the brain. The "corpus striatum" includes the caudate and lenticular nuclei. The "lenticular nucleus" is the putamen and globus pallidus. The "neostriatum" is the caudate-putamen, which is actually a continuous structure. The "paleostriatum" is the globus pallidus. Wilson's term "extrapyramidal" included all the nonpyramidal motor systems, including premotor cortex, corpus striatum, subthalamic nucleus, substantia nigra, red nucleus and other tegmental structures of the brain stem. In addition, the dentato-rubro-thalamic pathway was included as an ascending extrapyramidal motor system from the cerebellum.

In the radiological sense, "central cerebral" means the corpus striatum, internal capsule and dorsal thalamus. This is the common clinical usage and has the great advantage of simplicity. The insula lies laterally, and the floor of the lateral ventricle and wall of the third ventricle form the medial boundary. The central cerebral region thus lies between the angiographic sylvian triangle and the deep venous angle. The central cerebral region sits like a large head upon the brain stem. The internal capsule, in its passage between the cortex and the brain stem, splits the telencephalic corpus striatum. The lenticular nucleus lies lateral to the capsule, while the caudate head lies medially. The diencephalon remains entirely medial to the capsule, the dorsal thalamus lying just below and caudal to the caudate head. The caudate and thalamus form the floor of the lateral ventricle; the thalamus and hypothalamus form the wall and floor of the third ventricle. The subthalamus and zona incerta lie between the internal capsule and the hypothalamus; they lie beneath the dorsal thalamus. The zona incerta is the rostral continuation of the brain stem tegmentum into the diencephalon. Junctional structures which cross the hemispheral-midbrain boundary include the following:

1. Tegmentum—zona incerta.

2. Red nucleus.
3. Substantia nigra.
4. Cerebral peduncle.

Connections of the Central Cerebral Region

A. Corpus striatum
   1. Afferents.
      a. Corticostriate—wide regions of the cerebral cortex of each hemisphere (frontal, parietal, temporal, insular and cingulate) project to the ipsilateral corpus striatum.
      b. Thalamostriate—the dorsomedial, center median and ventral nuclei of the dorsal thalamus project to the corpus striatum. Some fibers loop through the caudate head and turn back into the putamen and globus pallidus.
      c. Reticulostriate—indirect projections from the reticular formation via the center median (an intralaminar nucleus) to the putamen; reticulosubthalamic projections are also prominent.
      d. Striopallidal projections—the globus pallidus is innervated largely by the caudate and putamen. Projections from the substantia nigra and subthalamic nucleus are also present.
   2. Efferents (fields of Forel).
      a. Thalamic fasciculus (H1)—from the globus pallidus to the VA-VL complex of the dorsal thalamus (transcapsular).
      b. Lenticular fasciculus (H2)—from the globus pallidus to the brain stem tegmentum (transcapsular).
      c. Ansa lenticularis—from the globus pallidus to the brain stem tegmentum (passes ventral to the capsule).
      d. Central tegmental tract—contains pallido-olivary, tegmento-olivary, rubro-olivary, and reticular fibers and innervates the inferior olive (in turn projecting to the cerebellum).
      e. Pallidohypothalamic and pallidosubthalamic projections—to these basal diencephalic centers.

B. Internal capsule (The anterior limb lies between the caudate head and the lenticular nucleus; the posterior limb lies between the thalamus and the lenticular nucleus.)
   1. Anterior limb.
      a. Frontopontine tract.
      b. Anterior thalamic peduncle—frontal projections from the medial thalamic nuclei and cingulate projections from the anterior thalamic nuclei.

2. Posterior limb.
    a. Corticobulbar tract—most rostral (face).
    b. Corticospinal tract—arm, trunk, and leg, rostrocaudally.
    c. Corticorubral and corticotegmental tracts—adjacent to corticospinal tract.
    d. Sensory radiations—thalamocortical projections in posterior half of the posterior limb.
    e. Sublenticular part—auditory radiations and temporal visual radiations.
    f. Retrolenticular part—visual radiations, posterior thalamocortical radiations and caudal-cerebral corticopontine, corticotectal and corticotegmental projections.

C. Thalamus

The dorsal thalamus is the major portion of the diencephalon (interbrain). The latter lies between the greatly expanded telencephalon (end-brain) and the mesencephalon (midbrain). The telencephalon and diencephalon comprise the forebrain. The telencephalon develops about the lateral ventricles, the diencephalon about the third ventricle, and the mesencephalon contains the aqueduct. The diencephalon consists of a smaller paleothalamus and a larger neothalamus. The neothalamus becomes massive and bidirectionally connected with the extensive neocortex of the telencephalon. The paleothalamus consists of more primitive mediobasal structures lying between the brain stem reticular core and the mediobasal "limbic system" of the cerebrum. The brain stem reticular core, paleothalamus and limbic system constitute the "old-brain." The specific systems (e.g. medial lemniscus, pyramidal tract), neothalamus and neocortex constitute the "new-brain." In the process of encephalization the massive new-brain buries the small, but widely distributed, old-brain within the cerebral midline and septobasal regions.

The paleothalamus includes the following:

1. Hypothalamus.
2. Ventral thalamus (subthalamus and zona incerta).
3. Epithalamus (habenula, posterior commissure, pineal).
4. Medial division of the dorsal thalamus.
    a. Midline nuclei (reuniens, rhomboid, paraventricular, parataenial).
    b. Medial nuclei (medial dorsal, submedian).
    c. Intralaminar nuclei (parafascicular, center median, paracentral, central medial and central lateral).
    d. Anterior nuclei (anterodorsal, anteroventral, anteromedial and lateral dorsal).

The dorsal thalamus has two other divisions, both larger and both neothalamic. These are the lateral and posterior divisions. This neothalamic mass is separated from the paleothalamic medial division by the internal medullary lamina. The neothalamic mass is separated from the internal capsule by the external medullary lamina and reticular shell of the dorsal thalamus. The reticular nucleus of the dorsal thalamus is a ventral thalamic derivative which covers the pole, lateral and ventral walls of the dorsal thalamus and is continuous with the subthalamus below. The neothalamic mass forming the bulk of the dorsal thalamus is continuous, the posterior division lying immediately behind the lateral division. The components of the neothalamus are as follow:

1. Lateral division of the dorsal thalamus.
   a. Ventrobasal complex.
      (1) VA—ventral anterior.
      (2) VL—ventral lateral.
      (3) VI—ventral intermediate.
      (4) VP—ventral posterior (VPL and VPM).
   b. Lateral posterior.
2. Posterior division of the dorsal thalamus.
   a. Pulvinar.
   b. Metathalamus.
      (1) Lateral geniculate body.
      (2) Medial geniculate body.

On the basis of extrathalamic and intrathalamic connections, the thalamic nuclei have been divided into the following four groups:

1. Primary sensory nuclei (e.g. VP and geniculate bodies).
2. Secondary relay nuclei (e.g. VL, VA, anterior nuclei).
3. Association nuclei (e.g. MD, pulvinar, LP).
4. Reticular nuclei (e.g. intralaminar nuclei and reticular pole).

In terms of cortical projection of thalamic nuclei, they may be grouped as follow:

1. Frontopolar—MD.
2. Frontodorsal and frontolateral—VL.
3. Parietal—VP, LP, pulvinar.
4. Caudal-cerebral—lateral geniculate (to primary visual cortex) and pulvinar (to parieto-occipital and temporo-occipital cortex).
5. Temporal—medial geniculate (to primary auditory cortex); the bulk of the temporal neocortex is associative and without specific thalamic projection.
6. Limbic (including orbital, insular, cingulate and parahippocampal cortex)—from the limbic nuclei of the thalamus (anterior nuclei, lateral and medial dorsal nuclei and ventral anterior nucleus).

The important connections of the dorsal thalamus are of two basic types: reticular and nonreticular. The brain stem reticular formation is distributed to all the thalamic nuclei by three routes.

1. Intrathalamic fasciculus—from the intralaminar nuclei.
2. Reticular shell—reticular projections from the thalamic pole and reticular shell turning back into the dorsal thalamus and brain stem.
3. Periventricular system—from hypothalamic and subthalamic regions to the medial division of the dorsal thalamus.

Significant nonreticular connections of the dorsal thalamus include the following:

1. Medial dorsal nucleus—from the amygdala, anterior hypothalamus, septum and orbitofrontal cortex; to the frontopolar and frontobasal cortex.
2. Anterior nuclei (the lateral dorsal nucleus is a posterior extension of the anterior group)—from the hypothalamus (mammillothalamic tract) and septum; projects widely to the cingulate gyrus.
3. Ventrobasal complex.
   a. VA—from the globus pallidus (fasciculus thalamicus); to the paraolfactory region and subcallosal cingulate gyrus.
   b. VL—from the globus pallidus (fasciculus thalamicus) and cerebellum (dentato-rubro-thalamic tract); to frontolateral and frontodorsal cortex.
   c. VI—border zone of the motor and sensory regions of the ventrobasal complex.
   d. VPL—from the nuclei of the posterior columns of the spinal cord and the anterior spinothalamic tract; only a minority of lateral spinothalamic fibers reach the sensory nuclei of the thalamus, most terminating in the brain stem reticular core; to the dorsal region of the postcentral gyrus (sensory—from the body).
   e. VPM—from the sensory nuclei of the cranial nerves (trigeminal and glossopharyngeal lemniscus); to the lateral region of the postcentral gyrus (sensory—from the face).
4. Pulvinar and lateral posterior nuclei—these are association nuclei of the dorsal thalamus; they receive from the primary sensory nuclei (VP) and the intrathalamic association nucleus (center median); they project to the postcentral parietal lobe; the pulvinar also projects to the posterior temporo-occipital region.
5. Geniculate bodies—the medial geniculate receives auditory fibers from the lateral lemniscus via brain stem relays; it projects to the primary auditory cortex (Heschl's gyri) of the temporal lobe via the sublenticular capsule. The lateral geniculate receives the visual component

of the optic tract; it projects to the primary visual cortex (calcarine area) of the occipital lobe via the optic radiation.

Blood Supply of the Central Cerebral Region

A. Arterial supply to the basal ganglia
   1. Middle cerebral artery, lenticulostriate branches—to the caudate head, putamen and lateral part of the globus pallidus.
   2. Anterior cerebral artery, Huebner's branch—to the caudate head and rostral putamen.
   3. Anterior choroidal artery—to the medial part of the globus pallidus and caudate tail.
   4. Posterior cerebral artery, posteromedial central branch—to the caudal part of the globus pallidus.

B. Arterial supply to the internal capsule
   1. Anterior cerebral artery, Huebner's branch—to the anterior limb.
   2. Posterior communicating artery—to the inferior part of the anterior limb.
   3. Middle cerebral artery, lenticulostriate branches—to the rostral two-thirds of the posterior limb.
   4. Posterior cerebral artery, posteromedial central branch—to the caudal third of the posterior limb and retrolenticular capsule.
   5. Anterior choroidal artery—to the sublenticular part of the internal capsule.

C. Arterial supply to the dorsal thalamus
   1. Posterior cerebral artery (chief artery of supply).
      a. Thalamoperforant branches—medial division.
      b. Thalamogeniculate branches—geniculate bodies and pulvinar.
      c. Posterior choroidal branches—lateral and posterior divisions.
   2. Posterior communicating artery, thalamotuberal branch—anterior nuclei and medial dorsal nucleus.
   3. Anterior choroidal artery—lateral and posterior divisions.
   4. Middle cerebral artery, thalamic branches--lateral dorsal and lateral posterior nuclei.

D. Venous drainage of the central cerebral region
   1. Lenticulostriate veins—drain the deep central cerebral region.
   2. Deep middle cerebral vein—drains the insula.
   3. Basal vein of Rosenthal—formed by the union of the lenticulostriate, deep middle cerebral and anterior cerebral veins; joins the internal cerebral vein to form the great vein of Galen.
   4. Septal vein and thalamostriate vein—drain the corpus striatum and

thalamus and unite to form the internal cerebral vein (lesser vein of Galen).

5. Great vein of Galen—formed by the union of the basal veins, internal cerebral veins, posterior vein of the corpus callosum, internal occipital veins and superior cerebellar veins.
6. Straight sinus—formed by the union of the great vein of Galen and the inferior longitudinal sinus.
7. Torcular—formed by the union of the straight, superior longitudinal, and transverse sinuses.

Infarction Syndromes of the Central Cerebral Region

A. Middle cerebral artery, proximal to the lenticulostriate branches
   1. Hemiplegia, contralateral.
   2. Hemisensory deficit, contralateral.
   3. Hemianopia, contralateral.
   4. Stupor or coma if acute.
   5. Aphasia, major hemisphere.

B. Anterior cerebral artery, Huebner's branch
   1. Hemiparesis, contralateral—greatest in the face, tongue and proximal arm.
   2. Ataxia.

C. Anterior choroidal artery—no clearly defined syndrome

D. Posterior cerebral artery
   1. Thalamogeniculate (or thalamoperforant).
      a. Transient hemiparesis—contralateral.
      b. Persistent hemihypesthesia—contralateral.
      c. "Thalamic pain"—deep pain in the hypesthetic regions which is not well localized ("anesthesia dolorosa").
      d. Homonymous hemianopia—contralateral.
   2. Mesencephalic artery (posterior cerebral arteries at the basilar bifurcation, with bilateral thalamoperforant occlusions).
      a. Akinetic mutism with hypersomnia.
      b. Internal and external ophthalmoplegia.
      c. Conjugate ocular palsies.
      d. Intention tremor—may be noted.
   3. Posterior choroidal artery—usually involved with more proximal posterior cerebral occlusion.
      a. Stupor or coma—with acute proximal occlusion.
      b. Homonymous hemianopia, contralateral.
      c. Visual agnosia and alexia.
      d. Receptive aphasia—dominant side.

Neurophysiology of the Central Cerebral Region

A. Central motor integration

Motor integration occurs at many levels of the nervous system. The cortical and spinal levels are critical for effective extrapyramidal and pyramidal integration. In addition, the extrapyramidal system affects motor activity at many central cerebral and brain stem levels in association with cerebellar influence. The compensatory abilities of these systems are so great that unilateral destructive lesions within the basal ganglia often go unnoticed unless the corticospinal system is also involved. The general physiological principles involved include the following:

1. The cerebral cortex widely innervates the corpus striatum; the chief motor output of the latter is the globus pallidus.
2. Electrostimulation of the corpus striatum has a tendency to inhibit cortically induced movement. Stimulation of the caudate may induce torticollis to the opposite side with movement of contralateral extremities.
3. Large lesions of the corpus striatum may result in forward movement to the side of neostriate destruction. Ablation of the globus pallidus may reduce contralateral tone. Hypokinesia may result from caudate lesions extending into the septum or from pallido-subpallidal lesions.
4. Experimental tremor produced at the striatal level tends to be faster (10-12 cps) than that resulting from brain stem lesions.
5. The substantia nigra innervates the putamen and globus pallidus. Nigral destruction can result in hypertonus. Focal lesions in the ventromesial tegmentum (nigrostriatal pathway) can produce resting tremor (4-5 cps). Similar tremor, often with ataxic elements, results from section of the brachium conjunctivum or destruction of the dentate nucleus of the cerebellum.
6. Midbrain transection results in decerebrate rigidity with extensor hypertonus of all extremities. Striatal rigidity results from bilateral destructive lesions at a higher central cerebral level. It consists of flexor hypertonus of the arms and extensor hypertonus of the legs. Pallidal rigidity results from bilateral destructive lesions of the nigro-pallidal systems. It consists of flexor hypertonus of all extremities, the neck and trunk.
7. The chief outflow tract of the striatum, the globus pallidus, projects to the VL. It is joined by the chief outflow of the cerebellum (dentato-rubro-thalamic) at the VL. The VL is the final common motor projection to the rolandic and premotor frontal cortex. A stereotactic lesion (thalamotomy) of the VL will reduce contralateral tremor and rigidity in parkinsonian man. The effect of the lesion is improved

by destruction of tremor-synchronous cells (in VI and VL). Focal stereotactic lesions in the globus pallidus (pallidotomy) or fields of Forel (campotomy) or cerebellum (dentatotomy) have also been employed to reduce hypertonus without inducing paralysis.

8. The globus pallidus also projects caudally into the brain stem tegmentum. The extrapyramidal spinal projections ultimately drive the gamma motoneuron, largely through the reticulospinal tract. The vestibulospinal system facilitates the reticulospinal system. The rubrospinal system does not proceed lower than the cervical cord in man. The extrapyramidal pathways integrate postural tone and the postural background of both automatic and voluntary movement. The pyramidal pathway, taking a more direct course to the spinal motoneuron pool through the corticospinal tract, projects upon the alpha motoneuron or spinal interneurons. Local spinal inhibition of alpha motoneurons allows for the phasic innervation necessary for the performance of skilled motor activities. Motor integration is continuously modified by proprioceptive sensory feedback derived from peripheral motor receptors.

B. Central sensory integration

The thalamus has been regarded as the "chief sensory ganglia" of the forebrain. Its development parallels that of parietal and caudal cerebral sensory cortex. The primary sensory nuclei of VPL and VPM act as subcortical relays to the postcentral gyrus. The geniculate nuclei relay visual and auditory information to the primary sensory cortices of the calcarine region and temporal operculum respectively. The lateral posterior nucleus and pulvinar integrate sensory data at the thalamic level and relay widely into the secondary sensory fields of the parietal, posterior temporal and occipital regions. Awareness of noxious stimulation is believed to enter consciousness at the thalamic level. The physiological role of the thalamus extends beyond the organization and transmission of sensory impulses from the periphery. Important motor integrators of the thalamus include the VL, MD and the center median nuclei. The VL is the final common path to rolandic and premotor cortex, mediating both cerebellar and striate influence to the frontomotor region. The MD may be important in the transmission of limbic-affective influence upon the prefrontal lobes, serving the elaborate motor behavior accompanying goal-directed activity. The center median nucleus sits at the bifurcation of the reticular formation. Reticular fibers pass directly into the nucleus, above the nucleus into the dorsal thalamus, and below the nucleus into the subthalamus and lateral hypothalamus. The center median projects widely to other thalamic nuclei and to the putamen. Reticular activation of motor activity may thus be organized at both the thalamic and cortical levels. The thalamus, like the cortex, is inherently sensorimotor. Beyond this level of physiological activity, the thalamic mesial and reticular elements play an important role in arousal and sleep mechanisms. Reticular activation, with behavioral arousal and electrographic desynchronization, can result from intralaminar reticular stimulation which is prevented by a midbrain-core lesion. Reticular suppression with behavioral sleep and electrographic synchronization can result from midline thalamic stimulation. The major experimental studies resulting in reticular activation or suppression from old-brain sites have been reviewed (Needham and Dila, 1968). Lesions of the thalamus (adjacent to the walls of the third ventricle) may result in coma, disorientation, memory loss and mutism. Since the thalamus develops in parallel with all parts of the cortex, including the limbic, it plays a physiological role in memory, in attention, in the symbolism related to speech and in complex affective behavior. Thus the thalamus acts as a complex multiple relay station with internal discriminating, sorting and integrating capacities.

NEUROSURGICAL SYNDROMES OF THE CENTRAL CEREBRAL REGION

Central cerebral syndromes are "neurosurgical" only in a restricted sense. Thalamic tumors are considered beyond the reach of successful operative resectability. They may, however, require a shunt to relieve intracranial hypertension prior to radiotherapy.

Hypertensive hemorrhage into the basal ganglia usually does not permit significant neurological recovery. This is especially true when the hemorrhage involves the major hemisphere. Evacuation of the central cerebral hematoma is not nearly as effective as evacuation of the lobar clot in terms of neurological recovery. However, hypertensive central cerebral hemorrhage is more common than subarachnoid hemorrhage due to ruptured aneurysm. The neurosurgeon called to see all cases of intracranial hemorrhage will commonly witness the central cerebral hypertensive form. The ruptured middle cerebral or carotid aneurysm may produce a similar picture with acute arterial hypertension secondary to elevated intracranial pressure. When intracranial hemorrhage is the result of chronic arterial hypertension, neurosurgical consultation is particularly important in the early diagnosis of the acute cerebellar hematoma which is a surgical emergency. The frontopolar and temporal hematomas may also mimic the more common central cerebral apoplexy.

The central motor or extrapyramidal syndromes, (i.e. Parkinson's disease) are only "neurosurgical" when the dyskinesia and hypertonus are medically intractable. The best stereotactic results are obtained for tremor and rigidity.

Development of the Central Cerebral Syndromes

A. Rapidly progressive central cerebral syndromes
    1. Hemorrhagic—hypertension, hemorrhagic infarction, ruptured aneurysm or arteriovenous malformation may be responsible for the acute syndrome commonly including headache, obtundation and hemiplegia. Traumatic intracerebral hematoma, often associated with lobar hematoma, cerebral contusion and brain swelling may similarly involve the central cerebral region. Intraneoplastic hemorrhage into a deep glioblastoma or oligodendroglioma may suddenly announce the tumor.
    2. Infarctive—thrombosis as a result of middle cerebral or carotid occlusive disease, or from basilar—posterior cerebral ischemia, can result in central cerebral infarction. The anterior border of the central region may be involved by anterior cerebral occlusion proximal to Huebner's artery. Central cerebral infarction may be the result of arterial spasm accompanying subarachnoid hemorrhage. Embolism from a carotid plaque or from a cardiac or noncardiac external source must be ruled out.
    3. Edematous—cerebral edema of relatively rapid onset often complicates metastatic carcinoma to the brain. The onset is not as sudden as seen in the embolic or hemorrhagic strokes. It may progress over several days. Cerebral edema may involve the central regions as a result of any supratentorial primary tumor. It is most marked with glioblastomas and often least pronounced with meningiomas, although exceptions occur. Cerebral edema complicating intracranial hemorrhage or trauma may be of rapidly progressive type.

B. Gradually progressive central cerebral syndromes—these are usually primary gliomas of the cerebrum and may occur in childhood or adult life. The duration of the history may be several weeks, several months or several years. In childhood, cerebral ependymomas and astrocytomas must be considered. In adult life, glioblastomas, astrocytomas and oligodendrogliomas may be responsible, although cerebral ependymomas also occur. Slowly enlarging deep cerebral arteriovenous malformations may produce a tumor syndrome. The spectrum of clinical signs includes progressive hemiparesis, personality change, papilledema and convulsions. Extensive unilateral involvement of the basal ganglia typically produces no full-blown extrapyramidal picture. However, tremor, subtle changes in tone and hypokinesia are not rare signs of central cerebral tumors.

Deficits of the Central Cerebral Syndromes

These signs include the following:

A. Central motor deficits—these are the motor signs usually designated extrapyramidal.

B. Capsular deficits—these are the motor and sensory signs of internal capsular involvement; the motor component is considered pyramidal.

C. Thalamic deficits—these are the varied signs indicating a dorsal thalamic lesion.

The central cerebral region with its basal ganglia and thalamus, pierced by the internal capsule, is of neurosurgical importance for several reasons.

1. The capsule, thalamus and central motor ganglia are often involved together in deep mass lesions (e.g. thalamic glioma, or capsular hematoma).
2. Central cerebral signs do not always indicate deep extension of a cerebral mass. They may occasionally result from the secondary central effects of a lobar mass (e.g. compression, edema).
3. Central cerebral tumors may occasionally simulate certain features of parkinsonism (e.g. poverty of movement, rigidity, tremor).
4. Stereotactic advances have increased the need for diagnostic acumen in the various movement disorders.

A. Central motor deficits

Extrapyramidal signs indicate a disturbance in the indirect motor system. Pyramidal signs result from a lesion in the direct motor system. The nonpyramidal motor complex includes cortical, central motor and cerebellar elements. The central motor components include telencephalic, diencephalic and junctional (diencephalic-mesencephalic) structures.

1. Telencephalic—caudate, putamen and globus pallidus.
2. Diencephalic—subthalamus, center median and ventral lateral nuclei.
3. Junctional—substantia nigra, red nucleus and tegmentum.

Central motor disorders express themselves in static (tonic) and mobile (kinetic) abnormalities. Tonic and kinetic defects may appear independently, as in rigidity without tremor and vice versa. While rigidity results in slowness of movement and postural fixation, bradykinesia and postural deficiencies may occur without rigidity. The motor deficits may be positive (hypertonia, hyperkinesia) or negative (hypotonia, hypokinesia).

1. Hypertonic signs.

Pathological increase in motor tone is demonstrated by resistance to passive stretch, a tendency toward postural fixation, and poverty of spontaneous movement. Spasmodically increased rigidity, with assumption of an abnormal posture, may occur. It is clinically useful to consider hypertonus as chronic or acute. Drug resistant chronic hypertonias may in some instances be relieved by stereotactic treatment; in this special sense they are "neurosurgical syndromes." The acute hypertonias occur as components of the syndromes of intracranial trauma, hemorrhage, pressure and mass lesion.

a. Chronic hypertonias.

(1) Spasticity (elastic or clasp-knife rigidity).

Resistance to passive stretch reaches a rapid peak at the onset, with sudden reduction in resistance during continued stretch. Spasticity is greatest in the flexors of the upper extremity and extensors of the lower extremity. In its most typical form it is associated with paralysis. It is preceded by and associated with hyperactive tendon reflexes. Clonus and the Babinski sign usually coexist. Adductor spasm may occur. While the responsible lesion may be of sudden or slowly progressive onset, spasticity is most often gradual in its development. In central cerebral lesions, spasticity represents a combined pyramidal-extrapyramidal deficit as a result of capsulolenticular involvement. It is also seen in frontal, brain stem and spinal cord disorders.

(2) Plastic rigidity.

There is a smoothly maintained resistance to passive stretch during the entire movement. Flexors and extensors at an involved joint are about equally affected. Early signs are rigidity of the neck, pronators-supinators of the forearm, and flexors-extensors of the wrist. Tendon reflexes are unchanged. Early spasticity at times has a plastic quality but can be differentiated by its hyperactive tendon reflexes. Parkinsonism is the most common source, but vascular and mass lesions of the basal ganglia should be ruled out.

(3) Lead pipe rigidity.

There is an immense and maintained rigidity of both flexors and extensors of the involved extremity. A stiff spine may occur on the same basis. This intense hypertonus is most often due to advanced parkinsonism.

(4) Cogwheel rigidity.

Intermittent release of an otherwise smoothly maintained plastic rigidity indicates actual or incipient tremor. This interrupted rigidity may be an early sign of parkinsonism when elicited by flexion and extension of the wrist. Clenching the opposite fist will reinforce the cogwheel effect.

(5) Flexion dystonia.

This is a generalized form of plastic rigidity in which postural fixation in flexion involves the neck, trunk, and extremities. There is adduction, flexion and pronation of all joints, with the exception of the fingers which are hyperextended. The dystonia is generalized, in contrast to tremor which tends to be distal. A lesser degree of rigidity is present in the extensors. A fetal position of total flexion represents the termanal stage of parkinsonism.

(6) Torsion dystonia.

This is an unequally distributed form of rigidity, the hypertonus reaching a crescendo during "torsion spasm." Exaggerated postures are maintained with extension of the lower limb and flexion or extension of the upper limb. Proximal torsion-rotation movements of the extremities occur during the spasm, differentiating it from the more distal, slow, writhing movements of athetosis. Both torsion spasm and athetosis may involve arm, leg and trunk, but in athetosis arm-hand movement is dominant. In torsion dystonia, rigidity is persistent, although increased during spasm. In athetosis, increased tone occurs during the movement, but tone is normal or reduced in the intervals. Torsion dystonia is also associated with scoliosis, lordosis and torticollis. Early signs include hyperpronation and inversion of the foot. These may be spasmodic and exaggerated by walking. Hyperextension of the fingers may be an early sign.

(7) Hemiplegic dystonia.

This is an asymmetrical rigidity in which there is flexion of the upper limb and extension of the lower limb. Fingers are flexed. The neck is extended (retrocollis) and may be turned (torticollis). The spine is extended. Pyramidal signs are absent, but grasp reflexes may be present. The facial immobility, dysarthria and dysphagia of parkinsonism (craniomotor rigidity) may coexist.

(8) Spastic dystonia.

This is similar to hemiplegic dystonia with the addition of spasticity and pyramidal signs. The state is extremely rigid with clonic rigidity and hyperactive reflexes. The limbs are fixed in the spastic position of flexed upper, and extended lower, extremities. Resistance to passive movement is more difficult to overcome than in ordinary spasticity, the clasp-knife effect becoming indistinct.

(9) Craniomotor rigidity.

Disease of the basal ganglia does not often spare the muscles supplied by the cranial nerves. In parkinsonism, the major cranial deficits are rigidity and poverty of movement. Examination of the eyes may reveal ocular bradykinesia, paucity of blinking and expressionless staring. Upward deviation of the eyes is not accompanied by the normal elevation of the eyebrows. There is general paucity of facial expression in the absence of paralysis. Labioglossal, pharyngeal and laryngeal rigidity contribute to the slow, monotonous, inarticulate speech which may be reduced to a whisper. Postural deficiencies, tremor of the tongue and respiratory rigidity contribute to the dysarthria. Dysphagia and an open mouth (visible tongue sign) contribute to the drooling of saliva (sialorrhea).

Spasmodic vertical ocular deviation (oculogyric crisis) suggests a postencephalitic state. The Kayser-Fleischer ring of brown pigmentation at the limbus of the cornea occurs in Wilson's disease. Facial grimacing occurs in chorea and athetosis. Explosive speech and inconstant facial tics suggest chorea. "Pathological laughter" suggests bilateral corticobulbar involvement (pseudobulbar palsy) which may be superimposed upon the basal ganglia signs. The "perpetual smile" may indicate Wilson's disease.

(10) "Paratonia" ("Gegenhalten").

This is a diffuse low-grade increase in muscle tone of the plastic type. It may occur in poorly relaxed or uncooperative patients. Generalized paratonic rigidity and a Babinski sign suggest a frontal tumor.

b. Acute hypertonias.

These are the rigidities of relatively sudden onset which accompany intracranial trauma, hemorrhage and mass lesion. They are characteristically associated with coma.

(1) Acute spasticity.

Following an acute capsulolenticular insult, flaccid hemiplegia usually evolves into a spastic form within a few weeks. If the lesion is capsulothalamic, the hemiplegia may remain flaccid. The responsible lesion may be a central infarct or hemorrhage. Acute spasticity, appearing within 48 to 72 hours of the onset of coma, suggests that the responsible lesion is hemorrhagic and that it has ruptured into the ventricle. The coma deepens and unilateral early spasticity is rapidly followed by generalized rigidity, fever and eventual decerebration.

(2) Decorticate rigidity.

This is a bilateral hypertonic state maintained in the posture of spasticity with rigid flexion of the upper extremities and extension of the lower extremities. There are hyperactive reflexes, and Babinski signs may be present bilaterally. The posture may be spontaneous or induced by noxious stimulation. The clasp-knife effect is indistinct due to the intensity of maintained hypertonus. This is an acute central cerebral deficit usefully considered as telencephalic-diencephalic (in contrast to the diencephalic-mesencephalic level of decerebrate rigidity).

(3) Decerebrate rigidity (extensor rigidity).

There is bilateral hypertonia of all extremities in a position of rigid extension. The upper limbs are hyperpronated, the lower hyperextended. Tendon reflexes are hyperactive and bilateral Babinski signs may occur. The posture may be spontaneous or induced. Midbrain decerebration indicates acute involvement of critical structures which cross the diencephalic-mesencephalic junction (reticular formation-tegmentum). In pontine decerebration, the arms are extended and hyperpronated, while the legs reveal a flaccid paraparesis.

(4) Acute nuchocrural rigidity.

This is a form of plastic paratonic generalized rigidity ("Gegenhalten"). There is an acute increase in resistance to passive movement most marked in the neck and legs. The patient is typically restless, confused or stuporous. It is an early sign of transtentorial herniation and may precede pupillary changes. With deepening coma, the nuchal rigidity may disappear only to reappear in the deeper coma of decerebration. The resistance to passive movement of the legs persists on the nonhemiplegic side during the tentorial hernation and converts to extensor rigidity at the time of decerebration. Any supratentorial mass may be responsible.

(5) Opisthotonic rigidity.

There is severe extensor rigidity of the extremities, neck and spine with retrocollis and marked lordosis. This may occur spontaneously and intermittently, associated with irregular respiration, blood pressure and pulse (tonic brain stem seizures). It may occur upon noxious stimulation of the decerebrate patient. Acute brain stem contusion or posterior fossa mass may result in opisthotonus. Severe hydrocephalus with hydrocephalic attacks and foraminal impaction (tonsillar herniation) may produce intermittent opisthotonus. The cerebellar tumor with tonsillar herniation through the foramen magnum may also produce spinal rigidity with marked lordosis and retrocollis in which the patient is fully conscious. Attempts to flex the neck result in extreme pain in the neck and head. The extremities may be maintained in a normal attitude during the alert phase. Sudden deterioration in vital signs with apnea and episodic bradycardia follow. The alert patient with foraminal impaction due to cerebellar mass may thus become deeply comatose with amazing rapidity, without passage through a stuporous or semicomatose phase.

(6) Nuchal rigidity.

Stiff neck is a most important sign in the neurosurgical patient. In some instances it has localizing value, but in most it is nonlocalizing. As a central cerebral sign, it is seen with the chronic hypertonias of parkinsonism and dystonia. There is obvious localizing significance if cervical disc or vertebral disease accounts for nuchal rigidity.

Stiff neck is the cardinal sign of meningitis. It is characteristically present in cerebral subarachnoid hemorrhage, although it may disappear during deepening coma. In spinal subarachnoid hemorrhage, nuchal rigidity is typically preceded by back pain and occasionally by sciatic pain. Traumatic subarachnoid hemorrhage occurs commonly in head-injured patients, especially in those rendered comatose. In addition, acute epidural, subdural or intracerebral hematoma may be responsible. Increased nuchal rigidity may herald the extension of hemorrhage into the ventricular system. Associated basilar skull fracture or cervical fracture-dislocation should be considered in the comatose patient with or without nuchal rigidity. Attempts at neck flexion in the traumatically comatose are fraught with hazard to the spinal cord due to the possibility of coexistent cervical fracture.

Stiff neck may result from tumors in various situations. Tumor of the foramen magnum and cerebellar tumor with tonsillar herniation are diagnostic considerations. Foraminal impaction during hydrocephalic attacks may produce intermittent nuchal rigidity. Supratentorial mass lesions with transtentorial herniation produce nuchal resistance. Central cerebral or frontal lobe tumors may result in hypertonus on neck flexion even in the absence of herniation. Stiff neck accompanies the acute hypertonias of decortication, decerebration, opisthotonus and nuchocrural rigidity.

2. Hyperkinetic signs.

Hyperkinesias of central motor origin are rhythmical (tremor) and nonrhythmical (chorea, athetosis, ballism). Tremor is especially amenable to stereotactic treatment. These movement disorders are characteristic of extrapyramidal disease.

a. Tremor.

The tremor of parkinsonism is a slow (4-8/sec), rhythmical, alternating contraction of antagonists. It may present as interrupted rigidity. It may not be obvious unless passive movement is attempted, the rigidity taking on a cogwheel release. It may be present only upon emotional stimulation. It may occur only when the hand is in certain positions (postural tremor). Tremor may occur entirely without hypertonia. It most commonly begins in one hand, occurring when the hand and arm are at rest (static tremor). It may produce characteristic movements of the thumb and fingers (pill-rolling tremor). It may be suppressed by voluntary activity, and in this way contrasts with cerebellar intention tremor. The latter is an ataxic action tremor in which dyssynergia is greatest at the termination of voluntary movement. The parkinsonian occasionally may have tremulous diffculty on voluntary movement. Under these circumstances (finger-to-finger, finger-to-nose, lifting a glass of water) this intentional tremor is nonataxic and is also associated with tremor at rest. Cerebellar ataxic tremors are not associated with rigidity and are also differentiated by hypotonia, dysmetria and nystagmus. Parkinsonian tremor is exaggerated by any external stimulation and is suppressed by sleep. Like the other extrapyramidal hyperkinesias, it is abolished by pyramidal paralysis. The usual manner of eventual spread is from the upper extremity to the lower on the same side, and then to the upper, then lower limbs of the opposite side. It is most marked distally. It may involve the tongue and masseters. Head tremor is a late sign and in parkinsonism always follows limb tremor. Isolated head tremor is seen in essential (hereditary) and senile tremors, in cerebellar titubation, hydrocephalus and aortic insufficiency.

b. Nonrhythmical hyperkinesias.

A spectrum of irregular dyskinetic movements results from diffuse or focal involvement of the basal ganglia. Degenerative, vascular or other neuromedical etiology is responsible (e.g. Huntington's chorea, subthalamic infarction with hemiballism). Ballism, hemichorea, chorea, choreo-athetosis, athetosis and torsion spasm are all nonrhythmical hyperkinesias with a specific relationship to background tone.

(1) Ballism—throwing, kicking and flailing movements are most commonly unilateral (i.e. hemiballism). There is background hypotonia during the excessive movements which are often continuous.

(2) Hemichorea—A term frequently applied to hemiballism to indicate its close relation to chorea. The irregular and sudden jerking movements of chorea may be superimposed on the throwing and kicking ballistic dyskinesia. Background tone is reduced.

(3) Chorea—sudden jerking irregular movements associated with facial grimacing. Bilateral and unilateral forms occur. Background hypotonia is most common, but in rare forms rigidity may be present.

(4) Choreo-athetosis—an intermediate mixture of explosive choreoform jerking with the elaborate hand and arm posturing of athetosis. The upper extremity movement may appear semipurposeful. Background tone is variable and may be much increased during athetoid posturing.

(5) Athetosis—slow, writhing movements of the arm, leg and trunk which are most marked distally and in the upper extremity. Various postures including hyperpronation of the hand and hyperextension of the fingers are assumed during the movement. Background tone may be normal between movements, but tone is elevated during the movements.

(6) Torsion spasm—the hyperkinetic phase of dystonia. The hypertonia often assumes postures of athetosis, and dystonia has been termed "frozen athetosis." Background tone is continually elevated and is even more increased during the torsion spasm. Exaggerated postures with proximal torsion—rotation movements of the arm, leg and trunk occur with scoliotic, lordotic and torticollic components.

3. Hypotonic signs.

These are postural deficiencies not associated with resistance to passive stretch. They are not due to paralysis or sensory loss, but rather to reduced tone. The abnormal posture is typically not fixed. It is accentuated by eye closure and diminished by voluntary effort. The postural deficit affects the head, limbs or trunk. The postural drift is in the general direction of flexion. These postural-hypotonic signs are readily differentiated from postural fixation due to rigidity. The postural-hypotonic signs of parietal lobe origin are associated with parietal sensory signs. Cerebellar hypotonia is differentiated by the presence of ataxia. The hypotonic central motor signs include the following:

a. Chin-chest sign—the postural stability of the head may appear normal until the patient shuts his eyes. The head then falls gently forward.
b. Arm-sag sign—the patient is able to alternatively touch the examiner's hands held above the patient at arm's length. Eye closure leads to an immediate downward drift of these to and fro movements.
c. Knee-sag sign—the patient fails to straighten his knee during leg elevation, walking or standing.
d. Cerebral rombergism—the patient is unable to maintain an upright position when standing especially with his eyes shut; in contrast to the cerebellar Romberg, there is no associated ataxia. These difficulties are also present when sitting and walking. There is a general forward sagging of the trunk.

4. Hypokinetic signs.

These deficits include slowness in the initiation of movement ("bradykinesia") and loss of normal associated movements. While these impoverished movements often result from rigidity, hypokinesia or akinesia may be present without rigidity. This poverty of movement should be differentiated from the paucity of motor activity of parietal neglect, apraxia or paralysis. These hypokinetic central signs include the following:

a. Loss of arm swing during walking.
b. Loss of facial expression.
c. Loss of blinking.
d. Impairment of rapid alternating movement.
e. Inability to start, to turn, or to arise from a chair.

B. Capsular deficits.

Capsular involvement is usually the result of infarction or hemorrhage resulting in capsular hemiplegia. The lesion produced by bleeding from Charcot's artery of hypertension (lenticulostriate) is typical (Figs. 53 and 54). The internal capsule may be involved with the lenticular nucleus (globus pallidus and putamen). The internal capsule may be compromised with the thalamus. The bulk of the lesion commonly involves the external capsule and putamen. In such cases, the internal capsule may be compromised by compression and ischemia while the hematoma lies more laterally in the central cerebral region. The clinical syndrome of capsular hemiplegia remains rather uniform. Coma is com-

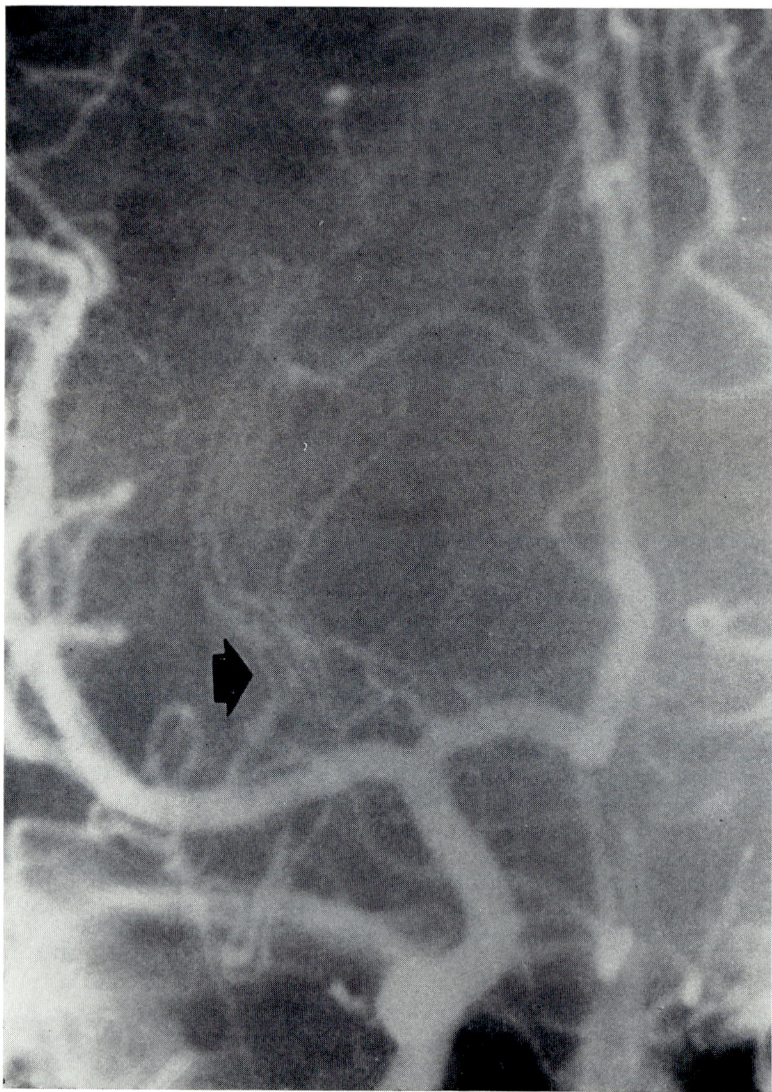

Figure 53. Normal lenticulostriate arteries. These fine vessels to the basal ganglia are not displaced. The central cerebral region is angiographically normal.

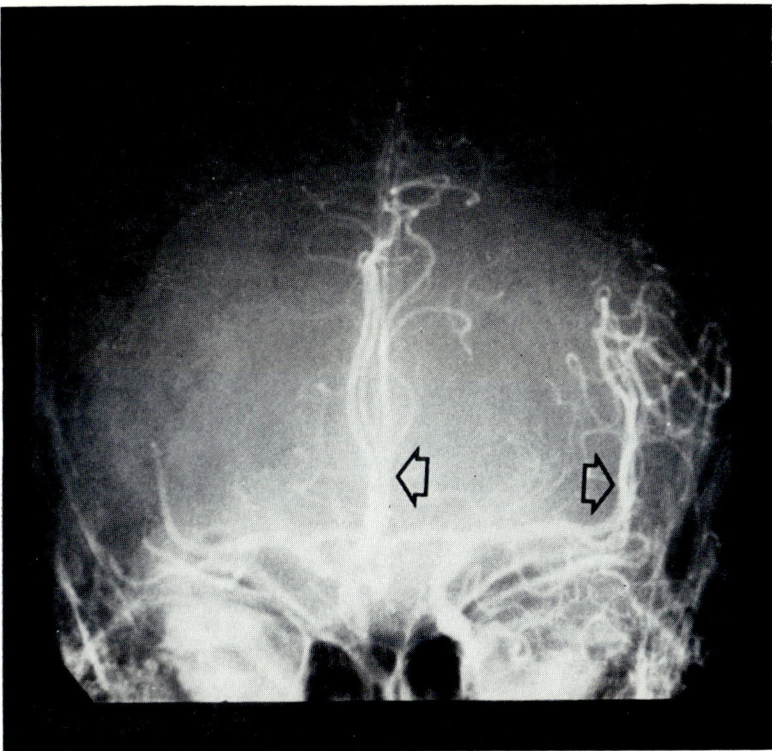

Figure 54. Central cerebral hemorrhage. There is "widening of the T" when compared to the anterior cerebral-middle cerebral distance of the opposite side. The lenticulostriate arteries are displaced by the hemorrhage.

mon, but occasionally the patient will remain alert and complain of severe bifrontal, vertex or generalized headache of sudden onset. Capsulobasal ganglia involvement in the dominant hemisphere results in aphasia and contralateral hemiplegia, hemisensory deficit and hemianopia. Obtundation obscures the aphasic, sensory and field defects. Nondominant involvement wil not result in aphasia, although speech may still be impaired by dysarthric disturbances. Capsular hemiplegia of sudden onset clinically evolves in one of four basic patterns.

1. Coma and "neurogenic shock" (i.e. arreflexic flaccidity) from which the patient does not recover.
2. Coma and early spasticity or decerebration (i.e. within 24 to 72 hours)—usually due to massive intraventricular hemorrhage (Fig. 55) ; extension of hemorrhage into the midbrain or central stem hemorrhage from midbrain compression commonly occur; the patient does not recover from these massive hemorrhagic extensions.

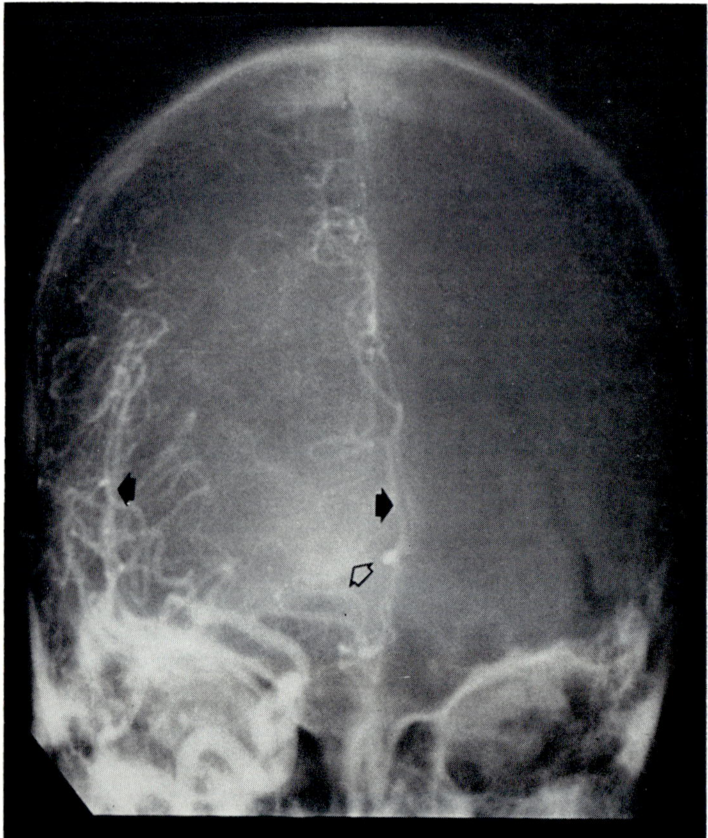

Figure 55. Intraventricular hemorrhage. "Widening of the T" between the two black arrows indicates the central cerebral hemorrhage. The white arrow points to opacification of the ventricle due to intraventricular extension of the hemorrhage. Intraventricular bleeding ordinarily occurs without such evidence of angiographic ventricular opacification.

3. The patient remains alert (or rapidly becomes alert from initial stupor) and the hemiplegia remains permanently flaccid; this has been termed "pure pyramidal flaccidity," spasticity being the result of associated basal ganglia involvement. However, dense persistent flaccidity is often the result of extensive thalamic (or parietal) destruction with marked sensory loss.
4. The patient remains or becomes alert and the flaccid hemiplegia eventually (i.e. usually about 2 to 3 weeks) becomes spastic; this is more common than the permanently flaccid form. Initially, all reflexes may be absent on the hemiplegic side. The Babinski sign tends to appear first in the presence of flaccid arreflexia and is commonly

present in the first day. Deep tendon reflexes may reappear in the lower extremity during the second or third day and in the upper extremity in several days. Eventually, the reflexes become hyperactive as hypertonia replaces flaccidity. Spasticity reveals an increased resistance to passive movement with an initial rise and rapid fall in resistance (clasp-knife phenomenon). The upper extremity eventually assumes the position of flexion and the lower of extension and contractures are prominent.

Capsular hemiplegia involves the face, tongue, arm and leg (corticobulbar and corticospinal tracts in the posterior limb of the internal capsule). Hemisensory defect results from involvement of the sensory radiations (or thalamus) behind the corticospinal tract. Homonymous hemianopia results from involvement of the geniculocalcarine tract in the retrolenticular capsule. A dilated and sluggish pupil (oculomotor palsy) on the side of the hemorrhagic lesion indicates transtentorial herniation or direct extension of hemorrhage into the midbrain tegmentum. Herniation can occur with or without massive intraventricular bleeding. A small pupil is sometimes seen on the side of the lesion in the first hours following intracerebral hemorrhage. It may be a misleading sign, since the opposite pupil is relatively larger although not dilated. As the mass effect increases, this initially small pupil may convert to the dilated pupil of oculomotor palsy. Bilaterally dilated pupils in the intracerebral hemorrhage case occur with massive intraventricular rupture, direct extension of bleeding from the cerebrum into the midbrain, or with transtentorial midbrain compression.

Monoplegia suggests a cortical rather than capsular lesion. Whenever the acute hemiplegia is not dense and uniformly distributed to both extremities, a lesion above the capsule should be suspected. Lobar hematoma in the frontal pole may be responsible for such differential hemiparesis. Facial weakness associated with capsular hemiplegia is usually readily detectable and central in type with sparing of the brow. At times a pseudoperipheral facial palsy can occur with loss of wrinkles over the forehead on the paretic side. Facial weakness may be difficult to detect in comatose patients. Flattening of the nasolabial fold, blowing out of the paretic cheek, and asymmetrical grimacing on retromandibular noxious stimulation indicate the side of facial palsy. Facial palsy on one side and hemiplegia on the other indicates a pontine lesion. Transtentorial herniation occasionally spares the face because of the medial position of corticobulbar fibers in the cerebral peduncle and associated coma obscuring minor paresis.

Sparing of the face in the presence of hemiparesis also can occur in cortical-subcortical lesions of the frontodorsal region. Sparing of the face is characteristic of spinal hemiplegia.

The internal capsule may also be involved by the extension of a tumor into the central cerebral region. This is particularly common in the primary cerebral gliomas. A slowly progressive spasticity of the contralateral extremities is typical, with hemiparesis converting to spastic hemiplegia. Spasticity and hyperreflexia may precede marked paralysis in tumors extending from frontal regions. Flaccidity with hypoactive reflexes can occur with tumors extending from parietal regions; these are less common than frontal tumors. Tumors involving the thalamus typically also involve the capsule and basal ganglia, so that spastic hemiplegia is often noted. Flaccidity and hypoactive reflexes in the tumor case should always suggest a cerebellar mass; however, even cerebellar tumors may produce spasticity and hyperreflexia by brain stem compression or obstructive hydrocephalus. Central cerebral gliomas may result in contralateral hemisensory deficits with hemihypesthesia as a result of extension to the thalamus, parietal lobe and posterior half of the internal capsule. Contralateral homonymous hemianopia indicates retrolenticular or caudal cerebral involvement by the tumor, the optic radiation being totally involved at, or distal to, the lateral geniculate body. Retrolenticular capsular field cuts are hemianopic rather than quadrantanopic, as a result of the close approximation of visual radiations within the posterior capsule. Capsular deficits can appear rather suddenly in metastatic carcinoma to the brain. The metastases are most commonly in the middle cerebral distribution. The marked cerebral swelling associated with secondary tumor deposits can involve the capsular region even if the tumor itself does not. Sudden capsular deficit in the primary brain tumor indicates intraneoplastic hemorrhage. Rapidly worsening hemiparesis due to compression of the cerebral peduncle at a level below the capsule is the result of transtentorial herniation common in brain tumors. It does not necessarily imply intraneoplastic hemorrhage.

C. Thalamic deficits

Just as a neoplasm involving the basal ganglia commonly does not result in extrapyramidal signs, so the thalamic tumor (Fig. 56) does not produce the classical thalamic syndrome of spontaneous central pain and hyperpathia. The thalamic tumor may present clinically in one of four patterns.

1. Mental disorder.
2. Progressive hemiparesis (or other focal neurological deficit).

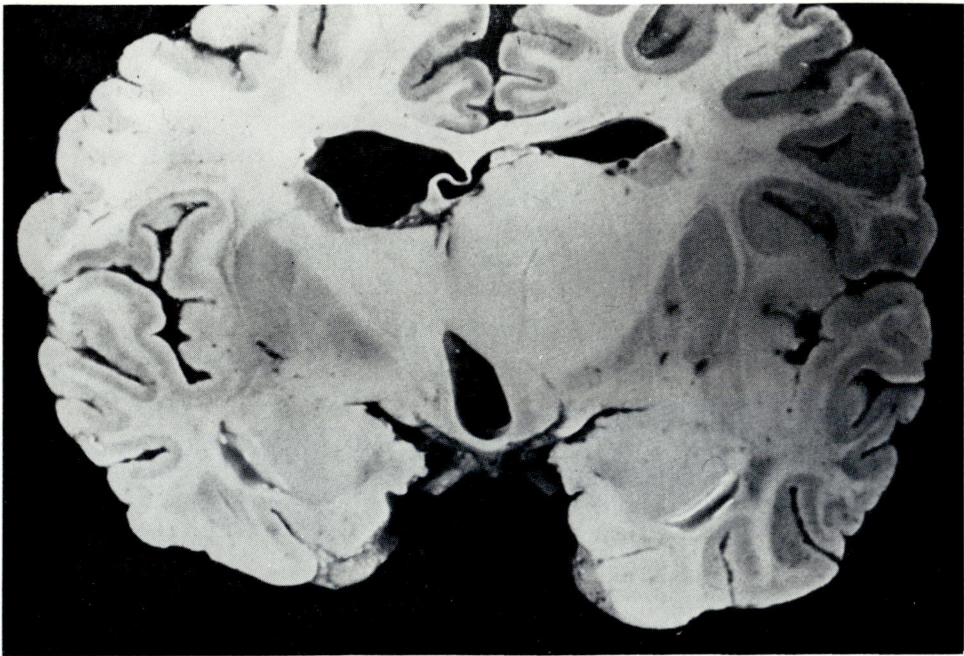

Figure 56. Thalamic astrocytoma. The thalamus on one side is expanded. Elevation of the floor of the body of the lateral ventricle on the tumor side is characteristic. The third ventricle is shifted and dilated, the hydrocephalus due to posterior third ventricular occlusion by the tumor.

3. Intracranial hypertension.
4. Convulsive disorder.

Thalamic tumors are uncommon neoplasms which can present in childhood, adolescence or later in adult life. The clinical signs are nonpathognomonic.

1. Mental disorder.

These disturbances may present as a loss of normal energy, apathy, memory loss and progressive dementia. Dementia may or may not be associated with elevated intracranial pressure in the presence of a thalamic tumor. Incontinence occurs and the demential syndrome resembles that of a frontal or corpus callosum tumor.

2. Progressive hemiparesis and other focal neurological deficits.
   a. Hemiparesis is the single most common focal sign. However, the paralysis may be minimal and in certain cases is entirely absent.
   b. Hemisensory deficits—may be in the primary, postural or discriminative modalities. Ataxia of the sensorially deficient extremities may be prominent.

c. Hemianopia—sometimes occurs; like hemiparesis, hemisensory deficits, the field cut is also contralateral to the mass.

d. Focal ocular signs—a variety of ocular signs occur, but they may be entirely absent.

(1) Nystagmus.

(2) Small pupil on the side of the mass.

(3) Vertical gaze palsy—suggests tectal compression.

(4) Abducens palsy—indicates intracranial hypertension.

3. Signs of intracranial hypertension.

Headache is a common initial complaint and may be bifrontal, generalized, occipital or vague in character. The cardinal signs of intracranial hypertension (headache, vomiting, papilledema and stupor) may be the sole indicators of the thalamic tumor. Hydrocephalus can result from the thalamic tumor (Fig. 57), usually from posterior third ventricular occlusion. When dementia is present, headache may not be prominent despite elevated intracranial pressure. Drowsiness can be a prominent feature of the thalamic tumor even in the absence of intracranial hypertension.

4. Convulsive disorder.

Seizures occur only in a minority of thalamic tumors at the time

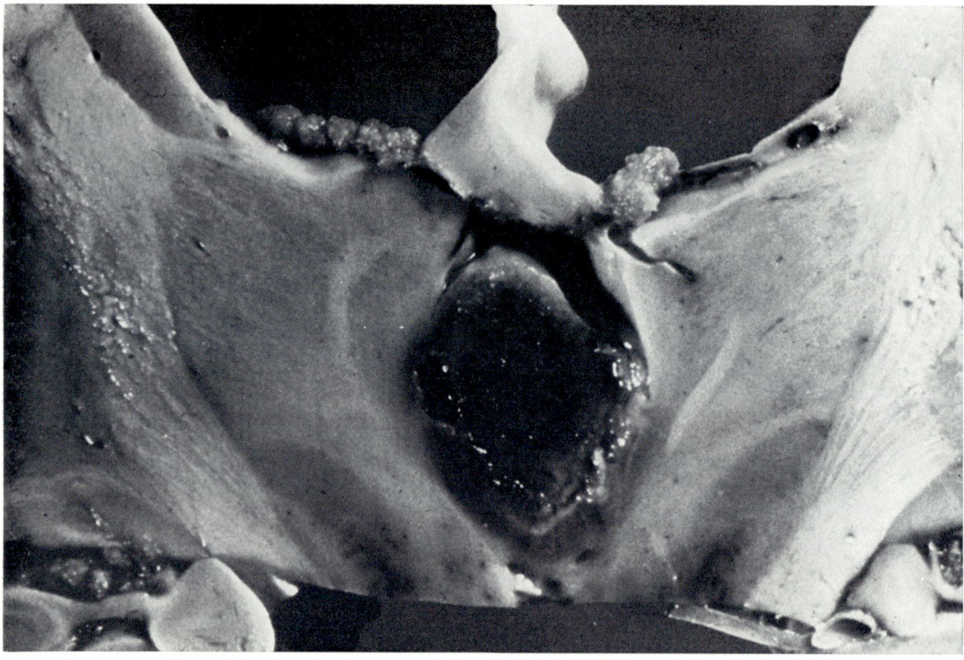

Figure 57. Thalamic glioblastoma. The glioblastoma extends into and occludes the third ventricle, resulting in marked lateral ventricular hydrocephalus.

of clinical presentation. A variety of attacks can occur, including grand mal (nonlocalized general attacks with loss of consciousness at the outset) and focal cerebral seizures. Focal motor or focal sensory attacks which vary in their site of origin suggest the deep source of the ictus. Focal sensory attacks may be accompanied by vague hemibody paresthesias. The focal seizures readily become generalized. Intermittent syncopal attacks may occur simulating epilepsy.

Deformities (Angiographic and Pneumographic) of the Central Cerebral Syndromes

A. Angiographic

1. Widening signs of the central cerebral mass.
   a. Widening of the T (frontal view)—on the side of a central cerebral mass there is increased distance between the middle cerebral artery and the anterior cerebral artery. The middle cerebral artery becomes straightened and the angiographic sylvian point is closer to the inner table than normal. The anterior cerebral-pericallosal artery may remain in the midline, but the internal cerebral vein is usually shifted to the opposite side.
   b. Widening of the lenticulostriate–midline distance—the lenticulostriate arteries (frontal view) are displaced laterally and downward.
   c. Opening of the venous angle (lateral view)—the thalamostriate vein in the floor of the lateral ventricle is elevated. While thalamic tumors almost always shift the internal cerebral vein across the midline, they may not elevate this vein.
   d. Widening of the basal–internal cerebral venous junction (lateral view)—the basal vein of Rosenthal may be displaced downward, while the posterior part of the internal cerebral vein is displaced upward.
   e. Widening of the curvature of the choroidal arteries (lateral view)—both the anterior and posterior choroidal arteries normally course around the posterior end of the thalamus, parallel to one another. If these arteries are visualized, their curve may be increased around a thalamic tumor.
   f. Widening of the posterior cerebral arteries (frontal view)—lateral displacement of the posterior cerebral arteries away from one another as they course around the midbrain, implies extension of tumor to the upper brain stem.
2. Downward displacement—vessels which may be displaced (lateral view) include the following:

a. Basilar vein.
b. Anterior choroidal artery.
c. Posterior communicating—posterior cerebral arteries.
d. Basilar bifurcation.

Note: Hydrocephalus can result in a widening of the T with straightening of the middle cerebral arteries on frontal view due to ventricular enlargement. On this view however, the thalamostriate vein is noted to be laterally deviated and depressed by the enlarged lateral ventricle. A central cerebral tumor, however, tends to elevate the thalamostriate vein. Widening of the anterior cerebral-pericallosal angle on lateral view with stretching of the pericallosal artery would favor hydrocephalus. Thalamic tumors themselves may ultimately result in hydrocephalus, the posterior third ventricle being the usual site of occlusion.

3. Opacification of a lateral ventricle (frontal view)—central cerebral hypertensive hemorrhages into the thalamus and capsule readily extend into the lateral ventricle. Occasionally, the frontal horn on the side of the mass will be opacified. The lenticulostriate arteries are deviated away from the bulk of the central hematoma.

B. Pneumographic

1. Elevation of the floor of the body of the lateral ventricle—indicates a mass in the region of the thalamus. A temporal mass may narrow the lateral angle of the lateral ventricle (AP view) by elevation of the angle from below; however, the main part of the floor of the ventricle is not elevated as much as it is with a central mass.
2. Narrowing of the third ventricle—this is common posteriorly. The anterior third may sometimes be enlarged as a result of posterior third occlusion by thalamic mass.
3. Shift and curvature of the third ventricle—this is common, the third ventricle being distorted and dislocated to the opposite side. The upper third ventricle has greater mobility than the floor of the third ventricle and tends to be shifted to a greater degree.
4. Septum—the septum pellucidum may remain in the midline. If shifted, the lower part of the septum tends to shift more than the upper in thalamic (or temporal) tumors.
5. Lateral displacement of the temporal horn—a central cerebral mass tends to dislocate the temporal horn laterally and downward while it displaces the third ventricle in the opposite direction across the midline.
6. Ventricular dilatation—mild to moderate ventricular enlargement with bilateral ventricular filling can occur in thalamic tumors. Abnormalities in the region of the third ventricle may suggest third ven-

tricular tumor. Upward deviation of the floor of the lateral ventricle, with narrowing of the posterior ventricular body close to its junction with the atrium (PA view), indicates a thalamic mass on that side. Occlusion of the foramen of Monro by a thalamic tumor is less common than ventricular enlargement due to posterior third ventricle occlusion by this tumor.

7. Tumors whose main bulk lies within the basal ganglia (i.e. lenticular region) are commonly regarded radiologically as "thalamic" because of similar deformities (in the floor of the body of the ventricle, the third ventricle and temporal horn). Posterior deep frontal gliomas commonly invade the central cerebral region and may deform the lateral wall and floor of the anterior horn.

Additional Diagnostic Studies

A. Plain skull x-rays

1. Plain skull x-rays in central cerebral tumors reveal little in terms of localizing evidence.
2. Pineal shift away from the side of a central cerebral mass is characteristic, but occurs in any unilateral supratentorial mass.
3. Pressure atrophy of the sella—may be evident in tumor cases with intracranial hypertension, but does not indicate the site of the mass.
4. Central cerebral tumor calcifications in infancy suggest cerebral teratoma; in childhood, the cerebral ependymoma is a likely diagnosis. Tumor calcifications in adult life may be the result of cerebral astrocytoma, oligodendroglioma or ependymoma. However, most cerebral gliomas do not reveal tumor calcification visible on plain x-rays.
5. Calcification in the region of the basal ganglia can occur with or without hypoparathyroidism. They are usually symmetrical.
6. Choroid plexus calcification—occurs normally, but may be somewhat asymmetrical or unilateral. Posterior displacement of a calcified glomus by a large central cerebral mass can occur.

B. EEG

1. The EEG does not absolutely differentiate a vascular lesion from a tumor.
2. The deep cerebral tumor may be associated with a normal EEG. The closer a cerebral tumor is to cortex the greater the chance of focal delta activity.
3. Abnormally increased theta activity of regular and bilaterally synchronous type may occur with thalamic tumors.
4. Frontal delta activity, more prominent on the side of the central cerebral tumor, may be evident in tumors close to the anterior part

of the third ventricle. Caudal delta activity may be noted with central cerebral tumors adjacent to the posterior third ventricle.

5. Generalized slowing may indicate intracranial hypertension which can occur in central cerebral tumors as well as with other space-occupying lesions in other sites.
6. Photically driven electrographic activity may be depressed on the side of a cerebral tumor when the EEG is otherwise poorly lateralizing.
7. Focal epileptiform activity is often present in supratentorial tumors of various types. This is particularly true of the gliomas of the cerebral hemisphere, tumors which commonly extend into deep cerebral regions.
8. Since most cerebral infarcts involve the cortex while most intracerebral hemorrhages spare the cortex, focal EEG signs are more common in ischemic than in hemorrhagic cerebral lesions.
9. Reduction of background activity is commonly seen on the side of a vascular lesion; it has some lateralizing value but is otherwise nonspecific.
10. While focal delta activity is more common on the side of an infarct, it can be seen in certain cases of intracerebral hemorrhage. Bilaterally synchronous delta or theta activity can be seen in vascular lesions of ischemic or hemorrhagic type involving the thalamus. A clinically ill patient with a basal ganglia hemorrhage may have a surprisingly intact appearing record, especially with regard to the absence of slow activity.
11. Epileptiform activity often associated with cerebral tumors is relatively less common in vascular lesions. It can be seen in the deep cerebral arteriovenous malformation which may mimic a deep cerebral tumor. It may accompany intracerebral hemorrhage and is less often seen in infarction.

C. Brain scan

1. The brain scan is often negative in low-grade cerebral gliomas, while the EEG is commonly abnormal.
2. The scan, like the EEG, is usually abnormal in glioblastoma multiforme. The uptake may be deep-seated in the central cerebral region; is may be diffusely increased when compared to the opposite hemisphere.
3. A positive central cerebral scan in the older age group should also suggest metastatic carcinoma.
4. A positive central cerebral scan in the adolescent or young adult should raise the possibility of arteriovenous malformation. The larger

and more superficial the malformation, the greater the incidence of a positive test. Hemorrhage is not required.

5. The initial scan in cerebral infarction is typically negative, while the scan in intracerebral hemorrhage may be positive. A negative scan does not rule out a hemorrhage.

CHAPTER 10

PERICHIASMATIC SYNDROMES

Neuroanatomy of the Perichiasmatic Region

A. Subhemispheric relationships

A variety of neurosurgical syndromes result from space-occupying lesions involving the optic pathway at the base of the brain. The deficits produced are closely dependent upon the anatomy of this subhemispheric region (Figs. 58 and 59). The basal optic system is a paired semidecussating brain tract and not a true cranial nerve. The intracranial optic nerves, chiasm and tracts can be considered together for several practical reasons.

1. Perichiasmatic tumors (e.g. chromophobe adenoma, craniopharyngioma, tuberculum meningioma, hypothalamic astrocytoma) often involve these basal optic structures in combination (e.g. optic nerve-chiasm; chiasm-optic tract).
2. The anatomical relationship of the basal optic pathway to the sella is variable.
   a. The chiasm itself usually lies above the dorsum or diaphragm. It may, however, lie at the tuberculum ("prefixed") or behind the dorsum ("postfixed").
   b. The height of the chiasm above the sellar diaphragm may vary between 0 and 10 mm.
   c. The angle of inclination of the chiasm is often as much as 45°, the basal optic pathway progressively ascending as it proceeds posteriorly.

   Thus a chromophobe adenoma expanding upwards in the usual fashion may compress optic nerve(s), nerve-chiasm, chiasm, or chiasm-tract depending upon optic-sellar anatomy in the individual case. The anterior chiasm (extramacular decussation) and posterior chiasm (macular decussation) when compressed also result in differing visual deficits.
3. Occasional eccentricity or invasive potential of tumor growth may produce less common syndromes (e.g. lateral chiasmal compression with shift of the chiasm against the opposite internal carotid artery; cavernous sinus invasion; anterior, middle or even posterior fossa extension).
4. The basal optic pathway is critically related to the circle of Willis.

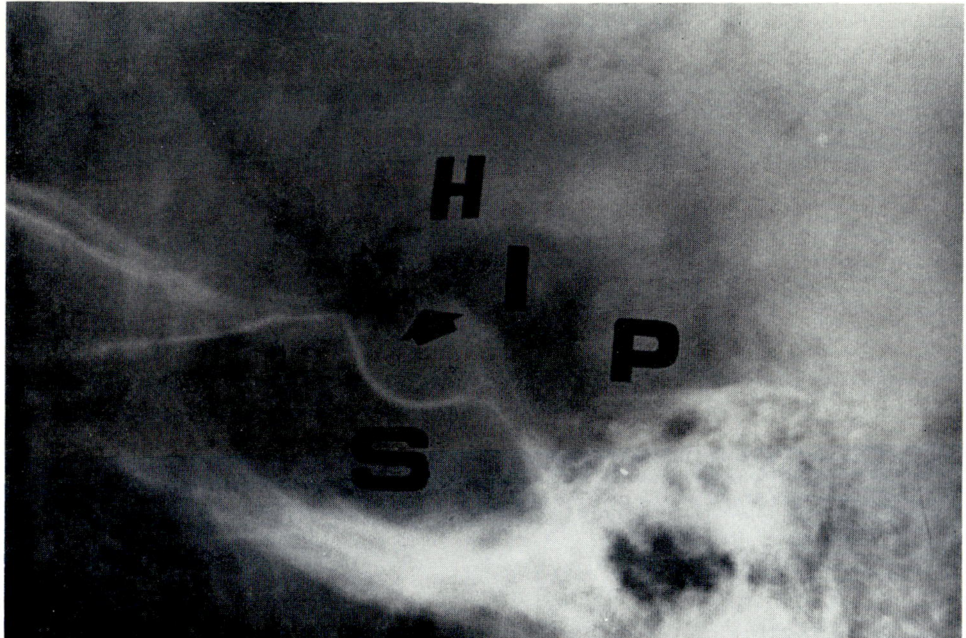

Figure 58. Normal perichiasmatic region. Pneumoencephalography reveals the position of the optic chiasm (white arrow) and infundibulum (black arrow) above the sella. "H" indicates the hypothalamus, "I" the interpeduncular cistern just in front of the cerebral peduncles and "P" the pons. "S" is the sphenoid sinus.

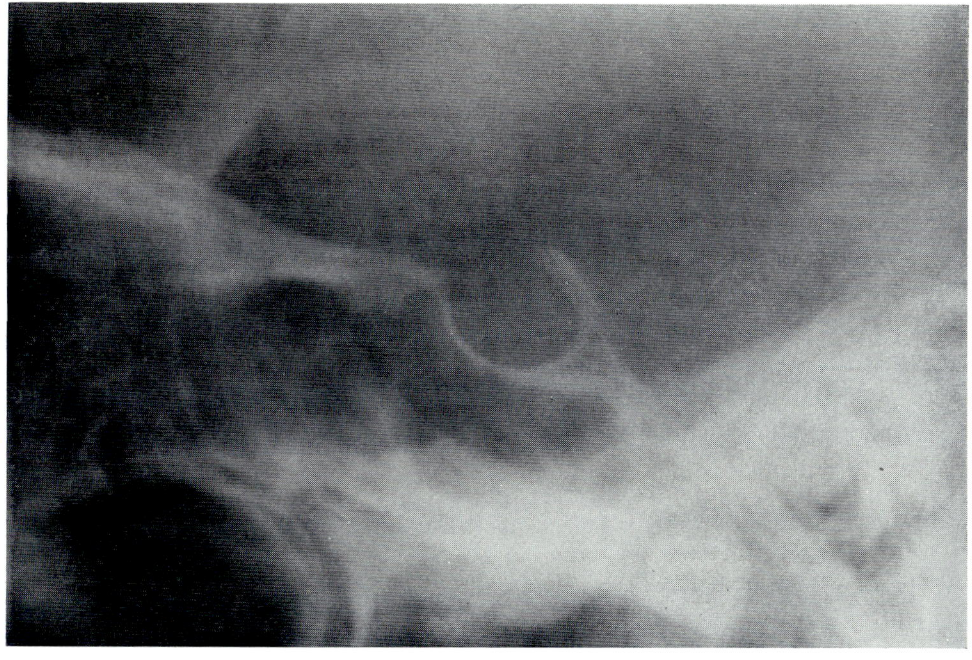

Figure 59. Normal sella.

Aneurysms therefore may produce perichiasmatic syndromes and may mimic pituitary tumors in every detail.

At the base of the brain, the hypothalamus lies immediately above the optic chiasm. The chiasm forms part of the anterior floor of the third ventricle. The hypothalamus forms the lateral walls of this ventricle and its remaining floor. The rostral wall of the third ventricle is the lamina terminalis, dividing telencephalon from diencephalon. This thin rostral wall proceeds up from the chiasm to the anterior commissure, just in front of the foramen of Monro at the thalamic pole. The hypothalamus becomes continuous with the frontobasal region rostrally and with the midbrain tegmentum caudally. The infundibular stalk descends just behind the chiasm through an opening of variable size in the sellar diaphragm to the intrasellar pituitary. The circle of Willis supplies the hypothalamus with arterial blood. These vessels (anterior cerebral-anterior communicating; internal carotid-posterior communicating; posterior cerebral-basilar bifurcation) form a polygon within the cisterna basalis. This basal expansion of the subarachnoid space is rostrally the suprasellar cistern and caudally the interpeduncular cistern. The rostral and caudal portions of this essentially continuous cistern may be partially divided by the membrane of Liliequist, extending from premammillary hypothalamus to posterior clinoids. The intracranial optic pathway ascends through this basal cistern as the circle of Willis descends through it. As the optic nerves merge to form the chiasm, they penetrate the circle of Willis from below, lying just beneath the anterior cerebral-anterior communicating arteries. The lateral pillars of the arterial circle, the internal carotids, become the lateral boundaries of the chiasm. As the optic tracts continue to ascend, they pass above the posterior communicating and posterior cerebral arteries. The visual pathways ascend through the arterial circle, narrowing at the chiasm in order to do so. The optic sensory system has a reverse relation to the oculomotor nerve. The optic tracts proceed caudally in the roof of the interpeduncular cistern, while the oculomotor nerve passes rostrally at its floor. The optic tracts round the lateral border of the cerebral peduncles as they first appear at the base of the cerebrum. The oculomotor nerves emerge at the medial border of the peduncles as they are about to penetrate the upper pons. While the optic tract passes above the posterior cerebral artery, the oculomotor nerve emerges below it. The oculomotor nerve then passes forward between the posterior communicating artery and the uncus of the temporal lobe. It pierces the dura lateral to the posterior clinoid process to enter the cavernous sinus. The oculomotor, trochlear, abducens and ophthalmic division of the trigeminal nerve all lie lateral to the carotid artery within the cavernous sinus, the latter constituting the lateral wall of the sella. These intracavernous cranial nerves enter the orbit through the superior orbital fissure as ophthalmic veins leave the orbit to enter the sinus. The optic nerve and ophthalmic artery traverse the medially adjacent optic foramen. The optic foramen and superior orbital fissure and their neurovascular contents constitute the "orbital apex" (see Chs. 2 and 8). The orbital apex is located at the juncture of the anterior, middle and pituitary fossae to each side of the midline.

The large central opening of the tentorium, the "oval door of the tent," the supratentorial-infratentorial passage, has a host of critical relationships and is the keystone in a variety of neurosurgical syndromes. The rostral portion of the oval door is the perichiasmatic region and the caudal portion is occupied by the midbrain. The insertions of the tentorium include its peripheral margin and the free margin of the oval door. The peripheral margin is attached to the posterior clinoid and upper edge of the petrous part of the temporal bone, forming the petroclinoid ligament over which the oculomotor nerve passes before its dural exit. The peripheral tentorial attachment passes caudally from the petrous ridge to the mastoid angle of the parietal bone and transverse ridge of the occipital bone. This peripheral tentorial attachment contains the superior petrosal sinus rostrally and the transverse sinus caudally. The central or free margin of the oval door crosses above the petroclinoid ligament of the attached margin to insert at the anterior clinoid process. On the medial side of the anterior clinoid process is the optic foramen; on the lateral side is the sphenoparietal sinus of the sphenoid ridge, while beneath it is the superior orbital fissure. The four clinoids are the attachments of the sellar diaphragm which is a fold of the inner layer of dura. The rostral extreme of the oval door is thus the tuberculum sella in the midline and the orbital apices just laterally. As the free edge of the tentorium proceeds caudally from the anterior clinoid, it lies lateral to the supracavernous carotid. The ophthalmic artery passes from the supracavernous carotid through the optic foramen beneath the optic nerve. The posterior communicating artery passes caudally, medial to the oculomotor nerve. The anterior choroidal artery passes superiorly along the uncus, lateral to the optic tract. Just at the point where the free edge of the tentorium is lateral to the supracavernous carotid, the free edge lies above the cavernous sinus with its neurovascular contents. Just caudal to the carotid pillars of the chiasm, the free edge is bounded medially by the extracavernous portion of the oculomotor nerve. The free edge at this point is bounded laterally by the gasserian ganglion of the trigeminal, lying in the medial portion of the middle fossa in Meckel's cave beneath a dural covering. Overhanging the free edge above, and notched by it, is the uncus of the temporal lobe.

The posterior cerebral artery emerges from the bifurcation of the basilar at the upper border of the pons. It passes around the cerebral peduncle, the oculomotor nerve lying between it and the superior cerebellar artery below. The posterior cerebral artery lies below the optic tract as it passes around the peduncle to gain the free edge of the tentorium. Just beneath the free edge is the trochlear nerve, proceeding forward toward the cavernous subhemispheric region, having passed around the cerebral peduncle from the dorsal midbrain region. The optic tracts, posterior cerebral arteries and basal veins all encircle the cerebral peduncle.

B. Hypothalamus

The hypothalamus is a small but critical region forming the walls and floor of the third ventricle below the hypothalamic sulcus. It extends from the lamina terminalis to the midbrain. Rostrocaudally are the preoptic, supraoptic, tuberal and mammillary regions. Mediolaterally are the periventricular, medial and lateral zones. The medial forebrain bundle connects the basal forebrain and midbrain tegmentum and passes through the lateral hypothalamic zone. Just lateral lies the zona incerta. Reticular projections from the brain stem reticular core (tegmentum) pass forward through the lateral hypothalamic zone and zona incerta (subthalamus) beneath the dorsal thalamus (the ventral bypass). These reticular projections terminate in hypothalamic, septal and basal forebrain regions. Most of the hypothalamic nuclei lie medially.

1. Periventricular nuclei (preoptic, suprachiasmatic, paraventricular, infundibular and posterior).
2. Medial nuclei (anterior, ventromedial, dorsomedial and premammillary).
3. Lateral nuclei (preoptic, lateral, tuberomammillary and supraoptic).

Afferent connections to the hypothalamus include the following:

1. Periventricular system—from the medial division of the dorsal thalamus and mesencephalic periaqueductal gray.
2. Inferior thalamic peduncle—from the dorsal thalamus.
3. Tegmentohypothalamic tract and mammillary peduncle—from the midbrain.
4. Medial forebrain bundle—from the basal forebrain and septum.
5. Fornix—from the hippocampus to the mammillary bodies.
6. Direct amygdalohypothalamic tract—from amygdala and piriform cortex.
7. Stria terminalis—from amygdala to medial hypothalamus.
8. Pallidohypothalamic tract—from the globus pallidus.

Efferent projections from the hypothalamus include the following:

1. Mammillothalamic tract—to the anterior nuclei of the dorsal thalamus.
2. Medial forebrain bundle—to the basal forebrain and septum.

3. Direct hypothalamoamygdalary tract—to the amygdala and piriform cortex.
4. Periventricular system—to the medial division of the dorsal thalamus and mesencephalic periaqueductal gray.
5. Diffuse hypothalamotegmental tract—to the mesencephalic tegmentum.
6. Mammillotegmental tract—to the mesencephalic tegmentum.
7. Hypothalamopretectal and tectal projections to pretectal and superior collicular areas.
8. Supraoptico-hypophysial tract—from the supraoptic and paraventricular nuclei to the neurohypophysis.
9. Tuberoinfundibular tract—from the tuberal nuclei to the median eminence and infundibular stem of the neurohypophysis.

C. Pituitary

The pituitary gland may be separated into a glandular division in vascular contact with the hypothalamus, and a neural division which is an extension of the hypothalamus. Further subdivision includes the following:

1. Adenohypophysis (glandular).
   a. Pars distalis (anterior lobe).
   b. Pars tuberalis.
   c. Pars intermedia.
2. Neurohypophysis (neural).
   a. Pars neuralis (posterior lobe).
   b. Infundibular stem.
   c. Median eminence.

The pars intermedia of the glandular division lies between the pars distalis and pars neuralis. The pars tuberalis of the glandular division surrounds the infundibular stem and median eminence. The median eminence of the tuber cinereum of the hypothalamus is a neurohypophyseal structure.

Blood Supply of the Perichiasmatic Region

A. Pituitary

1. Arterial.
   a. Superior hypophyseal arteries—these paired arteries arise from the supracavernous carotid (below the ophthalmic artery and just above the cavernous sinus). They supply the hypophyseal stalk.
      (1) Anterior branch.
      (2) Posterior branch.
      (3) Trabecular branch.

The anterior and posterior branches supply the upper stalk and median eminence. The trabecular branch supplies the lower part of the stalk and anastomoses with the ascending branch of the inferior hypophyseal artery upon the pars neuralis.

b. Inferior hypophyseal arteries—these paired arteries arise from the intracavernous carotid and supply the pars neuralis.
    (1) Ascending branch—forms a ring around the pars neuralis and anastomoses with the trabecular branch of the superior hypophyseal artery.
    (2) Descending branch—completes the anastomotic ring around the pars neuralis.

2. Portal.

The pars distalis (anterior lobe) receives no direct arterial blood; it is supplied by the hypophyseal portal system. The pars neuralis (posterior lobe) receives no portal blood. The hypophyseal portal system arises from capillary tufts in the median eminence and stalk. Portal blood is then distributed to the pars distalis.

3. Venous.

Venous drainage from both the pars distalis and pars neuralis is by way of twig veins to the cavernous, superior circular and subhypophyseal venous sinuses.

B. Hypothalamus
    1. Arterial—the hypothalamus has the most greatly concentrated blood supply of central nervous structure. Small arteries arise directly from the circle of Willis. The arterial supply of the hypothalamus is separate from that to the pituitary.
    2. Venous—to the cavernous sinus.

C. Subhemispheric optic pathway
    1. Optic nerve and retina—ophthalmic and central retinal arteries.
    2. Optic chiasm—anterior and posterior communicating arteries.
    3. Optic tract—anterior choroidal and posterior communicating arteries.

Infarction Syndromes in the Perichiasmatic Region

The arterial circle of Willis provides an extensive means of collateral supply to the hypothalamus. However, infarction may result from arterial spasm due to rupture of an aneurysm. Stupor, coma and akinetic mutism result from ischemia to the critical anterior or posterior hypothalamic regions. There are two clinical forms of akinetic mutism: vigilant coma and somnolent mutism. In coma vigil, the speechless immobile state is accompanied by an intact oculomotor system: gaze appears alert. The infarct lies in the field of supply of the anterior cerebral-anterior communicating arteries and vessels of the anterior perforated substance. Septoanterior hypothalamic infarction produces the syndrome. In contrast, somnolent mutism is a speechless immobile state accompanied by persistent lethargy with eye closure, requiring external stimulation to alert the patient's gaze. Ophthalmoplegia and vertical gaze palsy are common in this form of mutism. When stimulation is terminated, the patient soon closes his eyes and reverts to his previous somnolence. The responsible infarct is situated at the diencephalic-mesencephalic junction. Somnolent mutism is produced in the syndrome of the mesencephalic artery which is the first portion of the posterior cerebral artery at the basilar bifurcation. This is the posterior segment of the circle of Willis. Occlusion of perforating branches of the mesencephalic artery resulting in posterior periventricular and periaqueductal infarction result in somnolent mutism.

Other forms of brain stem infarction may simulate akinetic mutism. Pontine infarction with bilateral supranuclear motor paralysis preserving the oculomotor system can produce a mute akinetic state in which communication by blinking is possible. This has been referred to as the locked-in syndrome.

Neurophysiology of the Hypothalamo-Hypophysis

The physiology of these closely related structures is both endocrine and neural. Both the hypothalamus and adenohypophysis secrete hormones. The hypothalamic hormones include the following:

1. Vasopressin (ADH).
2. Oxytocin.
3. Releasing factors (corticotropic, thyrotropic and gonadotropic releasing factors for ACTH, TSH, LH and FSH).

The adenohypophyseal hormones include the following:

1. ACTH.
2. TSH.
3. Gonadotropic hormones-LH (ICSH), lactogenic hormone (prolactin) and FSH.
4. Growth hormone.
5. MSH—intermediate lobe hormone.

The physiology of these hormones is far beyond the scope of this text. Functional principles of importance to the neurosurgeon are as follow:

A. Antidiurectic hormone (ADH, vasopressin)

1. Secreted by the supraoptic and paraventricular nuclei of the hypothalamus and stored in the neurohypophysis after axonal migration along the supraoptic-hypophyseal tract.
2. Increased osmolality (e.g. dehydration) results in increased ADH

(osmoreceptors and volume receptors). Decreased osmolality (e.g. water intoxication) results in reduced ADH.

3. ADH acts upon the distal renal tubule which requires ADH in order to reabsorb water from urine at that level.
4. Normal serum osmolality range is 285 to 295 mOsm/liter.
5. Diabetes insipidis—insufficient ADH results in the following:
   a. Large urine output (4 to 10 or more liters per day).
   b. Urinary dilution (specific gravity consistently at 1.010 or below, usually 1.004 or less).
   c. Dehydration, polyuria, polydipsia, thirst and weight loss.
6. Experimental diabetes insipidis results from hypothalamic lesions of the supraoptic and paraventricular nuclei or section of the supraoptic-hypophyseal tract in the pituitary stalk.
7. Ancillary tests of value in the diagnosis of diabetes insipidis are as listed below:
   a. Water deprivation test.
   b. Response to pitressin.

B. ACTH

1. Secreted by the pars distalis and stimulates the production of adrenal cortical steroids.
2. Increased ACTH results from release of CRF (corticotropin releasing factor) from the hypothalamus (via the hypophyseal portal system to the pars distalis). Both physiological and stressful states may result in ACTH increase.
3. Adrenal cortical insufficiency—due either to primary adrenal deficiency or secondarily to hypopituitarism. The best differential test is the measurement of blood and urinary 17-hydroxysteroids and 17-ketosteroids before and after the administration of ACTH. Increased levels of these steroids result in cases of hypopituitarism, but not in cases of addisonian primary adrenocortical insufficiency. A screening test employing the measurement of blood 11-hydroxy corticoids before and after parenteral ACTH is valuable.
4. Pituitary insufficiency—endogenous ACTH production (reflected by urinary excretion of 17-hydroxycorticoids and 17-ketogenic steroids) can be assessed by the Methopyrapone (Metopirone®) test. This agent reduces the secretion of cortisol by the adrenal cortex, in turn producing a rise in endogenous ACTH by a normal pituitary, with resultant increased urinary steroid excretion. Hypopituitarism is indicated by failure to elevate the already reduced 17-hydroxy and 17-ketogenic steroid levels. Limited pituitary reserve (i.e. a milder degree

of pituitary insufficiency) is reflected by a failure to produce an increase in the control values of these steroids.

5. Ancillary tests of value in the assessment of adrenal cortical insufficiency (primary or secondary) include the following:
   a. Water loading test.
   b. Glucose tolerance test.

Note: Direct measurement of blood corticosteroid levels is of great value and may replace other tests of adrenocortical function. All endocrine studies related especially to diabetes insipidis or hypopituitary–hypoadrenal states must be carried out under rigidly controlled conditions for diagnosis and prevention of serious test complications. In the presence of diabetes insipidis the water deprivation test can aggravate an already present dehydration. Excessive pitressin may result in water intoxication as a result of its antidiuretic effect. In the presence of pituitary and adrenal insufficiency, the administration of mepyrapone, the water loading, insulin sensitivity or sodium deprivation tests may induce an acute adrenal crisis.

C. Results of hypophysectomy
   1. Secondary hypoadrenalism—may result in hypoglycemic-hypometabolic coma and hypotension.
   2. Secondary hypothyroidism.
   3. Secondary hypogonadism.
   4. Dwarfism, if growth is incomplete.
   5. Diabetes insipidis, if stalk transection is high.
   6. Greatly increased sensitivity to insulin (important when hypophysectomy is done for control of diabetic retinopathy).

D. Hypothalamic control of temperature regulation
   1. The main "thermostat" is the anterior hypothalamus—preoptic region. Electrostimulation results in heat loss and reduction of shivering. Hypothermia is produced.
   2. Electrostimulation of the posterior hypothalamus results in shivering with a resultant hyperthermia. A lesion here prevents shivering and vasomotor response to cold.

E. Hypothalamic control of feeding and drinking
   1. Stimulation of the lateral hypothalamus produces feeding and drinking responses. Destruction of the ventromedial nucleus also results in hyperphagia.
   2. Destruction of the lateral hypothalamus results in aphagia and adipsia. Stimulation of the ventromedial nucleus inhibits feeding.
   3. Stimulation of the amygdala inhibits feeding, while ablation pro-

duces hyperphagia (similar to the results of ventromedial hypothalamic studies).

4. Other limbic structures have both facilitatory and inhibitory influences upon feeding and drinking (e.g. medial forebrain bundle, midbrain limbic region).
5. Glucoreceptors in addition to the osmoreceptors and volume receptors of the hypothalamus play a role.

F. Hypothalamus and emotional behavior

The hypothalamus is a key region in old-brain integration. It is critically located between the brain stem core, the limbic system and the pituitary. It appears to play a major role in the translation of neural and hormonal activity into mood and expressional emotive behavior. The decorticate animal still exhibits such behavior. The cerebral substrate of emotional activity has traditionally been regarded as limbic-hypothalamic. The principle pathway mediating limbic influence to the hypothalamus is the medial forebrain bundle. By way of analogy, this bidirectional multiple fiber system is the internal capsule of the old-brain. It connects the frontoseptal region with the hypothalamus and midbrain tegmentum. It is joined by many descending systems as it passes into the lateral hypothalamic area. Included are fibers from the medial orbitofrontal, frontopolar and premotor cortex, cingulum, paraolfactory area (septum), caudate head and globus pallidus, amygdala and hippocampus (via the septum), and preoptic region. The hippocampus (via the fornix) projects to the mammillary body. The fornix has additional septal, hypothalamic and tegmental projections. These additional fornical fibers join with the medial forebrain bundle in the diffuse hypothalamo—tegmental tract which descends into the midbrain core (limbic midbrain region). Additional systems which play a role in hypothalamic-limbic integration are as listed below:

1. Mammillothalamic tract-mammillary body to anterior thalamic tubercle (in turn to cingulum; in turn to medial forebrain bundle).
2. Periventricular system-hypothalamus to medial dorsal nucleus (in turn to frontal lobe; in turn to the medial forebrain bundle).
3. Reticular formation, lateral hypothalamic projections. Reticular fibers terminate in the hypothalamus (pituitary activating system), septum and basal forebrain.

The limbic system thus funnels its influences into the hypothalamus from many sources, largely via the medial forebrain bundle. A telencephalic-diencephalic-endocrine substrate provides the background for emotive experience. Examples of experimental production of affective behavior include the following:

1. Stimulation.

a. Rage attacks—from anterior hypothalamic, amygdala and tegmental sites (periaqueductal limbic midbrain area).
b. Escape reactions—from intermediate hypothalamic and tegmental sites.
c. Pleasure reactions—from septal, hippocampal and lateral hypothalamic sites.

2. Ablation.
a. Decortication—rage is the usual emotive expression; pleasure reactions require an intact limbic—diencephalic system.
b. Ventromedian hypothalamic lesions result in rage attacks.
c. Bilateral amygdala destruction—these animals tend to be placid, and without evidence of fear or rage on appropriate stimulation. Hyperphagia, psychic blindness and hypersexual activity are notable (Kluver-Bucy preparation).

G. Hypothalamus and sleep—electrostimulation and focal lesions at many levels of the old-brain are productive of sleep. Arousal similarly has been experimentally produced at many levels of the brain stem reticular core, paleothalamus and limbic system. Focal lesions within the reticular core of the brain stem, and those along the lateral walls and floor of the third ventricle (i.e. hypothalamus) result in hypersomnia and coma. The neurophysiology of both reticular activation and suppression is included in the brain stem section (see Chapter 11).

NEUROSURGICAL SYNDROMES OF THE PERICHIASMATIC REGION

Development of the Perichiasmatic Syndromes

A. Pituitary apoplexy syndrome—acute visual disturbance, stupor-coma and shock; acute hypopituitarism; acute intrasellar-subarachnoid hemorrhage; usually due to hemorrhage into a chromophobe adenoma; may be due to intrasellar aneurysm.

B. Infraclinoid aneurysm—acute supraorbital-retroorbital pain, acute ophthalmoplegia and visual loss; exophthalmos; expansion of an intracavernous aneurysm laterally produces ophthalmoplegia (3,4,6) and pain; expansion medially produces an intrasellar aneurysm which may compress the chiasm and pituitary without ophthalmoplegia and supraorbital pain.

C. Supraclinoid aneurysm—visual loss usually derives from an anterior communicating-anterior cerebral aneurysm above the chiasm or from a supracavernous carotid aneurysm lateral to the chiasm; less often an intrasellar aneurysm; less often associated with ophthalmoplegia (3,4,6) than the infraclinoid type; acute diplopia with oculomotor paralysis but sparing the optic system is common in posterior communicating-carotid aneurysm.

D. Acute opticochiasmatic trauma—acute visual loss; may be associated with transection of the infundibular stalk and hypothalamic injury with early diabetes insipidis; intrasellar hemorrhage with acute hypopituitarism or infarction of the pars distalis with chronic post-traumatic hypopituitarism; coma out of proportion to the degree of head injury should suggest hypothalamo-hypophyseal trauma.

E. Acute hydrocephalus in the childhood craniopharyngioma—commonly associated with visual loss and hypopituitarism, and less often with hypothalamic endocrinopathy; usually due to third ventricular block at the foramen of Monro, less often to cisternal block.

F. Acute hydrocephalus in the childhood posterior fossa tumor—may produce a pseudochiasmatic syndrome with bitemporal hemianopia and even sellar enlargement due to intrasellar third ventricular herniation. Non-neoplastic obstructive hydrocephalus (e.g. aqueductal stenosis) may also be responsible.

G. Progressive pituitary tumor syndrome—sellar expansion and optic-chiasmatic compression are common. Hypopituitarism and chromophobe adenoma (Fig. 60) are commonest in the adult. Craniopharyngioma (Fig. 61) is the commonest intrasellar tumor in the child, although this tumor also occurs in the adult with hypopituitarism and visual loss. Eosinophilic adenoma with hyperpituitarism (gigantism in the child and acromegaly in the adult) may be responsible. Intrasellar aneurysm can mimic the sellar-chiasmatic-hypopituitary syndrome closely.

H. Optico-chiasmatic arachnoditis—the late result of previous traumatic, hemorrhagic or inflammatory basal meningitis; may mimic a progressive chiasmatic syndrome with visual loss, optic atrophy and a normal sella.

I. Basal glioma syndromes—the optic glioma of childhood is a relatively slow growing astrocytoma which may involve the optic nerve alone, or nerve-chiasm, tract and hypothalamus. It is commonly associated with von Recklinghausen's disease. Astrocytoma within the diencephalon may also compress the chiasm from above. A frontal astrocytoma may mimic the olfactory meningioma presenting optic atrophy and crossed papilledema.

J. Basal meningioma syndromes—the tuberculum and anterior clinoidal meningiomas, although slowly growing, compress the basal optic pathway earlier than the larger olfactory meningioma. The typical patient is an adult woman, although they occur in both sexes. These meniningiomas compress the optic nerve(s) and anterior chiasm, while the large middle sphenoid (alar) meningioma may compress the optic tract or lateral

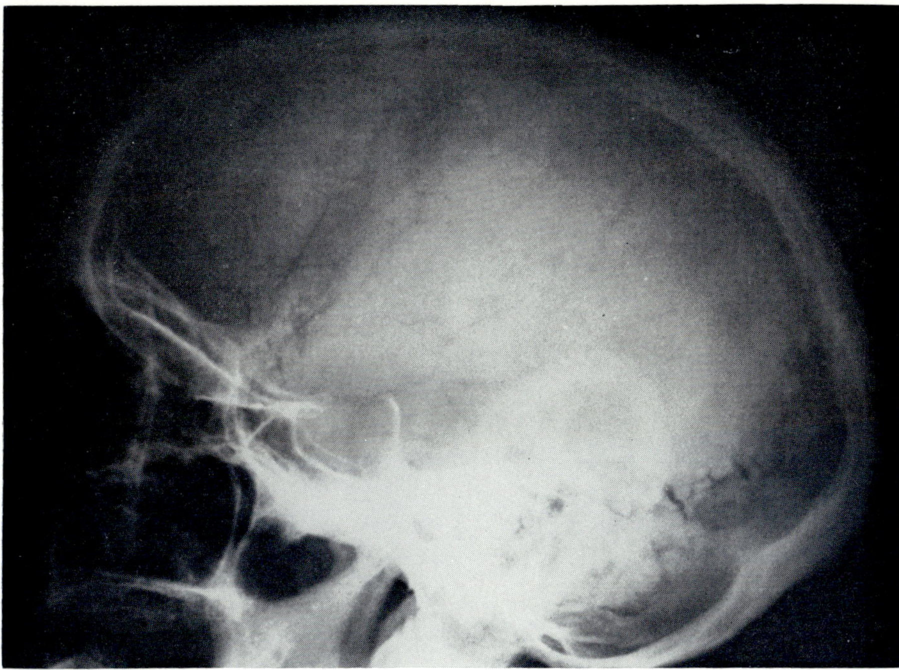

Figure 60. Chromophobe adenoma.

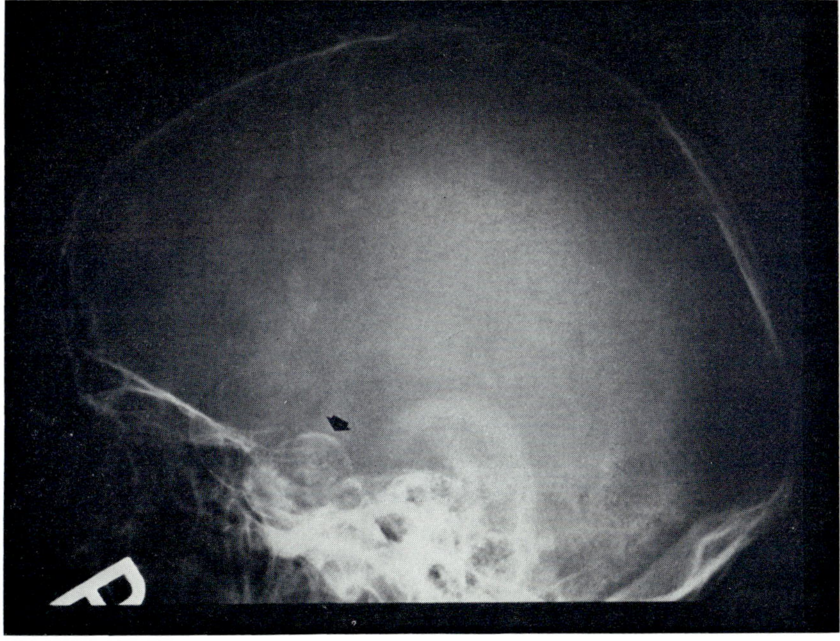

Figure 61. Intrasellar craniopharyngioma.

chiasm. Moderate to slowly progressive visual loss, optic atrophy and normal sellar size in the adult should suggest meningioma. Early oculomotor palsy and exophthalmos associated with these findings points to the inner sphenoid ridge. Anosmia and impaired mental acuity point to the anterior fossa where a large olfactory meningioma may be responsible for these signs as well as visual impairment.

K. Foster Kennedy syndrome—unilateral optic atrophy with crossed papilledema is an unusual combination, suggesting the anterior fossa basal meningioma or frontobasal glioma. The syndrome is not absolutely pathognomic for tumor, however.

Deficits of the Perichiasmatic Syndromes

Perichiasmatic syndromes are of six types.

1. Sellar-chiasmatic.
2. Rostrochiasmatic.
3. Ventriculochiasmatic.
4. Retrochiasmatic.
5. Laterochiasmatic.
6. Intrachiasmatic.

The intracranial optic nerve and optic tract syndromes are included with the rostro- and retrochiasmatic syndromes respectively. Most tumors (e.g. chromophobe adenoma, tuberculum meningioma) compressing the intracranial optic nerve are apt also to involve the chiasm. Tumors compressing the optic tract (e.g. craniopharygioma) commonly also involve the chiasm. The three visual signs of greatest importance in perichiasmatic diagnosis are deterioration in visual acuity, defects in visual fields and primary optic atrophy.

Deterioration in Visual Acuity

Failure of central visual acuity is the single most critical factor, for it brings the patient to medical attention even when other symptoms have failed. Visual acuity depends upon macular vision. Since all the macular fibers serving monocular central vision are contained within the optic nerve, compression of the optic nerve at any level virtually always produces central scotoma and acuity failure. Peripheral wedge-shaped defects or complete monocular blindness also occur. Even when both optic nerves are compressed, acuity failure is more prominent on one side first. Binocular vision begins with the chiasm. Macular fibers, like extramacular fibers, semidecussate. Central vision in the chiasm is thus served by both crossed and uncrossed macular fibers. While nasal extramacular fibers cross in the anterior chiasm, nasal macular fibers cross in the posterior chiasm. In order for central visual acuity to fail due to strictly chiasmatic compression, both crossed and uncrossed macular fibers of the same eye must be compromised. "Splitting" of the macula is not enough by itself to impair acuity. Even though the vertical hemianopic meridian passes through the fixation point, ocular compensation permits the intact macular half to preserve acuity. "Sparing" of the macula with peripheral field defects, similarly prevents acuity failure. In median chiasmatic compression of crossing macular fibers, visual acuity deteriorates (macular loss) only upon progressive involvement of uncrossed macular fibers in the lateral chiasm, or upon coincident compression of the optic nerve. The optic tract, in addition to its extramacular component, contains the crossed macular bundle of the opposite eye and the uncrossed macular fibers of the ipsilateral eye. The maximal lesion of the optic tract can only impair one-half of macular and extramacular vision for each eye. The tract lesion thus spares acuity until the chiasm is also involved. Acuity is also spared with unilateral lesions of the optic radiation or visual cortex, which must be bilaterally involved to produce acuity failure.

The chiasm is inclined as much as a 45° angle upward with regard to the sella (chiasmatic tilt). In fact, the entire basal optic pathway ascends toward the brain. The chiasm is usually centrally fixed over the dorsum or diaphragm. If the optic nerves are unusually short, the chiasm is prefixed at the tuberculum. If the optic nerves are excessively long, the chiasm is postfixed behind the dorsum sellae. The height of the chiasm above the diaphragm may vary from 0 to 10 mm. The optic nerves enter the cranial cavity just medial to the anterior clinoids of the sella. Despite the height of the chiasm, and despite the length of the optic nerves, the latter are always closer to the sellar content and to the dome of the typical pituitary tumor than are the optic tracts. The anatomical relationship of optic nerves and chiasm to the sella sets the stage for central visual failure. The intracranial tumors producing relatively early loss of central acuity are perichiasmatic, usually benign and extracerebral. In the adult, pituitary adenomas are most common. Space-occupying perichiasmatic aneurysms must always be ruled out. Malignant intracerebral tumors of the caudal half of the brain, even though they may destroy the optic radiation, tend to spare central visual acuity until secondary optic atrophy consequent to papilledema occurs. Malignant gliomas of the frontal lobe, even though they spare the optic radiation, nonetheless may produce central blindness by optic-chiasmatic compression with primary atrophy, or later acuity loss due to secondary atrophy after papilledema.

Defects in Visual Fields

Cushing noted that the "signature" of chiasmatic involvement is bitemporal hemianopia. This results from median compromise of crossing naso-retinal fibers which occurs only in the chiasm. This highly localizing sign has no counterpart in the optic nerve or tract. Purely monocular blindness results from ocular, intraorbital or intracranial optic nerve involvement. Homonymous hemianopia results from a tract, geniculate, radiation or visual cortical lesion. The commonest cause of bitemporal hemianopia is tumor, while the commonest source of homonymous hemianopia is stroke. Despite the great localizing value of the bitemporal defect, tumor diagnosis may yet be delayed with blindness the result. The reasons include the following:

1. Bitemporal defects may be asymptomatic until central visual acuity failure.
2. Bitemporal defects may be subtle and early defects readily escape gross confrontation.
3. Early bitemporal defects are often scotomatous and will be missed by formal perimetry at 3/330, but can be elicited by tangent screen testing using small (1/2000) white objects.
4. Bitemporal scotomas identified on tangent screen evaluation may then be misinterpreted as the scotomas of demyelinating or other nonsurgical optic involvement.
5. Bitemporal scotomas can be due to a rapidly advancing pituitary tumor already beyond the confines of the sella.
6. Unusual field defects other than bitemporal hemianopia also occur with chiasmatic lesions, again simulating nonsurgical disease.

Bitemporal hemianopia is only complete when the entire median chiasm is compromised (i.e. a functional longitudinal transection). A partial peripheral bitemporal hemianopia occurs with anterior median chiasmatic compression (i.e. extramacular decussation). To this may be added the central scotoma of optic nerve involvement at the anterior chiasmatic angle. The central scotoma of the chiasmatic lesion is unilateral or bilateral. The unilateral central scotoma of chiasmatic origin is differentiated from that of intraorbital optic origin by the presence of bitemporal peripheral field loss. Junctional scotoma with a central scotoma and crossed temporal peripheral field loss points to the intracranial segment of the optic nerve just before joining the chiasm. This "optic root" of the chiasm contains fibers of the opposite optic nerve which have crossed ventrally in the anterior chiasm, looped into the optic root and then turned back toward the optic tract. In contrast, a posterior median chiasmatic compromise produces central bitemporal hemianopic scotomas (i.e. macular decussation). These scotomas stop at the vertical midline as long as uncrossed fibers escape. To these bitemporal scotomas may be superimposed the incongruous homonymous hemianopia of optic tract involvement at the posterior chiasmatic angle.

When the chiasm is involved from below, quadrant loss proceeds from the superior temporal field; when suprachiasmatic pressure is exerted, quadrant loss proceeds from the inferior temporal field. Nasal and binasal hemianopias indicate lateral chiasmatic compression. Still more bizarre and irregular field defects indicate intrachiasmatic tumor.

Primary Optic Atrophy

This is the least dependable of the three major signs of perichiasmatic tumor. At the time the patient with visual failure is initially seen, the fundi may appear deceptively normal. Primary atrophy takes a number of weeks before it is apparent on fundoscopy. It appears earliest and is most prominent with optic nerve involvement, then in chiasmatic involvement, and appears latest and least when due to a tract lesion. Once apparent, optic atrophy roughly parallels visual acuity impairment. However, in certain instances of extramacular atrophy with partial macular fiber escape, white discs may accompany surprisingly good central vision. Formal perimetric and tangent screen examinations are thus imperative in all cases of acuity failure, despite the presence of normal discs. Despite its limitations, primary optic atrophy remains an important sign. When present with homonymous hemianopia, it indicates an optic tract lesion, rather than an optic radiation or cortical lesion. When optic atrophy is due to a lesion compressing the median chiasm, it is bilateral. At first it may appear that normal bitemporal pallor is increased, while the temporal disc edges are sharpened. This appears as a paradoxical sign in view of concurrent bitemporal hemianopia. When atrophy results from a lesion at the anterior chiasmatic angle, involving one optic nerve, the atrophy of the ipsilateral disc is greater, especially in its temporal portion. The signs of primary optic atrophy include the following:

1. Pallor, whiteness or slight blueness of the disc.
2. Unusually sharp definition of the disc.
3. Flatness of the disc.
4. Persistence of the spots of the lamina cribrosa.
5. Obliteration of some or all of the "ten small vessels." circumferentially crossing the disc edge.
6. Persistence of the four to five larger arteries and four to five larger veins which also cross the disc edge.

Papilledema is relatively uncommon in the perichiasmatic syndromes. Bitemporal hemianopia combined with papilledema suggests craniopharyngioma. Cerebellar tumor with papilledema and third ventricular hydrocephalus can produce a false-localizing bitemporal cut. A large basal meningioma or large chromophobe tumor with third ventricular obstruction can produce choked discs with bitemporal cuts, but pale atrophic discs are much more common at this late stage.

A. Deficits of the sellar-chiasmatic syndrome

This syndrome is the result of an expanding mass, usually a chromophobe adenoma, originating within the sella turcica. The neurosurgical syndrome is "sellar-chiasmatic" because of the following reasons:

1. Both the initial and late symptoms of the pituitary adenoma are most commonly visual.
2. Visual impairment is a clear indication for neurosurgical intervention.

The sellar mass is often well beyond the actual confines of the sella at the time of its clinical emergence. The suprasellar extension may be as much as 2 cm before chiasmatic compression sufficient to produce visual symptoms occurs. Headaches are often negligible at the time of the onset of visual symptoms. The symptoms and signs of pituitary endocrinopathy are typically gradual in their development. The significance of amenorrhea may have been overlooked. Even bitemporal visual loss may have escaped notice especially when restricted to the superior temporal quadrants. In contrast, the onset of unilateral central blindness, due either to optic nerve or chiasmatic compression by the rising tumor, is dramatic. While unilateral visual loss is the common presenting complaint, occasionally bilateral acuity failure is noted at the outset. The patient typically describes cloudy vision or a veil before the eye, perhaps only noted upon fatigue or in a dimly lit room. He thinks he needs new glasses. The bitemporal hemianopia, when complete, reveals itself when the patient reports bumping into objects at his sides; the need to turn his head more frequently to the sides is noted especially when driving. Reading may suffer as a result of either central loss or inability to clearly see the left side of the page. The lateral skull x-ray reveals the typical "ballooned" sella turcica characterizing intrasellar origin of the mass. When the sella is ballooned, but visual symptoms are absent, it is not safe to assume sparing of the visual pathway. Normal acuity, normal fundi and normal confrontation fields do not prove that the optic system is spared. Formal perimetry and formal tangent screen testing is indicated. Any visual deficiencies obtained should be regarded as evidence of optic pathway compression by the sellar mass, even though the classical morphology of bitemporal hemianopia may not be detected.

Headaches of the sellar tumor are nonpathognomonic. While nonspecific, they are often bifrontal or retro-orbital. They are not the headaches of elevated intracranial pressure. The headaches of intracranial hypertension with associated vomiting occur in a small proportion of sellar tumors with third ventricular extension and should always raise the possibility of craniopharyngioma. Irritability may replace headache in the craniopharyngioma of childhood. In the adult, unusually severe headaches occur with the eosinophilic adenoma of acromegaly even when the tumor is not very large. Rupture of a pituitary tumor through the sellar diaphragm may temporarily relieve headaches. Unusually severe headaches always suggest aneurysm. Severe unilateral supraorbital or ocular pain should suggest intracavernous aneurysm or neoplastic invasion of the cavernous sinus. Bifrontal headache with transient diplopia is common in chromophobe adenoma and is due to lateral pressure on the wall of the cavernous sinus without actual invasion. Rupture into the sphenoid sinus may produce the congested sensation of the sinus headache, sometimes associated with CSF rhinorrhea. Headaches associated with fever and purulent nasal discharge in the patient with an enlarged sella may be due to sphenoiditis with sellar abscess. A sphenoid mucopyocele may be present.

1. Differential diagnosis of the sellar mass.
   a. Pituitary tumor.
      (1) Chromophobe adenoma.
         (a) Most common expanding intrasellar mass in the adult.
         (b) Usually associated with hypopituitarism.
      (2) Eosinophilic adenoma.
         (a) Produces hyperpituitarism in the adult in the form of acromegaly.
         (b) Produces hyperpituitarism in the child in the form of gigantism.
         (c) Frequently, the pituitary tumor associated with acromegaly proves to be a chromophobe adenoma on routine pathological study.
      (3) Basophilic adenoma.
         (a) Rarely expand the sella.
         (b) Associated with Cushing's syndrome.
         (c) May produce a sellar-chiasmatic mass after adrenalectomy for Cushing's syndrome.
      (4) Mixed pituitary adenoma.
      (5) Primary pituitary carcinoma.
   b. Craniopharyngioma.
      (1) May be extrasellar, intrasellar or both.
      (2) Usually in childhood, but also in adult life.
      (3) The most common intrasellar mass of childhood.
      (4) The most common perichiasmatic tumor to produce signs of elevated intracranial pressure.

(5) Associated with endocrinopathic signs in many but not all cases.

(6) Visual symptoms may be the only manifestations of craniopharyngioma in adult life (Fig. 62).

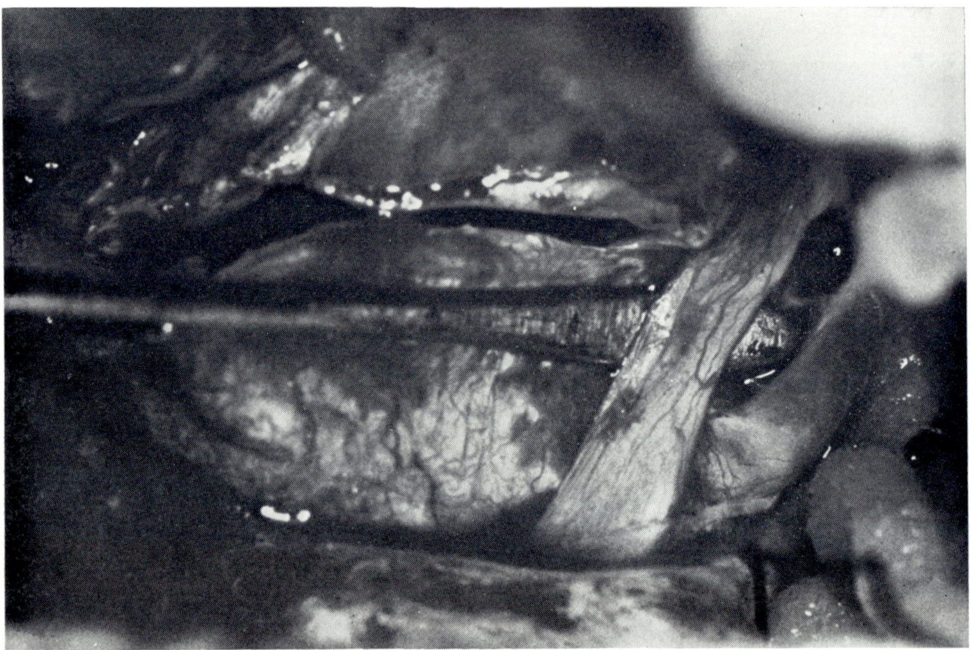

Figure 62. Intrasellar-extrasellar craniopharyngioma with optic nerve compression.

c. Intrasellar aneurysm.
   (1) Usually due to infraclinoid carotid aneurysm, but may occur with supraclinoid aneurysms.
   (2) May enlarge the sella.
   (3) May produce hypopituitarism.
   (4) May compress the basal optic pathway just like a pituitary tumor.

d. Sellar abscess.
   (1) Uncommon.
   (2) Associated with sphenoidal sinusitis or sphenoidal mucocele.

e. Pseudosellar mass syndrome.
   (1) Empty sella syndrome—intrasellar subarachnoid cyst (Fig. 63).
   (2) Third ventricular hydrops syndrome—intrasellar herniation of the hydrocephalic third ventricle (Fig. 64).
   (3) Suprasellar mass with apparent enlargement of sella turcica—erodes the clinoids from above rather than from beneath.

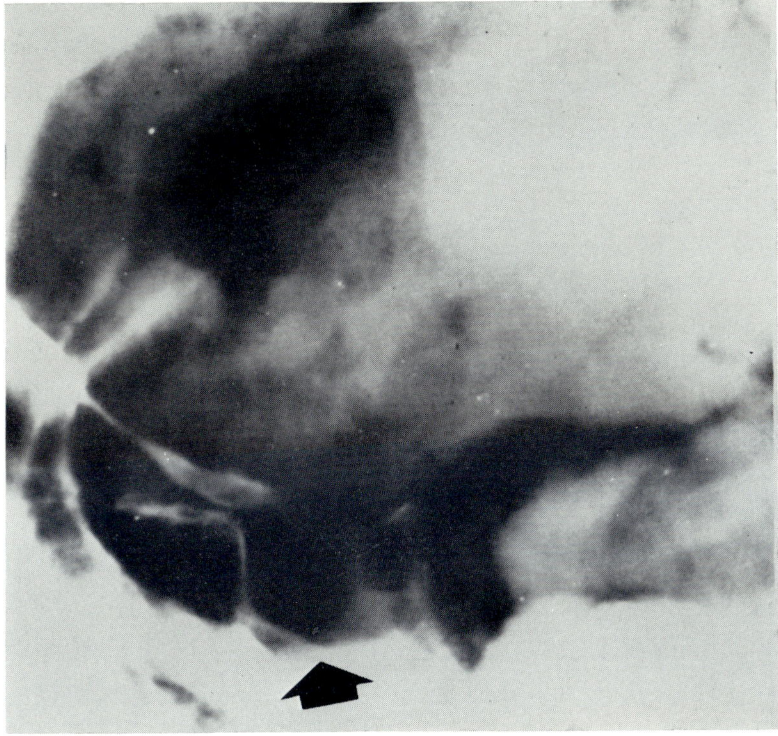

Figure 63. Empty sella. The enlarged sella fills with air on pneumography.

(4) Diffuse increase in intracranial pressure with apparent enlargement of the sella—erodes the dorsum, posterior clinoids and floor of the sella from above (pressure atrophy of the sella).

(5) Pseudo-double floor—calcification in the carotid wall suggests the double floor sign of expanding intrasellar tumor.

2. Ophthalmological signs of the sellar-chiasmatic syndrome.
   a. Bitemporal field defects which begin in the upper temporal quadrants—in the very early stage the quadrant loss may be limited to only one eye.
   b. Sellar mass sequence—quadrant involvement proceeds from the upper temporal to lower temporal to lower nasal to upper nasal. Complete bitemporal hemianopia may appear to be stationary for a long period before spread to the inferior nasal quadrant begins. This does not indicate cessation of tumor growth. In median tumors, the lateral chiasmatic fibers (i.e. subserving nasal visual fields) are laterally displaced before being more directly compressed.

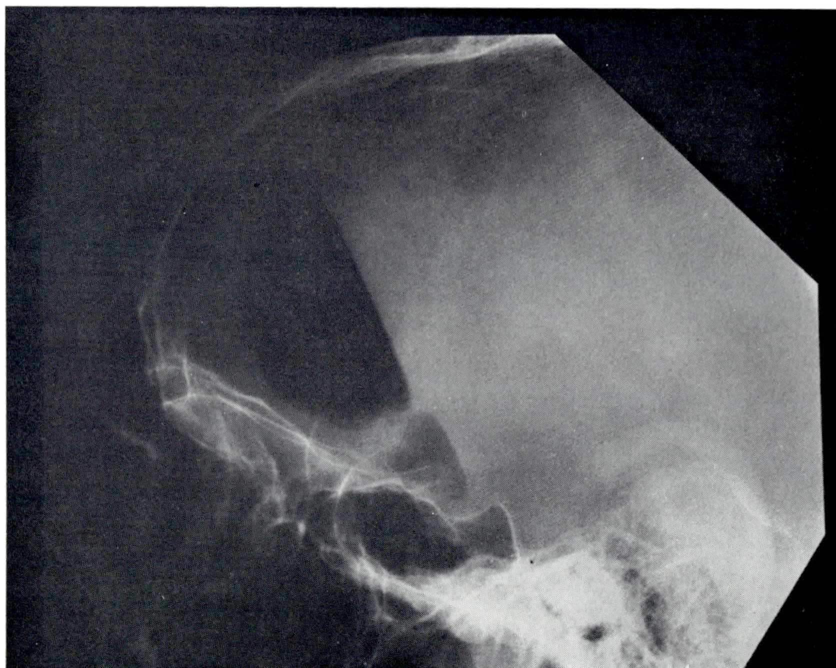

Figure 64. Intrasellar hydrops of the third ventricle. Hydrocephalus including the third ventricle is present. The posterior sellar elements are obliterated. The floor of the expanded third ventricle lies within the sella.

c. Relative symmetry of bitemporal hemianopia—this is more common in the sellar-chiasmatic syndrome than in chiasmatic compression due to a strictly extrasellar mass.

d. Central scotoma (macular loss) and poor visual acuity on one side—involvement of one optic nerve at the anterior chiasmatic angle is common.

e. Complete monocular blindness with contralateral temporal hemianopia—this occurs both with the sellar mass as well as with extrasellar tumors in which the sella is not enlarged. This visual field deficit is almost as common as bitemporal hemianopia due to pituitary tumors. It can result from anterior lesions which compress the optic nerve and chiasm, or from posterior lesions of the chiasm and optic tract.

f. Homonymous hemianopia without other visual deficit is uncommon in the sellar mass. It may occur with prefixation of the chiasm with compression limited to the optic tract. Eccentric tumor growth to the lateral chiasm or middle fossa tumor extension to the temporal lobe may produce homonymous defects.

g. Sudden onset of unilateral blindness should suggest an aneurysm.
h. Optic atrophy—may or may not be present.
i. Papilledema—usually absent in the sellar-chiasmatic syndrome.

3. Endocrine signs of the sellar-chiasmatic syndrome.
   a. Hypopituitarism and sellar mass in the adult.
      (1) The commonest mass is the chromophobe adenoma.
      (2) Typical endocrine syndrome is as follows:
         (a) Amenorrhea is an early sign. Decreased pubic and axillary hair is common; galactorrhea, either spontaneous or induced by nipple compression, may occur.
         (b) In the male, loss of libido and impotence are common. Decreased body hair and infrequency of shaving are noted. Testicular atrophy may occur.
         (c) Symptomatic hypoglycemia, hypotension, easy fatigue and poor stress tolerance are common. Addisonian hyperpigmentation is absent.
         (d) Mild cold intolerance, constipation, dry skin and brittle nails are not uncommon.
      (3) Atypical endocrine syndromes are as follow:
         (a) Pituitary myxedema—full-blown severe hypothyroidism may rarely be due to pituitary tumor. The full spectrum of symptoms and signs includes loss of mental acuity, lethargy, hearing loss and hoarseness. Precordial pain and distal extremity pain and paresthesia may occur. A puffy face with loss of nasolabial folds, loss of the outer parts of the eyebrows, brittle hair with alopecia, thickened lips and sallow color is characteristic. Cardiomegaly, distant heart sounds, hypotension and bradycardia occur. Deep tendon reflexes are "hung-up" (i.e. delayed relaxation). Hypothermia is typical in the rare instances of myxedema coma.
         (b) Late acromegaly—in well-advanced acromegaly due to eosinophilic adenoma, late onset hypopituitarism may replace previous hyperpituitary function. Generalized weakness, weight loss, hypotension and hypothyroidism are then superimposed upon the prominent acromegalic features.
         (c) Acute hypopituitarism—this may occur as a result of hemorrhage into a chromophobe adenoma (pituitary apoplexy). Acute diplopia or blindness followed by stiff neck, retinal hemorrhage and stupor or coma may occur. Shock with circulatory collapse ensues. This contrasts with the progressive

systemic hypertension which usually accompanies the other acute comas associated with intracranial hemorrhage.

b. Hypopituitarism and the craniopharyngioma.
   (1) The commonest intrasellar mass in the child is the craniopharyngioma, pituitary tumors and aneurysms being rare.
   (2) The usual extrasellar craniopharyngioma is accompanied by an intrasellar extension with sellar enlargement in approximately half the childhood cases.
   (3) The typical presentation of the childhood craniopharyngioma is with elevated intracranial pressure due to third ventricular (and cisternal) block.
   (4) Pituitary dwarfism—when due to a craniopharyngioma, skeletal growth is arrested at the stage when the pars distalis is destroyed. Body proportions remain normal and sexual infantilism persists. Primary amenorrhea results. Birth size is normal.
   (5) Skin is pale, smooth and hairless.
   (6) Loss of normal childhood energy is common.
   (7) Slight weight gain with relative anorexia and other signs of mild hypothyroidism are common. Obesity with hyperphagia is uncommon even when the hypothalamus is compressed by the craniopharyngioma.
   (8) Severe reduction in weight (pituitary cachexia) is also uncommon; the similarity of such severe wasting to that seen in the hypothalamic astrocytoma (diencephalic syndrome) is great.
   (9) Hypotension, bradycardia and hypothermia may be present.
   (10) Diabetes insipidis is an uncommon presenting sign at the time of clinical diagnosis.
   (11) Drowsiness and stupor are usually due to increased intracranial pressure with extension into the third ventricle, rather than to hypothalamic involvement without elevated pressure.
   (12) Craniopharygioma is also a tumor of adult life, when it is much less common than pituitary tumor. Visual failure with or without endocrine deficit is the presenting complaint, rather than symptoms of intracranial hypertension of the childhood craniopharyngioma.

c. Hyperpituitarism and the sellar mass—this combination almost invariably indicates the presence of a pituitary adenoma with excessive growth hormone production. The pituitary tumor may prove to be the classical eosinophilic adenoma, a mixed adenoma, or what appears to be a chromophobe without chromophilic components. Several syndrome variants occur.

(1) Acromegaly—this occurs after epiphyseal closure. While growth is generalized, it is appositional rather than linear. Such growth excess is most prominent at the "acra" or terminal body points (e.g. jaw, hands, feet).

(2) Gigantism—this occurs before normal epiphyseal closure and results in excessive linear growth in the youth. Following closure of epiphyseal lines, the hyperpituitary giant may develop typical acromegalic features.

(3) Acromegalism—this refers to cyclic spurts of increased hormonal activity in the acromegalic. Such cycles occur relatively independently of growth in bulk of the tumor. Smaller tumors which do not compress the chiasm may produce extensive growth distortion. Following cessation of such a phase of acromegalism, the tumor may continue its expansion and ultimately compress the chiasm.

(4) Fugitive acromegaly—this is a partial or early form in which few acromegalic features are present, in spite of an expanding eosinophilic adenoma.

(5) Late acromegaly—in the advanced stage, signs of hypopituitarism (hypothyroidism, generalized weakness, weight loss, hypotension) may be superimposed upon the acromegalic features.

(6) Symptoms and signs of acromegaly—a normal intact sella is uncommon in eosinophilic adenoma. However, while an expanded sella is present in the great majority of cases, the basal optic pathway often escapes compression by this tumor. While both headache and visual loss occur in both tumors, severe headaches are more characteristic of the eosinophilic adenoma, while visual loss more typically occurs in the chromophobe adenoma. Diagnosis of the acromegalic is often made earlier. The severe analgesic-resistant headaches, the presence of malocclusion of the teeth, and diabetes mellitus may bring the patient to medical attention before visual failure. As in the chromophobe adenoma, amenorrhea and loss of libido are early signs. The development of typical acromegalic features is a gradual process which may escape early recognition. Larger rings, gloves, shoes, collars and hats are required. The fully developed syndrome reveals prognathism of the lower jaw. The teeth are widely spaced and leave their impressions on the upper surface of an enlarged tongue. The voice is hoarse. The lips and nose are thickened. The brow is prominent and may even result in a superior altitudinal defect on visual field test-

ing. The scalp is wrinkled. There is hypertrichosis and hyperpigmentation of the skin. The skin is coarse, thick and oily. Perspiration is excessive and malodorous. The neck is thick, and goiter, usually nonfunctional, is often present. The shoulders are stooped and there is dorsal kyphosis of the chest. Evidence of cardiomegaly is common, while splanchnomegaly often escapes detection on abdominal examination. Testicular atrophy may be present, along with loss of pubic and axillary hair. The extremities reveal moderate muscular wasting, but findings are most marked distally. The palm and fingers are broadened and thickened. The hand cannot be completely clenched shut. The feet are long, wide and flat. At the time these patients present visual symptoms, the acromegalic syndrome may be partial or complete. Previously severe headaches may have subsided with rupture of the tumor through the sellar diaphragm. However, the cephalic pains are replaced by the spinal pain accompanying osteoporosis, kyphosis and arthritis. Extremity pains and paresthesias are also common.

(7) Nonacromegalic hyperpituitarism—excessive pituitary secretion apart from growth hormone, with tumor mass sufficient to produce a sellar-chiasmatic syndrome, is unusual.

- (a) The basophilic adenoma—these do not produce a sellar mass; they are usually asymptomatic; they are found in approximately half the cases of Cushing's syndrome with adrenocortical hyperplasia.
- (b) The basophilic carcinoma—these are rare tumors which secrete excess ACTH; they are found in patients with Cushing's syndrome who have an unusual degree of hyperpigmentation.
- (c) The chromophobe adenoma—following bilateral adrenalectomy for Cushing's syndrome, an ACTH-producing pituitary tumor may balloon the sella and compress the chiasm. The tumor consists of agranular cells which may be degranulated basophils. These patients also develop unusually marked hyperpigmentation.
- (d) The presence of hyperpigmentation in Cushing's syndrome of hyperadrenocorticalism should raise the possibility of chromophobe adenoma or basophilic carcinoma. In contrast, the absence of hyperpigmentation in an otherwise typical case of addisonian hypoadrenocorticalism should raise the question of hypopituitarism (and chromophobe adenoma if the sella is expanded).

(e) Symptoms and signs of Cushing's syndrome— these hyper-adrenocortical manifestations may be associated with adrenal hyperplasia, with adrenal and pituitary tumors, and less often with tumors of the ovary, lung, thymus and pancreas. The typical patient is an adult woman. The onset is insidious with weight gain, hypomenorrhea and relatively early amenorrhea. Primary amenorrhea and retarded linear growth affect the young female. Loss of libido, impotence and testicular atrophy occur in the adult male. Diabetes mellitus is characteristic, but may be latent in the early stages of the syndrome. The face becomes rounded, reddened and oily with acne and hirsutism. "Buffalo neck" is present. Obesity is trunkal with sparing of the extremities. Examination of the chest reveals purplish striae over the breasts, kyphosis and hypertensive cardiomegaly. The abdomen is particularly obese and striae are most prominent. The striae affect the proximal thighs and leg; ecchymoses and ankle edema are notable.

4. Neurological signs of extension in the sellar-chiasmatic syndrome.
   a. Generalized seizures—indicate tumor (e.g. chromophobe adenoma) extension to the anterior fossa (frontobasal) or to the middle fossa (temporal) ; the presence of homonymous hemianopia usually indicates optic tract compression rather than temporal extension.
   b. Supraorbital hypesthesia—in the absence of intracavernous aneurysm, this indicates actual invasion of the cavernous sinus by tumor.
   c. Supraorbital-infraorbital-mandibular hypesthesia—indicates extension to the middle fossa (Meckel's cave) or to the posterior fossa (sensory root) by invasive tumor.
   d. Oculomotor, trochlear and abducens palsy—complete ophthalmoplegia usually indicates intracavernous aneurysm, but it may be due to invasive pituitary tumor. Sudden ophthalmoplegia favors aneurysm. Transient diplopia without obvious ophthalmoplegia is common in chromophobe adenoma which has not extended beyond the confines of the sella. In the great majority of cases the pituitary adenoma responsible for a sellar-chiasmatic syndrome does not invade the cavernous sinus or the anterior, middle or posterior fossae.
   e. Isolated oculomotor palsy with sellar ballooning.
      (1) Infraclinoid (cavernous) carotid aneurysm.
      (2) Extrasellar extension of pituitary tumor.
      (3) Intrasellar-extrasellar craniopharyngioma.

Note: Isolated oculomotor palsy without sellar ballooning.

(1) Supraclinoid (posterior communicating) aneurysm more commonly than infraclinoid aneurysm.
(2) Intraorbital tumor.
(3) Inner sphenoidal (clinoidal) meningioma.
(4) Gassero-petrosal meningioma or neuroma.
(5) Extrasellar craniopharyngioma.
(6) Chordoma.
(7) Nasopharyngeal carcinoma or metastatic carcinoma of the cranial base.
(8) Any supratentorial mass during transtentorial herniation.
(9) Hydrocephalic attack.
(10) Periaqueductal glioma of the brain stem.

f. Isolated abducens palsy—usually due to third ventricular extension of tumor with hydrocephalus and elevated intracranial pressure. Papilledema is typically absent in pituitary tumor even when intracranial hypertension due to ventricular block exists.

g. Cerebrospinal fluid rhinorrhea, meningitis—these complications indicate tumor extension to the sphenoid sinus.

h. Loss of mental acuity—may accompany advanced visual loss, subfrontal and hypothalamic compression, or ventricular block with hydrocephalus.

i. Coma—extension of tumor to the third ventricle with acute block of the foramen of Monro and hydrocephalus; hemorrhage into chromophobe adenoma (pituitary apoplexy); rupture of an aneurysm.

B. Deficits of the rostrochiasmatic syndrome

Cushing's classical chiasmatic syndrome consisted of bitemporal field defects, primary optic atrophy and an unexpanded sella. This triad is due to the suprasellar lesion which compresses the anterior-superior (i.e. rostral) chiasm and optic nerve(s). In contrast, the lesion below the chiasm commonly expands the sella, while the lesion behind the chiasm is less apt to result in early marked optic atrophy. Meningiomas are the most frequent source of rostral chiasmatic compression with an unexpanded sella. Mass lesions producing the syndrome may erode the anterior clinoid process (meningioma or aneurysm). The anterior clinoid and tuberculum sella may be hyperostotic as a result of regional meningiomas. The anterior cerebral and anterior communicating arteries lie just dorsal to the optic nerves at the anterior chiasmatic angle. The optic nerves and anterior chiasm lie within the subarachnoid space, in contrast to the posterior-superior chiasm within the third ventricular floor. The tumors (and aneurysms) responsible for the rostrochiasmatic syndrome are most common in adult life.

1. Differential diagnosis of the rostrochiasmatic syndrome.
   a. Meningiomas.
      (1) Tuberculum meningioma—may compress the anterior angle of the chiasm while still relatively small (in contrast to the olfactory meningioma).
      (2) Clinoidal meningioma—similarly will compress the optic nerve while still relatively small.
      (3) Large olfactory meningioma—this is usually an asymmetrical growth which can compress an optic nerve before it reaches the anterior chiasmatic angle.
   b. Frontal lobe glioma—large frontobasal gliomas can result in optic atrophy from direct optic compression.
   c. Anterior cerebral or anterior communicating aneurysm—may present as a suprachiasmatic mass and less often as an intrasellar mass. Visual loss can be gradual or can occur suddenly. There may be marked fluctuation in headaches and visual symptoms. Sudden visual loss suggests hemorrhage, but can occur with a "minor leak" preceding the major bleeding.
   d. Opticochiasmatic arachnoiditis—traumatic or inflammatory basal meningitis can involve the optic nerves and anterior chiasm within the subarachnoid space. Arachnoidal adhesions may involve the nerve, the chiasm, or both. Most cases of post-traumatic opticochiasmatic arachnoiditis result in visual failure a number of months or years after an injury.
   e. Acute chiasmatic trauma—immediate blindness may result. Head injuries in which the skull is distorted and the optic canals separated can result in a median chiasmal lesion. A classical chiasmatic syndrome with bitemporal hemianopia, optic atrophy and a normal sella results, the atrophy appearing several weeks after the head injury.
   f. Massive sellar tumor with dorsal indentation of the optic nerves and anterior chiasm by the anterior cerebral arteries—this accounts for the paradox of the large sella with an inferior altitudinal field defect. Altitudinal hemianopias are rarely due to chiasmatic lesions.
2. Ophthalmological signs of the rostrochiasmatic syndrome.
   a. Bitemporal field cuts which begin in the inferior temporal quadrants.
   b. Central scotoma (macular loss) with poor acuity on one side is common in addition to the bitemporal cuts.

c. Junctional scotoma due to "optic root" involvement—central scotoma with contralateral peripheral field loss.

d. Optic atrophy—common in meningiomas and in opticochiasmatic arachnoiditis. Any aneurysm compressing the optic nerve or chiasm may be responsible. Unilateral optic atrophy with contralateral papilledema (Foster Kennedy syndrome) suggests an olfactory meningioma or frontal glioma.

e. Involvement of one or both eyes with central or paracentral scotomas and inconstant visual field deficits suggests opticochiasmatic arachnoiditis. Visual loss is usually progressive, but may be sudden. Headaches are common, and with visual loss, may suggest tumor.

f. Visual field testing may be difficult in patients with large frontal gliomas or olfactory meningiomas due to inattention.

g. Clinoidal meningioma—unilateral blindness with a central scotoma is common. There may be greatly asymmetrical bitemporal hemianopia. Unilateral exophthalmos and oculomotor palsy may occur.

3. Endocrine signs of the rostrochiasmatic syndrome—meningiomas and aneurysms compressing the anterosuperior optic nerve and chiasm are typically not associated with any endocrinopathy.

4. Neurological signs of extension in the rostrochiasmatic syndrome—tuberculum and clinoidal meningiomas tend to reach diagnosis relatively early, while olfactory and more laterally situated sphenoidal meningiomas may escape diagnosis until advanced intracranial hypertension is present. Anterior communicating aneurysms, like other berry aneurysms, usually reach diagnosis at the time of subarachnoid hemorrhage.

C. Deficits of the ventriculochiasmatic syndrome

The posterosuperior border of the optic chiasm is incorporated into the anterior third ventricular floor. The posterior chiasm is tilted upward. The macular fibers decussate in this posterior portion of the chiasm. The lateral walls and remaining floor of the third ventricle constitute the hypothalamus which spans the chiasm in its suprachiasmatic portion. This syndrome occurs more often in childhood than in adult life.

1. Differential diagnosis of the ventriculochiasmatic syndrome.

a. Third ventricular hydrocephalus—from intraventricular craniopharyngioma, hypothalamic astrocytoma, pinealoma, posterior fossa tumor, aqueductal stenosis or fourth ventricular outlet obstruction.

   b. Hypothalamic astrocytoma with direct suprachiasmatic compression by tumor mass.
   c. Craniopharyngioma with direct suprachiasmatic compression by tumor mass.
2. Ophthalmological signs of the ventriculochiasmatic syndrome.
   a. Bitemporal hemianopia which begins in the inferior temporal quadrants.
   b. Central visual acuity may remain intact despite macular splitting.
   c. Bitemporal hemianopic scotomata may be especially difficult to detect in childhood.
   d. Papilledema—this is more common than in the usual perichiasmatic syndromes. Papilledema with bitemporal hemianopia usually indicates a craniopharyngioma. Papilledema is quite characteristic of posterior fossa tumors, but bitemporal field cuts in these cases are most unusual.
   e. In the great majority of instances, hydrocephalus, including enlargement of the third ventricle, does not result in visual field deficits of the chiasmatic type despite the relationship of the chiasm to the third ventricle. The posterior fossa tumor characteristically results in obstructive hydrocephalus, but visual field changes are more compatible with papilledema than bitemporal hemianopia. Falsely localizing visual field deficits can occur in unusual cases of posterior fossa tumor, however. Homonymous hemianopia due to upward compression of the occipital pole above a cerebellar tumor can occur. Bitemporal hemianopia due to a ventriculochiasmatic syndrome can be produced; bitemporal hemianopic scotomata due to posterosuperior chiasmatic compression are typically asymptomatic and may be undetected. Direct suprachiasmatic compression by a tumor mass within the third ventricle (i.e. craniopharyngioma, hypothalamic astrocytoma) more often results in bitemporal hemianopia than does third ventricular hydrocephalus.
3. Endocrine signs of the ventriculochiasmatic syndrome.
   a. Hypopituitarism—pituitary dwarfism and sexual infantilism may occur as a result of craniopharyngioma. Aqueductal stenosis and other forms of hydrocephalus without neoplasm may also result in hypopituitarism.
   b. Obesity with sexual infantilism—also seen with craniopharyngiomas.
   c. Diencephalic syndrome—cachexia and failure to grow; autonomic

instability; the appearance of brightness rather than stupor; optic atrophy is common; usually due to hypothalamic astrocytoma.

d. Precocious puberty—pinealoma, teratoma and hypothalamic astrocytoma in the third ventricular floor may be responsible.

4. Neurological signs of extension in the ventriculochiasmatic syndrome.
   a. The craniopharyngioma may be intrasellar or extrasellar or both. It may extend into the third ventricle and compress the hypothalamus. It may extensively involve the cisterna basalis. The chief signs of extension are the symptoms and signs of increased intracranial pressure. The foramen of Monro may be totally obstructed. Abducens palsy may result from intracranial hypertension, while oculomotor palsy may be due to direct third nerve compression by tumor in the interpeduncular cistern.
   b. The hypothalamic glioma may extend widely into the cerebrum, brain stem and subhemispheric optic pathways without producing intracranial hypertension until relatively late. Bizarre bilateral visual field changes suggest intrachiasmatic extension. Ophthalmoplegia and gaze palsies suggest extension into the midbrain. As in thalamic tumor, ventricular obstruction ultimately involves the posterior third (and periaqueductal) region; the anterior third ventricle may be occluded by tumor or dilated by more posterior obstruction.

D. Deficits of the retrochiasmatic syndrome

The posterior angle of the optic chiasm at its juncture with the optic tract is typically involved by retrochiasmatic tumors. Compression is directed upon the posteroinferior surface of the chiasm due to progressive ascent of the basal optic pathway. Tumors of this region characteristically compress both the optic tract and posterior chiasm at the time of diagnosis. Optic tract compromise, sparing the chiasm, leads to homonymous hemianopia, but spares visual acuity. Homonymous hemianopia with primary optic atrophy is pathognomonic of an optic tract lesion. However, optic atrophy of tract origin is a late sign. Involvement of the chiasm with the optic tract results in more progressive visual loss. The retrochiasmatic syndrome may appear in childhood or adult life and is virtually always the result of direct compression by tumor. It, too, is not as common as the sellar-chiasmatic syndrome.

1. Differential diagnosis of the retrochiasmatic syndrome.
   a. Craniopharyngioma—within the interpeduncular cistern; most common in childhood with signs of intracranial hypertension. The tumor may, however, appear even in late adult life, at which time

visual field and visual acuity deficits without intracranial pressure are prominent.

b. Chordoma—the clivus chordoma may result in progressive visual disturbance as a result of abducens and oculomotor palsies and retrochiasmatic compression. Young or middle-aged adults are typical patients.

c. Pituitary adenoma with prefixation of the optic chiasm—the patient is virtually always an adult.

Note: Compression of the optic tract against the anterior free edge of the tentorium by supratentorial mass—the homonymous hemianopia resulting from this form of tract compression is masked by progressive obtundation due to transtentorial herniation and does not present the features of the retrochiasmatic syndrome.

2. Ophthalmological signs of the retrochiasmatic syndrome.
   a. Bitemporal hemianopia—may be complete or partial; bitemporal upper quadrantic scotomata in the presence of sellar enlargement in the adult indicates pituitary adenoma with prefixation of the chiasm.
   b. Central visual acuity often remains intact until tumor compression extends from the posterior chiasmatic angle to the subschiasmatic region (i.e. central visual acuity is more rapidly impaired by anterior chiasmatic angle-optic nerve involvement than by posterior chiasmatic angle-tract compression). This occurs despite "splitting" of the macula in posterior angle tumors.
   c. Homonymous hemianopia—may be scotomatous or nonscotomatous, and results from optic tract compression. When the optic tract is compressed by a medial mass (i.e. posterior chiasmatic angle pressure) an incongruous homonymous hemianopia occurs with the greatest field loss on the side opposite the involved tract. When the optic tract is involved by a lateral (i.e. temporal) mass, the incongruous homonymous hemianopia is greater on the same side as the involved tract.
   d. Monocular blindness with contralateral temporal hemianopia—involvement of the optic tract and body of the chiasm, like compression of the optic nerve and chiasm, will lead to marked visual loss on the side of the tumor with a contralateral temporal cut.
3. Endocrine signs of the retrochiasmatic syndrome—endocrinopathic signs of pituitary adenomas and craniopharyngiomas have already been itemized. When a craniopharyngioma presents later in adult life, visual disturbances are often the only clinical features. The chordoma typically does not produce clinical endocrinopathy.

4. Neurological signs of extension in the retrochiasmatic syndrome—extension into the posterior fossa can occur in unusual cases of craniopharyngioma or chromophobe adenoma. A meningioma of Meckel's cave (and other "saddle tumors") characteristically extend from the middle to the posterior fossa, and when sufficiently large may compress the optic tract. A chordoma of the clivus may extend forward from the posterior fossa to the dorsum sella, middle fossa and orbital apex. The middle ridge sphenoid meningioma typically reaches large size before diagnosis. This is especially true on the nondominant side. An optic tract hemianopia may be superimposed upon the peripheral field defects of chronic papilledema in these large alar meningiomas. A variety of cranial nerve palsies, due either to direct compression or to intracranial hypertension, can thus accompany the retrochiasmatic syndrome.

E. Deficits of the laterochiasmatic syndrome

The lateral boundary of the optic chiasm is the intracranial carotid artery. The laterochiasmatic syndrome is unusual, but when it occurs, carotid aneurysm or tumor is responsible.

1. Differential diagnosis of the laterochiasmatic syndrome.
   a. Internal carotid aneurysm.
   b. Pituitary adenoma with eccentric lateral growth.
   c. Sphenoid meningioma—middle ridge tumors of large size may compress the lateral chiasm or optic tract (clinoidal-inner ridge meningiomas compress the optic nerve and diagnosis is relatively early due to loss of central vision).
2. Ophthalmological signs of the laterochiasmatic syndrome.
   a. Nasal hemianopia—results from lateral compression of visual fibers serving the ipsilateral temporal retina.
   b. Binasal hemianopia—this is a rare form of heteronymous hemianopia which can result from a lateral chiasmatic mass which shifts the chiasm against the carotid artery of the opposite side. Prolapse of the preoptic recess of a hydrocephalic third ventricle can produce the same effect; in this case, the optic nerves are separated and laterally compressed by the pulsating carotid arteries on each side.
   c. Lateral chiasmatic homonymous hemianopia—homonymous hemianopia is most commonly due to a lesion of the optic radiation or visual cortex. It is most often a result of ischemic vascular disease. Homonymous hemianopia of optic tract origin is less common. When it occurs, a tumor is almost always responsible. Like cerebral hemianopia, the homonymous hemianopia of tract origin

spares visual acuity (until chiasmatic compression is pronounced). Rarely, a homonymous hemianopia may be due to a lateral chiasmatic mass. The hemianopia is contralateral and is associated with ipsilateral loss of central visual acuity. This is the most rostral and most rare source of homonymous hemianopia.

3. Endocrine signs of the laterochiasmatic syndrome—the presence of hypopituitarism and ballooning of the sella with lateral chiasmatic compression favors the diagnosis of an eccentrically growing chromophobe adenoma. A carotid aneurysm however, can produce the same combination of optic, endocrine and radiological features. Sphenoid meningiomas do not produce evidence of endocrinopathy.
4. Neurological signs of extension in the laterochiasmatic syndrome—the sudden onset of supraorbital pain and ophthalmoplegia favors an intracavernous aneurysm (Fig. 65). A large intracavernous aneurysm may result in an orbital apex syndrome combined with lateral chiasmatic compression. First division trigeminal sensory loss with reduction in corneal sensitivity is an important sign. Exophthalmos accompanies orbital apex block. A small minority of chromophobe adenomas may invade the cavernous sinus with resultant first division

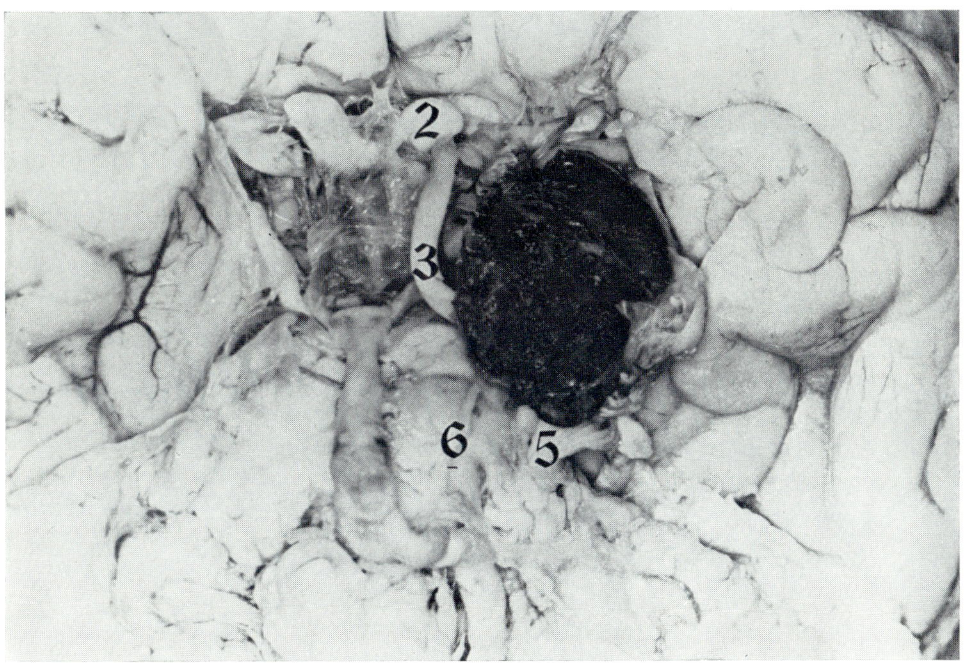

Figure 65. Parasellar cavernous aneurysm. This giant aneurysm arose from the intracavernous carotid artery and is seen here at the base of the brain. The optic, oculomotor, trigeminal and abducens nerves are identified by number.

pain and sensory loss plus ophthalmoplegia. Pituitary carcinoma should be considered in the older age group. A sphenoid meningioma may obstruct the superior orbital fissure and produce a similar syndrome. Extension of tumors laterally from the sella to the region of Meckel's cave results in a wider distribution of trigeminal pain and sensory loss.

F. Deficits of the intrachiasmatic syndrome

Intrinsic chiasmatic glioma is a syndrome of childhood. Stigmata of von Recklinghausen's disease may be present. Glioma of the optic nerve may extend caudally to involve the chiasm. Hypothalamic glioma may extend rostrally into the chiasm. An intrachiasmatic syndrome in the adult should suggest demyelinating disease. Chiasmatic trauma results in an intrinsic lesion at any age. Chiasmatic trauma is less common than optic nerve trauma. Transtemporal transection of the chiasm can result from a gunshot wound or other penetrating injury. Median longitudinal trauma to the chiasm may result from severe closed trauma with cranial distortion and separation of the optic nerves.

1. Ophthalmological signs of the intrachiasmatic syndrome.
    a. Bizarre bilateral field defects are characteristic of an intrachiasmatic lesion.
    b. The field defects are irregular.
    c. Bilateral central visual loss can occur.
    d. An optic nerve glioma may be visible on funduscopic examination; exophthalmos may be prominent; the hallmark of an extension of tumor into the chiasm is binocular visual defect.
    e. Complete transverse transection of the chiasm results in complete blindness with loss of light reflexes; light reflexes are preserved in bilateral central (i.e. cortical) blindness.
    f. Complete longitudinal midline transection of the chiasm results in bitemporal hemianopia in addition to the other field defects due to intrachiasmatic trauma. Light reflexes may be preserved.
    g. Associated transection of an optic nerve leads to complete monocular blindness with loss of the direct light reflex on that side.
2. Endocrine signs of the intrachiasmatic syndrome.
    a. Hypothalamic astrocytoma with extension into the optic chiasm may result in a diencephalic syndrome with failure to thrive, cachexia and optic atrophy.
    b. Trauma to the optic chiasm may be associated with traumatic diabetes insipidis and hypothalamic-upper brain stem contusion with deep coma and autonomic instability. Traumatic infarction of the

adenohypophysis resulting from occlusion of the portal venous system produces hypopituitarism, shock and obtundation.

Aneurysms and the Subhemispheric Optic Pathway

A major role of carotid angiography in the study of the perichiasmatic tumor suspect is the ruling out of an aneurysm. An aneurysm may closely mimic the clinical picture of a pituitary tumor. Ballooning of the sella may result from an intrasellar aneurysm. Erosion of a single anterior clinoid process may be due to an aneurysm rather than an inner sphenoidal meningioma. Erosion of an anterior and posterior clinoid on one side may be due to a parasellar aneurysm. The sudden onset of blindness should always suggest an aneurysm. The same applies to the sudden onset of ophthalmoplegia. However, blindness and ophthalmoplegia may be slowly progressive when due to aneurysmal compression of optic and cranial nerve structures. Slowly progressive visual loss without ophthalmoplegia may result from an anterior cerebral-anterior communicating aneurysm. Slowly progressive oculomotor palsy without visual loss may result from a posterior communicating-carotid aneurysm.

Carotid-Cavernous Aneurysm with Fistula

The carotid-cavernous aneurysm with fistula provides a special case in which progressive blindness and ophthalmoplegia occur together as the result of an aneurysm. These are traumatic, arteriosclerotic or congenital aneurysms within the cavernous sinus. The traumatic source of fistula is most common, while the congenital aneurysm responsible for the arteriovenous shunt is least frequent. Hence, the nontraumatic carotid-cavernous fistula is usually the result of rupture of an arteriosclerotic intracavernous carotid. The patient without trauma is thus typically middle-aged or older, while the head-injured patient with a traumatic aneurysm and fistula may be of any age. Symptoms and signs may begin within hours, weeks or months following development of the fistula. Once begun, the clinical picture is progressive. The symptoms include the following:

1. Bruit—the patient is usually aware of a "noise in the head."
2. Proptosis—the patient may note a unilateral ocular protusion or it may be called to his attention by relatives.
3. Diplopia—double vision is common.
4. Headache—ocular, retro-ocular or supraorbital pain on the side of the fistula is common.
5. Paresthesiae—may be noted in the ipsilateral trigeminal distribution.
6. Visual loss—progressive blindness in the ipsilateral eye is often noted by the patient.

7. Epistaxis—this is most unusual but can result from rupture of the aneurysm into the sphenoid sinus.
8. Symptoms of subarachnoid hemorrhage—these are unusual in the spontaneous intracavernous carotid fistula since it is extradural and rarely ruptures intracranially. In head trauma cases, evidence of subarachnoid blood may of course be due to associated traumatic subarachnoid hemorrhage or cerebral contusion.

The signs of a carotid-cavernous fistula include the following:

1. Obliteration of the bruit by ipsilateral carotid compression; the bruit is audible over the eye and neck.
2. Exophthalmos which may be pulsatile; the exophthalmos is ipsilateral to the fistula and may become bilateral (i.e. patent circular sinus). Periocular conjunctival swelling may be prominent.
3. Ophthalmoplegia—abducens and oculomotor palsy are common, and are often combined with trochlear palsy. Abducens or oculomotor palsy may appear in isolation.
4. Corneal anesthesia—loss of corneal sensitivity and keratitis may be present.
5. Optic atrophy and decreased visual acuity due to optic nerve compression and stretching occur. Retinal veins are congested. Retinal and preretinal hemorrhage may be noted. Hemorrhage in the region of the macula produces a more sudden visual loss.

Radiological Deformities in the Perichiasmatic Syndromes

A. Angiographic findings

1. Carotid siphon, intracavernous portion—lateral displacement (frontal view) is common in pituitary adenomas; elevation of the intracavernous carotid can be seen in locally invasive adenomas (lateral view) and is an uncommon sign of pituitary tumor; aneurysm is readily ruled out in pituitary tumor suspects by bilateral carotid angiograms.
2. Carotid siphon, supraclinoid portion—elevation (lateral view) is termed "opening of the siphon" and is common in pituitary adenomas. "Closing of the siphon" and a tumor blush characterize suprasellar meningiomas. Even large craniopharyngiomas often reveal little angiographic abnormality. The hypothalamic glioma of low grade may show slight angiographic evidence, while glioblastoma invading the hypothalamus may present pathological vessels with A-V shunts.
3. Anterior cerebral artery, horizontal portion—this is commonly elevated by pituitary adenomas (frontal view); there may be elevation and caudal displacement by the tuberculum meningioma or other rostrochiasmatic tumor (lateral view). Glioma of the optic chiasm may produce a similar effect.

4. Anterior cerebral artery, pericallosal branch—stretching of the distal segment of the anterior cerebral-pericallosal occurs with hydrocephalus. This is uncommon in pituitary adenomas and should suggest craniopharyngioma with obstruction of the foramen of Monro.

B. Pneumographic findings
1. Upward bulging of the diaphragm of the sella—an early sign of an intrasellar tumor.
2. Absence of cisternal air within the sella—cisternal air may enter the sella in normals, but does not in pituitary tumors.
3. Signs of suprasellar mass or suprasellar extension of pituitary tumor are as follow:
   a. Occlusion of the suprasellar cistern.
   b. Elevation of the anterior floor of the third ventricle.
   c. Elevation of the floors of the anterior horns of the lateral ventricles—indicates a large suprasellar mass.

Note: Assorted additional angiographic and pneumographic deformities may be present indicating extension of tumor to involve middle fossa, anterior fossa or even posterior fossa structures. Such extensions occur in a small minority of pituitary tumors: "the invasive adenoma."

C. Plain skull x-rays and sellar views in the perichiasmatic syndromes

Plain sellar views of good quality are essential in perichiasmatic diagnosis. In the pituitary tumor suspect, these plain x-ray studies are supplemented by pneumography to delineate the outline of the tumor, its suprasellar and third ventricular extension, and to rule out an empty sella syndrome. This is supplemented by angiography to rule out aneurysm and to further delineate both the suprasellar and parasellar extent of the mass. Plain sellar findings include the following:

1. Intrasellar tumor.
   a. Ballooning of the sella—this intrasellar expansion is characteristic of the great majority of pituitary adenomas of neurosurgical significance. Seventeen millimeters is the upper limit of normal for the greatest anteroposterior dimension of the pituitary fossa.
   b. Undercutting of the clinoids—the undersurface of the anterior and posterior clinoids is eroded and these processes are pointed upward.
   c. Double floor—eccentric erosion of the floor of the sella by tumor. The tumor shadow may at times extend into the sphenoid air sinus.
2. Suprasellar tumor.
   a. The clinoids.
      (1) The clinoids are eroded from above and may point downward.

(2) A single clinoid may be eroded or absent.

(3) Erosion of a single anterior clinoid should suggest meningioma or aneurysm.

(4) Hyperostosis of an anterior clinoid points to a meningioma of the inner sphenoidal wing.

(5) Erosion or hyperostosis of both anterior clinoids and tuberculum indicates a midline meningioma.

(6) Erosion of both an anterior and posterior clinoid on one side suggests a parasellar carotid aneurysm. Occasionally, eccentrically growing pituitary tumors may result in this appearance.

b. Sellar enlargement and suprasellar tumor.

(1) The sella may be secondarily enlarged by direct pressure from above, or by intracranial hypertension due to ventricular obstruction by tumor.

(2) Direct pressure by a suprasellar tumor tends to be relatively localized, initially affecting one or two clinoids from above. The sellar enlargement which may accompany this process does not have the generalized ballooning appearance of the intrasellar tumor, the latter usually affecting all the clinoids from below.

(3) The suprasellar tumor with obstruction of the foramen of Monro may produce sellar enlargement (pressure atrophy) by virtue of intracranial hypertension. This affects the posterior elements (dorsum and posterior clinoids) of the sella before it affects the anterior elements (anterior wall, anterior clinoids, tuberculum). Thus, this can also be differentiated from the ballooning of the intrasellar tumor.

c. The "J-shaped" sella.

(1) Flattening of the anterior elements of the sella in the region of the chiasmatic groove and tuberculum give the sella a pear or J-shape.

(2) A J-shaped sella occurs in hydrocephalus, gargoylism, neurofibromatosis, optic nerve glioma and also idiopathically in infancy. Blindness indicates an optic glioma, with or without associated neurofibromatosis, as the primary diagnosis. Visual involvement may be unilateral or bilateral.

(3) A J-shaped sella due to an optic glioma is usually associated with enlargement of one or both optic foramina. An optic foramen greater than 6.5 mm in diameter is abnormal; the foramen is also abnormal if it is 2 mm or more greater than its mate. A foraminal meningioma may produce enlargement,

erosion or hyperostosis about the optic foramen. Neurofibromatosis may also result in enlargement of the foramen without blindness (i.e. without an associated optic glioma).

3. Perichiasmatic tumor calcification.
   a. Suprasellar tumor calcification is the hallmark of the craniopharyngioma. The tumor, and its calcifications, can also be intrasellar. A significant minority of craniopharyngiomas have no visible calcifications, however.
   b. A small minority of chromophobe adenomas are visibly calcified.
   c. Calcification may also occur in meningiomas and in the walls of an aneurysm. The calcification of a nonaneurysmal arteriosclerotic carotid artery may be mistaken for tumor calcification. This common form of calcification may also mimic a double-floored sella.

Additional Diagnostic Studies in the Perichiasmatic Syndromes

The basic diagnostic approach in the perichiasmatic tumor syndromes is neurological with an emphasis on neuro-ophthalmology, radiological with emphasis on the sella and its surroundings, and endocrinological. By comparison, additional studies such as EEG and brain scan are relatively low in positive yield. The EEG may be abnormal in those cases with intracranial hypertension and in those with middle or anterior fossa extension. These events occur in a small minority of pituitary tumors and therefore the EEG is usually normal. Bilateral theta may be prominent in craniopharyngiomas or other large extrasellar masses. With third ventricular obstruction and intracranial hypertension, the EEG is commonly, although not invariably, abnormal. Generalized slowing in the delta range may be prominent, or bifrontal delta activity may be noted alone. Extension into the middle fossa may result in lateralized abnormalities. The brain scan may be of value in terms of the subhemispheric meningioma. However, those perichiasmatic meningiomas in or close to the midline produce early blindness. The small size at the time of diagnosis of these mediobasal tumors contributes to resultant negative scans in a significant number of tuberculum and clinoidal meningiomas.

CHAPTER 11

POSTERIOR FOSSA SYNDROMES

Neuroanatomy of the Posterior Fossa

The Brain Stem and Cranial Nerves

THE MAJOR NEURAL STRUCTURES of the posterior fossa are the brain stem, its cranial nerves and the cerebellum (Fig. 66). The brain stem consists of

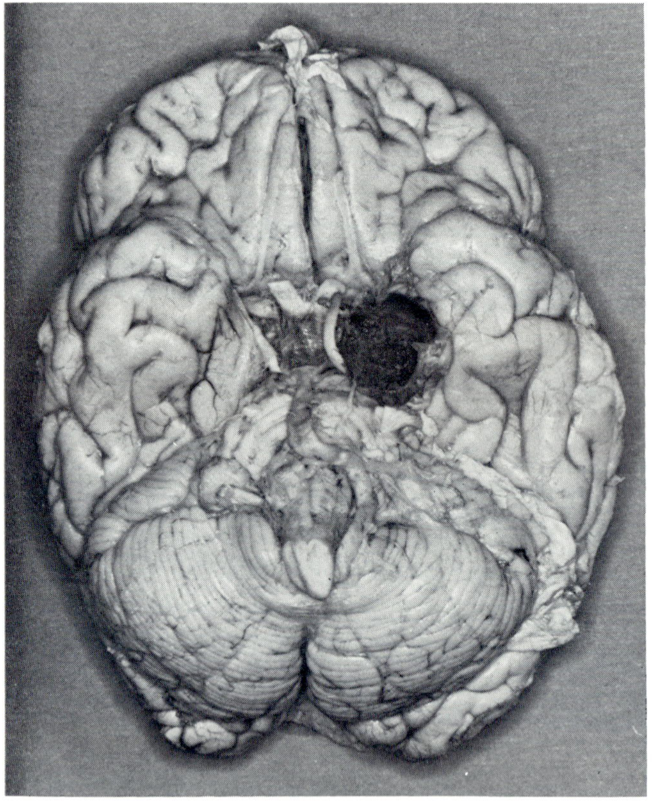

Figure 66. Base of the brain. The relation of the brain stem and cerebellum to the cerebral base is shown. The giant aneurysm (Fig. 65) is seen.

the midbrain, pons and medulla oblongata, extending from the tentorial opening above to the foramen magnum below. The quadrigeminal plate is the roof (i.e. "tectum") of the midbrain, lying dorsal to the aqueduct. The cerebellum is the roof of the pons and medulla, lying dorsal to the fourth ventricle.

The true cranial nerves are the peripheral nerves which emerge from the brain stem. They include cranial nerves three through twelve. The first (olfactory) and second (optic) "cranial nerves" are subhemispheric brain tracts rather than true cranial nerves. They do not arise from the brain stem. The olfactory tract lies in the anterior fossa, while the subhemispheric optic pathway lies above the pituitary fossa. While the true cranial nerves are widely distributed, at their points of emergence from the brain stem they traverse the posterior fossa.

All true cranial nerves emerge from either the ventral or lateral surfaces of the brain stem, with the exception of the fourth (trochlear). The latter cranial nerve is unique in that it is both dorsal and decussating, emerging just below the tectum. The ventral cranial nerves are the third (oculomotor), sixth (abducens) and twelfth (hypoglossal). The oculomotor nerves emerge closest to the midline of the ventral group, lying medial to the cerebral peduncle at their points of origin. The abducens nerves emerge from the ventral pontomedullary junction; they pierce corticospinal bundles at the base of the pons just before they appear at the pontine surface. The hypoglossal nerves emerge in rootlets from the ventral upper medulla; they lie just lateral to the pyramids. The first cervical nerves arise in line, just lateral to the pyramidal decussation of the lower medulla. This ventral group, the third, sixth and twelfth, are all motor nerves. They lie closely adjacent to the pyramidal system as it descends through the brain stem.

All the remaining cranial nerves emerge laterally from the pontomedullary brain stem. They have both sensory and motor components. They are conveniently grouped in three.

1. Trigeminal (fifth)—motor and sensory roots.
2. Nerves of the cerebellopontine angle (seventh and eighth)—the facial and intermediate nerves; the cochlear and vestibular nerves.
3. Vagal group (ninth, tenth and eleventh)—the glossopharyngeal, vagus and accessory nerves.

There are seven characteristic brain stem transverse sections of major anatomical importance. Two are mesencephalic, two are pontine, one is the pontomedullary junction and two are medullary.

1. Level of the superior colliculus (oculomotor).
   a. Centromedial—aqueduct and periaqueductal gray, oculomotor nuclei and medial longitudinal fasciculus.
   b. Paramedian—central tegmental tract and red nucleus.
   c. Lateral—medial and lateral lemnisci; medial geniculate body.

d. Ventral—substantia nigra and basis pedunculi of the cerebral peduncle.

Note: the "tectum" or "colliculi" or "quadrigeminal plate" lies dorsal to the aqueduct of the midbrain. The "tegmentum" lies ventral to the aqueduct and fourth ventricle at midbrain and pontine levels. The tegmentum is the central core of the brain stem and includes centromedial and paramedian structures and reticular formation.

2. Level of the inferior colliculus (trochlear).
   a. Centromedial—aqueduct and periaqueductal gray, trochlear nuclei and medial longitudinal fasciculus; decussation of the brachium conjunctivum (i.e. superior cerebellar peduncle).
   b. Paramedian—central tegmental tract and mesencephalic trigeminal nucleus.
   c. Lateral—medial and lateral lemnisci.
   d. Ventral—substantia nigra and basis pedunculi.
3. Level of mid-pons (trigeminal).
   a. Centromedial—upper fourth ventricle, medial longitudinal fasciculus, tectospinal and tectobulbar tracts.
   b. Paramedian—central tegmental tract and medial lemniscus.
   c. Lateral—sensory and motor trigeminal nuclei and lateral lemniscus.
   d. Dorsolateral—brachium conjunctivum (superior cerebellar peduncle); the extreme lateral position is occupied by the brachium pontis (middle cerebellar peduncle).
   e. Ventral—pontine nuclei, pyramidal bundles and transverse pontine fibers of the basis pontis.
4. Level of the lower pons (abducens and facial).
   a. Centromedial—fourth ventricle, medial longitudinal fasciculus, tectospinal and tectobulbar tracts and medial lemniscus.
   b. Paramedian—the abducens and facial nuclei (with facial colliculus in the floor of the fourth ventricle), central tegmental tract, superior olive and lateral lemniscus.
   c. Lateral—the spinal trigeminal nucleus and tract, and ventral spinocerebellar tract.
   d. Dorsolateral—the superior vestibular and dorsal cochlear nuclei; the brachium pontis occupies the extreme lateral position.
   e. Ventral—pontine nuclei, pyramidal bundles and transverse pontine fibers of the basis pontis.
5. Level of the pontomedullary junction (cochlear and vestibular).
   a. Centromedial—fourth ventricle, medial longitudinal fasciculus, tectospinal tract and medial lemniscus.

b. Paramedian—medial vestibular nucleus, inferior salivatory nucleus, and central tegmental tract.
c. Lateral—the spinal trigeminal nucleus and tract, ventral spinocerebellar and spinothalamic tracts.
d. Dorsolateral—lateral vestibular nucleus, restiform body (inferior cerebellar peduncle) and ventral cochlear nucleus.
e. Ventral—pontine nuclei and the pyramidal tract.

6. Level of the upper medulla (hypoglossal and vagal group).
   a. Centromedial—lower fourth ventricle, hypoglossal nucleus, medial longitudinal fasciculus, tectospinal tract, and medial lemniscus.
   b. Paramedian—dorsal motor nucleus of the vagus, nucleus solitarius and tractus solitarius, nucleus ambiguus, dorsal and medial accessory olives and the inferior olive.
   c. Lateral—spinal vestibular nucleus, spinal trigeminal nucleus and tract, ventral spinocerebellar and spinothalamic tracts.
   d. Dorsolateral—dorsal spinocerebellar tract and restiform body (inferior cerebellar peduncle).
   e. Ventral—medullary pyramid.
7. Level of the lower medulla (spinal accessory).
   a. Centromedial—central canal and pericentral gray, medial longitudinal fasciculus and tectospinal tract. The "sensory decussation" forming the medial lemniscus lies in the ventral midline cephalad to the pyramidal decussation. Adjacent to the dorsal midline is the nucleus gracilis, which along with the nucleus cuneatus, contributes internal arcuate fibers to the sensory decussation.
   b. Paramedian—spinal accessory nucleus.
   c. Lateral—lateral corticospinal tract, beginning at the pyramidal decussation; the dorsal spinocerebellar tract lies lateral to the lateral corticospinal tract; the ventral spinocerebellar tract lies lateral to the spinothalamic tract.
   d. Dorsolateral—nucleus and tractus cuneatus, lying just lateral to nucleus and tractus gracilis, and just medial to the spinal trigeminal nucleus and tract.
   e. Ventral—the anterior (direct) corticospinal tract composed of uncrossed pyramidal fibers.

The cranial nerves are conveniently considered in conjunction with the brain stem level to which each relates.

A. Cranial nerves afferent to the brain stem.
   1. Trigeminal—facial sensation.

      This lateral pontine (fifth) cranial nerve consists of two roots, the larger sensory root lying lateral to the smaller motor root. The sensory portion consists of three divisions, which converge in the gasserian ganglion of Meckel's cave in the middle fossa. The retrogasserian trigeminal root passes from the middle fossa through the porus trigemini into the posterior fossa to penetrate the lateral pons.

a. Peripheral branches.
   (1) Ophthalmic (first) division—lies lateral to the intracavernous carotid with the nerves serving ocular motility in the cavernous sinus; passes through the superior orbital fissure with these nerves. Terminal ophthalmic branches include the following:
      (a) Lacrimal nerve.
      (b) Frontal nerve—supraorbital and supratrochlear branches.
      (c) Nasociliary nerve—ethmoidal, external nasal and long ciliary branches.
   (2) Maxillary (second) division—enters the cranial cavity through the foramen rotundum. Terminal branches include the following.
      (a) Infraorbital nerve and superior dental branches.
      (b) Zygomatic nerve.
      (c) Sphenopalatine nerves.
   (3) Mandibular (third) division—the motor trigeminal root passes with this sensory division through the foramen ovale. Terminal sensory branches include the following:
      (a) Auriculotemporal nerve.
      (b) Lingual nerve.
      (c) Long buccal nerve.
      (d) Inferior dental nerve.

b. Central trigeminal connections—there are three brain stem sensory nuclei related to the trigeminal.
   (1) Mesencephalic nucleus—proprioception.
   (2) Main sensory nucleus of the pons—touch.
   (3) Nucleus of the spinal trigeminal tract—pain and temperature.

2. Intermediate nerve—taste, anterior two-thirds of the tongue.

The intermediate nerve is the sensory root of the facial (seventh) nerve. It joins with the facial, cochlear and vestibular nerves in the cerebellopontine angle. It passes with these nerves from the internal auditory meatus to the lateral pontomedullary junction.

a. Peripheral branches—taste fibers from the anterior two-thirds of the tongue pass in the lingual nerve to the chorda tympani to the facial nerve in the facial canal. The sensory ganglion is the geniculate.

b. Central sensory connections—to the nucleus of the tractus solitarius.

Note: Taste from the posterior third of the tongue is mediated by the glossopharyngeal nerve, vit the petrosal ganglion to the nucleus of the tractus solitarius. Taste from the epiglottis is mediated by the vagus nerve, via the nodose ganglion to the nucleus of the tractus solitarius.

3. Cochlear nerve—auditory sensation.

   At the internal acoustic meatus, the cochlear (eighth) nerve lies in the anteroinferior quadrant. The facial (seventh) nerve lies in the anterosuperior quadrant. The intermediate (seventh) nerve lies between the facial and cochlear nerves at the meatus. The intermediate nerve may become adherent to the cochlear nerve in its passage toward the brain stem. The superior vestibular (eighth) nerve lies in the posterosuperior quadrant, and the inferior vestibular (eighth) in the posteroinferior quadrant at the meatus.

   a. Peripheral branches—the cochlear nerve is formed from branches ending upon the organ of Corti. The sensory ganglion is the spiral.
   b. Central connections—to the dorsal and ventral cochlear nuclei.

4. Vestibular nerve—static and kinetic equilibrium.
   a. Peripheral branches—the vestibular nerves are composed of branches from the semicircular ducts, utricle and saccule of the labyrinth. The sensory ganglion is the vestibular.
   b. Central connections—to the superior, medial, lateral and spinal vestibular nuclei.

5. Glossopharyngeal nerve.

   The ninth, tenth and eleventh (glossopharyngeal, vagus and accessory) nerves constitute the "vagal group." Like the trigeminal and facial, the glossopharyngeal and vagus carry both sensory (afferents to the brain stem) and motor (efferents from the brain stem) components. The sensory components of the glossopharyngeal mediate both taste (posterior third of the tongue) and common sensation.

   a. Peripheral branches—the afferents are as follow:
      (1) Lingual branches.
      (2) Pharyngeal branches.
      (3) Tonsillar branches.
      (4) Tympanic branch.
      (5) Carotid sinus branch.

      The sensory ganglia include the following:
      (1) Petrosal.
      (2) Superior.
   b. Central sensory connections are as follow:

(1) Nucleus of the tractus solitarius.
(2) Nucleus of the spinal trigeminal tract.

6. Vagus nerve.

The tenth cranial nerve, in the company of the ninth and eleventh (vagal group), passes to the lateral medulla from the jugular foramen. Afferents to the brain stem traversing the vagus are largely visceral in origin. They mediate autonomic sensation and taste from the epiglottis. The vagus also carries somatic sensory fibers in its auricular branch.

a. Peripheral branches—the afferents include the following:
(1) Pharyngeal branches.
(2) Posterior glossal branches.
(3) Superior laryngeal branch.
(4) Thoracic and abdominal visceral branches.
(5) Auricular branch.
The sensory ganglia include the following:
(1) Nodose.
(2) Jugular.

b. Central sensory connections include the following:
(1) Nucleus of the tractus solitarius.
(2) Nucleus of the spinal trigeminal tract.

B. Cranial nerves efferent from the brain stem

1. Nerves of ocular motility.

a. Oculomotor nerve.
(1) Central—from the oculomotor nuclei and nucleus of Edinger-Westphal of the midbrain.
(2) Peripheral.
(a) All extraocular muscles except the superior oblique and lateral rectus.
(b) Levator palpebrae.
(c) Ciliary ganglion—postganglionic fibers to the pupillary sphincter.

b. Trochlear nerve.
(1) Central—from the trochlear nucleus of the midbrain.
(2) Peripheral—to the superior oblique.

c. Abducens nerve.
(1) Central—from the abducens nucleus of the pons.
(2) Peripheral—to the lateral rectus.

2. Motor root of the trigeminal nerve—mastication.

The motor root is smaller than, and lies medial to, the sensory root. The motor root leaves the cranial cavity with the mandibular division, through the foramen ovale.

a. Central—trigeminal motor nucleus of the pons.
b. Peripheral.
   (1) Muscles of mastication—temporal, masseter and pterygoids.
   (2) Tensor veli palatini.
   (3) Tensor tympani.

3. Facial nerve—facial expression.

The facial nerve can be usefully divided into segments.

a. Proximal—facial nerve from its brain stem emergence to the geniculate ganglion. The proximal segment is associated with a separate intermediate nerve (sensory root) and with the cochlear and vestibular nerves. It is one of the nerves of the cerebellopontine angle and internal auditory canal.
b. Middle—facial nerve in the facial canal from the geniculate ganglion to the stylomastoid foramen. The greater superficial petrosal nerve emerges at the level of the geniculate ganglion. The chorda tympani separates from the main facial trunk before it emerges from the stylomastoid foramen. The nerve to the stapedius arises between the above branches of the middle segment.
c. Distal—facial nerve beyond the stylomastoid foramen, including the postauricular branch and the branches within the parotid gland, terminating in the muscles of facial expression.

The efferent fibers from the brain stem employing facial pathways include the following:

a. Central.
   (1) Motor facial nucleus of the pons.
   (2) Superior salivatory nucleus.
b. Peripheral.
   (1) Greater superficial petrosal nerve—supplies visceral efferents to the lacrimal gland for tear secretion.
   (2) Nerve to the stapedius.
   (3) Chorda tympani—mediates salivary secretion as well as taste sensation from the anterior two-thirds of the tongue. The chorda tympani joins the lingual branch of the trigeminal (mandibular division). Preganglionic fibers from the superior salivatory nucleus reach the submandibular ganglion by this route; postganglionic fibers innervate sublingual and submandibular salivary glands.
   (4) Terminal facial branches—to the ipsilateral muscles of facial expression, stylohyoid and posterior belly of the digastric.

4. The vagal group.

The efferent fibers in the vagal group include the following:

a. Glossopharyngeal nerve.

(1) Central.
(a) Nucleus ambiguus.
(b) Inferior salivatory nucleus.

(2) Peripheral.
(a) Pharyngeal branches.
(b) Stylopharyngeal branch.
(c) Lesser superficial petrosal nerve—preganglionic fibers from the inferior salivatory nucleus pass via the glossopharyngeal nerve and its tympanic branch to the lesser superficial petrosal nerve. The latter terminates in the otic ganglion, from which postganglionic fibers innervate the parotid gland.

b. Vagus nerve.
(1) Central.
(a) Nucleus ambiguus.
(b) Dorsal motor nucleus of the vagus.
(2) Peripheral.
(a) Palate, pharynx and larynx—from the nucleus ambiguus, distributed by pharyngeal and laryngeal branches (recurrent and superior laryngeal).
(b) Thoracic and abdominal viscera—preganglionic fibers from the dorsal motor nucleus.

c. Accessory nerve.

The accessory (eleventh) nerve is a motor nerve composed of cranial and spinal roots. The cranial root is an aberrant vagus and is derived from the nucleus ambiguus along with the motor ninth and tenth. The spinal root ascends from the lateral margin of the cervical cord through the foramen magnum, joins the vagal group and emerges from the skull through the jugular foramen. The accessory nerve supplies the sternocleidomastoid and, joining with the third and fourth cervical nerves, innervates the trapezius.

5. Hypoglossal nerve.

The twelfth nerve is derived from the hypoglossal motor nucleus of the medulla. The rootlets emerge between the pyramid and the olive of the ventral medulla. The hypoglossal nerve passes through the hypoglossal canal to innervate the tongue.

a. Intrinsic muscles of the tongue.
b. Hyoglossus, genioglossus and styloglossus.

Note: The "ansa hypoglossi," derived from upper cervical motor fibers, innervates the infrahyoid muscles: sternohyoid, omohyoid and sternothyroid.

Cerebellar Anatomy

The cerebellum consists of a median vermis, the lateral hemispheres, the deep cerebellar nuclei and the cerebellar peduncles. The hemispheres and vermis are composed of three lobes.

1. Anterior lobe.
2. Posterior lobe.
3. Flocculonodular lobe.

The great bulk of the cerebellum consists of the large posterior lobe. The small anterior lobe lies beneath the apex of the tentorium. Its vermis bounds the anterior wall of the fourth ventricle at the upper pons. The small flocculonodular lobe lies inferocentrally, deep to the massive posterior lobe. The nodulus, the vermian component of the flocculonodular lobe, lies behind the posterior wall of the fourth ventricle.

The chief input of the cerebellum is through the middle cerebellar peduncle (brachium pontis) to the hemispheres of the large posterior lobe (neocerebellum). This input is mediated by the pontine nuclei and is largely derived from rostral (cerebral and upper brain stem) sources. An input to the cerebellum from spinal sources is mediated via the inferior cerebellar peduncle (restiform body) to the anterior lobe. The anterior lobe and its vermis (spinocerebellar input) and the posterior vermis of the posterior lobe (vestibular input) are considered the "paleocerebellum." The flocculonodular lobe is a vestibular structure and constitutes the "archicerebellum."

The deep cerebellar nuclei consist of the large dentate, the globose, emboliform and fastigial nuclear masses. The dentate receives input from the bulk of the cerebellar hemisphere. The output of the dentate nucleus constitutes the major component of the superior cerebellar peduncle (brachium conjunctivum), the major outflow tract of the cerebellum. The globose nucleus receives from the paravermian portion of the posterior lobe, the emboliform from the paravermian anterior lobe, and the fastigial (roof) nucleus from the vermis.

A. Cerebellar afferents

1. Pontocerebellar tracts—the pontine nuclei constitute the main afferent source to the cerebellum. The cerebellar hemispheres receive crossed pontocerebellar projections. The vermis receives both crossed and uncrossed pontocerebellar projections. Afferents to the pontine nuclei are listed below.
    a. Corticopontine tracts—from ipsilateral frontal, parietal, temporal and occipital cortex.
    b. Tectopontine tract.
    c. Spinopontine tract.
2. Olivocerebellar tract—the inferior olive projects widely to the oppo-

site cerebellum by fibers passing through the restiform body of the contralateral side. The hemisphere and deep cerebellar nuclei receive projections from the inferior olive, while the vermis receives from the accessory olive. The afferents to the inferior olive reach it by way of the central tegmental tract, the sources of which are as follows:

a. Periaqueductal gray.
b. Cerebral cortex.
c. Caudate.
d. Globus pallidus.
e. Red nucleus.

The spino-olivary projections are relayed to the vermis of the anterior lobe.

3. Dorsal spinocerebellar tract—this is an ipsilateral projection arising in Clarke's column of the thoracic and upper lumbar spinal cord. The projection is to the vermis of the anterior lobe, via the restiform body.
4. Ventral spinocerebellar tract—this arises in the gray matter of the spinal cord, in which it crosses to the opposite side, to recross at the level of the anterior lobe vermis. The projection bypasses the restiform body and enters the cerebellum in the superficial part of the brachium conjunctivum.
5. Afferents from the external cuneate nucleus—these arise from the posterior column at cervical cord levels and terminate in the vermis of the anterior lobe, via the ipsilateral restiform body. These fibers complement the dorsal spinocerebellar input from the thoracic and lumbar segments.
6. Reticulocerebellar projections—from the pontomedullary reticular formation to the hemisphere and vermis.
7. Trigeminocerebellar projections—from the nucleus of the spinal tract and main sensory nucleus of the trigeminal to the dentate nucleus, via the restiform body.
8. Vestibulocerebellar projections.
   a. Primary vestibular root fibers—to the flocculonodular lobe and fastigium; ipsilateral.
   b. Secondary vestibular projections from the vestibular nuclei of the brain stem—to the flocculonodular lobe, fastigium and posterior vermis; both ipsilateral and contralateral.

B. Cerebellar efferents

1. Brachium conjunctivum.

   The superior cerebellar peduncle is the chief outflow tract of the cerebellum. It contains efferents from all the deep cerebellar nuclei, but none directly from the cerebellar cortex. The major component is the dentatorubral tract. The brachium conjunctivum has three branches.

a. Ascending—crossed; major branch.
b. Descending—crossed.
c. Descending—uncrossed.

The ipsilateral dentate, globose and emboliform nuclei, along with the contralateral fastigial nucleus, project in the brachium conjunctivum. Fastigial fibers from the roof nucleus are the only projections which decussate within the cerebellum (see below, "Uncinate fasciculus"). The ascending portion of the brachium conjunctivum crosses to the opposite side to terminate as follows:

a. Red nucleus—major termination (e.g. dentatorubral tract); some fibers synapse in the red nucleus (e.g. dentato-rubro-thalamic) and some continue directly through the nucleus to the thalamus.
b. Tegmental and reticular terminations in the brain stem core.
c. Cerebellothalamic projections.
   (1) VL—a major cerebellar projection site from the dentate.
   (2) Subthalamus and zona incerta.
   (3) Center median—an important projection of the emboliform nucleus.

2. Uncinate fasciculus.

   The "hook bundle" of Russell is composed of crossed fastigial fibers passing over the brachium conjunctivum, and then between it and the restiform body. These projections terminate in the pontomedullary vestibular nuclei and reticular formation. The "uncrossed" descending limb of the brachium conjunctivum is derived from the uncinate projections of the opposite fastigial nucleus.

3. Direct vestibular projections.

   While the inferior cerebellar peduncle is largely afferent to the cerebellum, direct fastigiobulbar projections leave the cerebellum by this route. While all cerebellar nuclei project through the superior peduncle, only the fastigial nucleus projects through the inferior peduncle. These direct fastigiobulbar fibers terminate in vestibular nuclei of the brain stem. The flocculonodular lobe similarly has direct vestibular projections. The nodulus projects to the fastigium and vestibular nuclei. The flocculus projects to the vestibular nuclei via the juxtarestiform body.

Fourth Ventricular and Cisternal Anatomy

The fourth ventricle lies between the pontomedullary brain stem and the cerebellum. A line through the floor of the fourth ventricle passes through the center of the foramen magnum. A line from the tuberculum sella to the torcular (Twining's line) should have its midpoint within the fourth ventricle. The fastigium (roof nucleus) is the apex of the fourth ventricle. The ventricle begins from the termination of the aqueduct just caudal to the colliculi, and it ends at the obex. The anterior wall is the superior medullary velum, indented by the lingula, the first portion of the anterior lobe vermis. The posterior wall is the inferior medullary velum indented by the nodulus. The foramen of Magendie is a midline opening in the roof of the ventricle, connecting it with the vallecula of the cisterna magna. The vallecula is the anterior part of the cisterna magna, extending forward within the posterior cerebellar notch. The foramina of Luschka are the lateral openings of the fourth ventricle into the lateral recesses of the pontomedullary cistern. The cisterna magna, pontomedullary and lateral cisterns are continuous around the brain stem and cerebellum with the transtentorial cisterns above (i.e. interpeduncular, crural, ambient and quadrigeminal cisterns) . The cranial nerves and major vessels lie within the cisterns to their points of exit. The cisterna magna is continuous through the foramen magnum with the cervical subarachnoid space.

Blood Supply of the Brain Stem and Cerebellum

A. Arterial

The brain stem and cerebellum receive their arterial supply through the vertebrobasilar system. Paramedian, short circumferential and long circumferential arteries all supply the brain stem at midbrain, pontine and medullary levels. Long circumferential (i.e. cerebellar) arteries also supply the cerebellum and its peduncular brain stem attachments. Major trunks include the following:

1. Posterior cerebral artery—supplies the midbrain and its cerebral peduncles, in addition to diencephalic and telencephalic posterior cerebral supply.
2. Mesencephalic artery—this is the proximal segment of the posterior cerebral artery at the basilar bifurcation. Penetrating vessels from the bifurcation and mesencephalic trunks supply the midbrain, entering between the cerebral peduncles (i.e. "posterior perforated substance"). The mesencephalic arteries constitute the posterior segment of the circle of Willis.
3. Superior cerebellar artery—arises from the upper basilar artery just below its bifurcation. It supplies the dorsolateral midbrain and upper pons, superior and middle cerebellar peduncles, superior cerebellar hemisphere, vermis and dentate.
4. Basilar artery—arises at the pontomedullary junction from the union of the vertebral arteries; terminates at the mesencephalic—pontine

junction by its bifurcation into the mesencephalic segments of the posterior cerebral arteries. It supplies the pons with penetrating vessels and short circumferential branches. Its major branches are the posterior cerebrals, superior cerebellars and anterior-inferior cerebellars.

5. Anterior-inferior (middle) cerebellar artery—this supplies the pontine tegmentum and upper medulla, the middle and inferior cerebellar peduncles and the inferior cerebellar hemisphere. The anterior-inferior cerebellar artery commonly supplies most of the inferior cerebellum on one side, while the posterior-inferior branch of the vertebral supplies most of the inferior cerebellum of the opposite side. The vermis and dentate may receive arterial blood from either inferior cerebellar vessel, in addition to their superior cerebellar supply. The internal auditory artery is most often a branch of the anterior-inferior cerebellar artery rather than the basilar.
6. Posterior-inferior cerebellar artery—this arises from the vertebral artery and supplies the lateral medulla, fourth ventricular choroid plexus and inferior cerebellum.
7. Posterior spinal arteries—these paired arteries arise from the intracranial vertebral artery and supply the lower posterior medulla and spinal cord.
8. Anterior spinal rami—these paired arteries arise from the intracranial vertebrals and join in the midline as the anterior median spinal artery. This supplies the lower anterior medulla and spinal cord.
9. Intracranial vertebral arteries—these supply perforating branches to the anterolateral medulla, give rise to anterior and posterior spinal arteries, posterior-inferior cerebellar arteries, and unite to form the basilar artery.

B. Venous

1. Central mesencephalic vein—to the basal vein of Rosenthal (in turn to the vein of Galen) .
2. Lateral mesencephalic vein—to the basal vein and superior petrosal sinus.
3. Medial and lateral pontine veins—connect the basal vein above with the petrosal vein laterally and the medullary veins caudally.
4. Medullary venous plexus—to the pontine veins above, petrosal and cerebellar veins, and vertebrospinal plexus below.
5. Anterior cerebellar veins—from the inferior cerebellum to the pontine venous plexus; the petrosal vein runs from the flocculus to the superior petrosal sinus.
6. Superior cerebellar veins—from the superior cerebellum to the vein

of Galen medially; lateral superior cerebellar veins empty into the transverse and superior petrosal sinuses.

7. Posterior cerebellar veins—arise from the posterior cerebellum and empty into the transverse, straight and occipital sinuses.

C. Dural venous sinuses

The venous drainage of the brain stem and cerebellum is distributed in two general directions.

1. Tentorial venous sinus system—ultimately leading to the internal jugular vein.
2. Basilar plexus—leading to the vertebrospinal venous plexus.

Brain stem and cerebellar veins may empty directly into the basal vein or great vein of Galen as previously described. The great vein joins with the inferior longitudinal sinus to form the straight sinus. This sinus in the tentorial apex contains blood derived largely from deep cerebral and posterior fossa structures. At the internal occipital protuberance, the straight sinus usually forms the left transverse sinus, with variable connection with the torcular Herophili (confluence of the sinuses). In most cases, the superior sagittal sinus turns largely to the right, becoming the right transverse sinus, again with variable communication in the torcular. Both cerebral hemispheres are drained by the large superior sagittal sinus; the right transverse and sigmoid sinuses and right internal jugular vein are commonly larger than their counterparts on the left. The right internal jugular system is largely a cerebral venous channel. The left internal jugular is both a cerebral and infratentorial system in most instances. At the juncture of the straight and transverse sinuses, a tentorial sinus of Gibbs may be present. The occipital sinus in the falx cerebelli may also enter the torcular at this point. Other tentorial venous sinuses enter the transverse sinus as it courses along the tentorial attachment. The transverse sinus receives the superior petrosal sinus just as it turns downward to become the sigmoid sinus. The superior petrosal sinus connects the transverse sinus with the cavernous sinus; the superior petrosal receives the petrosal vein and veins from the middle ear. Just as the sigmoid sinus becomes the jugular bulb of the internal jugular vein, it receives the inferior petrosal sinus. The latter connects the sigmoid with the cavernous sinus and basilar plexus. The basilar plexus is an extensive group of venous channels in the dura over the clivus. It connects the cavernous and inferior petrosal sinuses with the vertebrospinal venous sinuses. The basilar plexus, like the tentorial sinus system (straight and left transverse), also receives venous drainage from the brain stem and cerebellum. The marginal sinus encircling the foramen magnum is the connection between the basilar plexus and vertebrospinal venous complex.

Infarction Syndromes of the Brain Stem

The following principles should be considered before making a diagnosis of brain stem infarction:

1. Brain stem infarction most commonly involves the medulla oblongata, somewhat less often involves the pons, and only occasionally is mesencephalic. Therefore, the higher the brain stem disorder, the greater the incidence of neurosurgical mass lesions. The typical midbrain syndrome is more apt to be the result of a supratentorial mass than a nonsurgical infarct.
2. Brain stem infarction is most common in older age groups. A "typical brain stem infarct" occurring in younger patients should be regarded with suspicion.
3. As in other vascular events, a sudden onset is characteristic. A tendency to improve following the initial neurological insult is a point in favor of vascular etiology. Neither sign is pathognomonic. Sudden onset with consequent improvement may occur as well with intracranial hemorrhage as with infarction.
4. A history of previous ischemic episodes favors a diagnosis of vascular infarction.
5. A history of neurological deficit occurring during sleep is compatible with infarction, but is less likely in intracranial hemorrhage.
6. The presence of coma is compatible with either infarction or hemorrhage. Retention of an alert state is common in infarction, is present in many cases of intracerebral hemorrhage and in the early stages of intracerebellar hemorrhage, and even occurs in some cases of intrapontine hemorrhage in the early phase.
7. The presence of acute arterial hypertension in patients with any sudden neurological deficit should be interpreted as due to intracranial hypertension until proven otherwise. This would favor intracranial mass or intracranial hemorrhage over infarction. Large cerebral infarcts are occasionally associated with sufficient cerebral edema to produce shift and intracranial hypertension. This is not the case in brain stem infarction.
8. The presence of chronic arterial hypertension (e.g. left ventricular hypertrophy, hypertensive retinopathy) is a point in favor of intracerebral, intrapontine or intracerebellar hemorrhage rather than infarction. Intracerebral hemorrhage is about three times more common than intrapontine hemorrhage; intracerebellar hemorrhage is the least common of these, but is always a surgical emergency. Any of these hemorrhages may occur in the normotensive patient (rule out arteriovenous malformation). Infarction obviously can occur in a hypertensive, as can hypertensive encephalopathy.

9. In the majority of instances, the spinal fluid is clear in infarction; however, hemorrhagic infarcts can result in bloody spinal fluid. In the great majority of intracerebral hemorrhages, the spinal fluid is blood-tinged. This is true even in patients retaining consciousness. The fluid may be clear, however, in one of five intracerebral hemorrhages. The CSF is virtually always bloody in the cerebellar hemorrhage, due to rupture of clot into the fourth ventricle.
10. If cerebellar infarction accompanies a brain stem infarction, the brain stem signs are usually more prominent. The presence of ataxia does not necessarily mean cerebellar infarction, as it occurs with lesions limited to the brain stem. If cerebellar hemorrhage occurs, consciousness is often retained for a period of a few or many hours; ocular and other brain stem signs may be prominent, while cerebellar signs may not be marked. Persistent vomiting is common.
11. The chronic subdural hematoma may present acutely with obtundation and hemiplegia, without history or evidence of trauma. A history of chronic alcoholism suggests possible remote trauma. Fluctuating signs may point to the diagnosis. Midline shift (pineal or echo) in the unilateral subdural, or downward depression of the pineal in the bilateral subdural, indicate the presence of supratentorial mass.
12. Hemorrhage into a brain tumor or acute ventricular obstruction by tumor may present a vascularlike syndrome of sudden neurological deficit.
13. Intrinsic brain stem tumors are more common in childhood, and in such cases intracranial hypertension is late. Cerebellar tumors are also more common in childhood; they are more common than intrinsic brain stem gliomas. Cerebellar tumors may present brain stem signs due to compression or invasion of the brain stem. Intracranial pressure elevation occurs early due to obstructive hydrocephalus.
14. Compressive hemorrhages of the upper brain stem ("Duret hemorrhages") involve the central parts of the midbrain and pons. They rarely extend into the medulla. They result from transtentorial herniation due to supratentorial mass. Impairment of consciousness is progressive.
15. Brain stem infarction syndromes are typically crossed hemiplegias with ipsilateral cranial nerve palsy.
    a. Midbrain syndromes.
        (1) Ipsilateral oculomotor palsy with crossed hemiplegia (Weber's) —more apt to be a supratentorial mass than a midbrain infarct.
        (2) Ipsilateral oculomotor palsy with crossed extrapyramidal signs

—hemichorea, tremor or rigidity (Benedict's) ; a relatively uncommon syndrome.

(3) Ipsilateral oculomotor palsy with crossed hemiataxia (Claude's) —a rare infarct. Systemic hypertension or bloody spinal fluid suggests simulation of these signs by cerebellar hematoma.

(4) Ophthalmoplegias and somnolence (syndrome of the mesencephalic artery)—somnolent mutism with ophthalmoplegia may be mimicked by the supratentorial mass resulting in stupor with impoverished movements.

(5) Internuclear ophthalmoplegia—paralysis of the adducting eye on attempted lateral gaze but preservation of convergence; horizontal nystagmus most marked in the abducting eye; usually with multiple ocular deficits including skew deviation, paralysis of vertical gaze and ptosis. Usually bilateral and often associated with vertical nystagmus (medial longitudinal fasciculus syndrome)—indicates an intra-brain stem lesion.

(6) Intracranial hypertension with vertical gaze palsy, frequent convergence palsy and occasional pupillary palsy (Parinaud's) —indicates a pineal tumor with aqueductal obstruction and dorsal midbrain compression.

b. Pontine syndromes.

(1) Ipsilateral horizontal gaze palsy with crossed hemiplegia (Foville's)—brain stem infarct (or hemorrhage) is likely. Marked head turning suggests an intracerebral rather than pontine lesion.

(2) Ipsilateral combined abducens and peripheral facial palsy with crossed hemiplegia (Millard-Gubler's)—clearly a brain stem lesion which could be infarct or hemorrhage. It is often nonvascular. This relatively common intrinsic brain stem syndrome can be simulated by the cerebellar clot with dorsolateral pontine compression. An ipsilateral abducens or facial palsy with nausea, vomiting, stiff neck and obtundation should suggest cerebellar hemorrhage.

(3) Cerebellar hemiataxia with crossed hemihypesthesia (Raymond-Cestan's)—rare, may or may not be vascular; hemihypesthesia may occur with brain stem lesions at other levels.

(4) Pontine apoplexy—classical intrapontine hemorrhage is usually fatal. Initial crossed hemiplegia occurs, with ipsilateral facial palsy being common; this rapidly converts to quadriplegia. There is horizontal conjugate gaze palsy to the side of the lesion; there may be complete loss of conjugate gaze in all

planes. "Ocular bobbing" may occur spontaneously, with random vertical eye movements in the absence of lateral eye movements. The pupils may be small, but light reflexes are often preserved until coma is deep. An ipsilateral loss of the corneal reflex is common; a bilateral loss accompanies deepening coma. The patient may be comatose from the outset. At times, consciousness may be retained for some hours during the hemiplegic phase; stupor and coma are progressive as the patient becomes quadriparetic.

c. Medullary syndromes.

(1) Lateral medullary syndrome (Wallenberg's)—relatively common; almost invariably, a vascular infarct, usually vertebral, sometimes posterior-inferior cerebellar, arterial occlusion. Symptoms include acute vertigo, nausea, vomiting, dysphagia, dysarthria, instability, hiccoughing, hoarseness and occasionally hemiparesthesias of the face or body. Diplopia or blurred vision may accompany the sense of instability and vertigo, but extraocular motor palsy is not present. The patient may fall to the side of the lesion, but consciousness is ordinarily not disturbed. The signs are all ipsilateral with the exception of hypesthesia to pain and temperature on the opposite half of the body. The ipsilateral signs include hemihypesthesia of the face with diminished corneal reflex, nystagmus most marked on gaze toward the lesion, miosis and ptosis, hemipalatal, pharyngeal and vocal cord paralysis and hemiataxia of the ipsilateral extremities. Partial lateral medullary syndromes are common, while other medullary infarctions are rare.

(2) Anterior medullary syndrome (preolivary)—ipsilateral hypoglossal palsy with crossed hemiplegia; crossed hemianesthesia with sparing of the face may be associated.

(3) Posterior medullary syndrome (postolivary)—this consists of a group of unusual disorders involving the bulbar cranial nerves and sparing the pyramidal tract. Crossed hemihypesthesia sparing the face may be associated. The glossopharyngeal, vagus, and accessory nerve may be involved in various combinations.

Neurophysiology

A. The brain stem

The brain stem is an elaborate reflex center. It is the site of integration of many suprasegmental (cerebral), segmental (cranial) and infrasegmental (spinal) influences. The brain stem is also an organ of passage from higher to lower levels and vice versa. It is a site of collateralization of information, with sensory and motor integrators in series and in parallel. The brain stem also exerts vital autonomic controls. However, altered brain stem physiology presents itself most commonly to the neurosurgeon as an impairment of consciousness. This is often due to upper brain stem compression by supratentorial space-occupying mass with transtentorial herniation. Intracranial hypertension is superimposed upon the signs of brain stem compromise. The infratentorial mass may have the same effect, with intracranial hypertension and eventual deterioration in consciousness. The structure which mediates the alert state is the mesencephalic–pontine reticular core: the "reticular activating system" (Fig. 67) . Because of its great complexity, the neurophysiology of the brain stem will be limited to key points regarding reticular activation and reticular surpression of importance to the neurosurgeon.

1. Reticular activation–this is behavioral and electrographic arousal. There is a generalized, low voltage, fast asynchronous rhythm recorded from the cerebral hemispheres.
   a. Electrostimulation.
      (1) High frequency stimulation of the mesencephalic and rostral pontine reticular core produces cortical activation and behavioral arousal.
      (2) The same effect can be produced by high frequency stimulation of the dorsal thalamus in its reticular portions, which can then be prevented by midbrain coagulation caudally.
      (3) Similar effects can be produced by stimulation at high rates in caudal hypothalamic and subthalamic regions.
      (4) Hippocampal activation (low frequency theta) can be obtained by nonspecific alerting stimuli or by electrostimulation of the septum. The septum receives the terminations of brain stem reticular projections which have reached beyond the diencephalon. The septum is a relay from the reticular core of the brain stem to the hippocampus.
      (5) Unspecific thalamocortical system mediates activating influence from diencephalic reticular centers to the neocortex.
   b. Transection–while transection of the midbrain or rostral pons results in coma, a midpontine pretrigeminal transection produces a "tonically vigilant" preparation with persistent electrographic arousal and alert-appearing gaze responses. Caudal pontine transection has resulted in a similar picture. This may be compared to

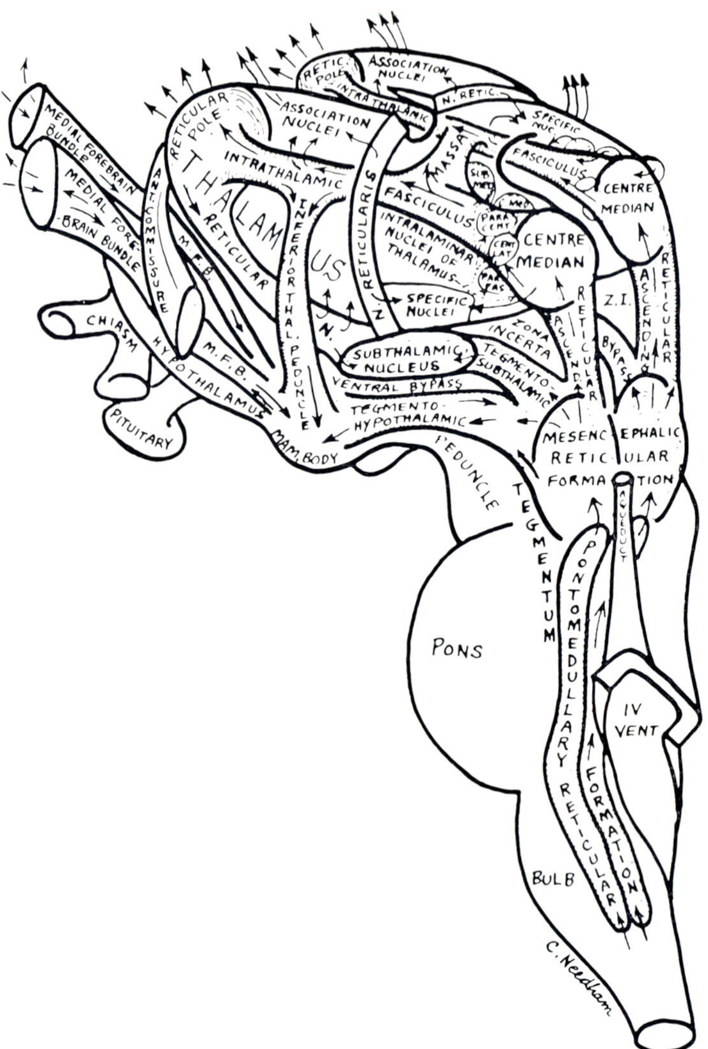

Figure 67. Reticular activating system. The brain stem reticular formation projects rostrally into the dorsal thalamus, subthalamus and hypothalamus. Reticular projections also terminate in the septum and basal forebrain.

the "locked-in syndrome" sometimes seen in human midpontine infarction. The patient is speechless and immobile due to bilateral supranuclear motor cranial nerve and spinal palsy, but an alert oculomotor system with ability to communicate through blinking persists. The akinetic mute, in contrast, although he may have an alert oculomotor system (vigilant coma), does not communicate.

2. Reticular suppression—this occurs with hypersomnia, stupor and coma. There is often a generalized, high voltage, slow, relatively synchronized rhythm recorded from the cerebral hemispheres. Sleep contains patterns similar to both reticular suppression and activation (e.g. "REM sleep"), and appears to be an active rather than passive phenomenon.
   a. Electrostimulation—stimulation, usually at low frequencies, at nearly any level of the central neuraxis (Fig. 68) from the basal forebrain to the medullary reticular formation can result in behavioral and electrographic sleep. Stimulation of midline thalamic and limbic structures can produce this picture.
   b. Focal lesions.
      (1) A relatively small lesion within the mesencephalic or rostral

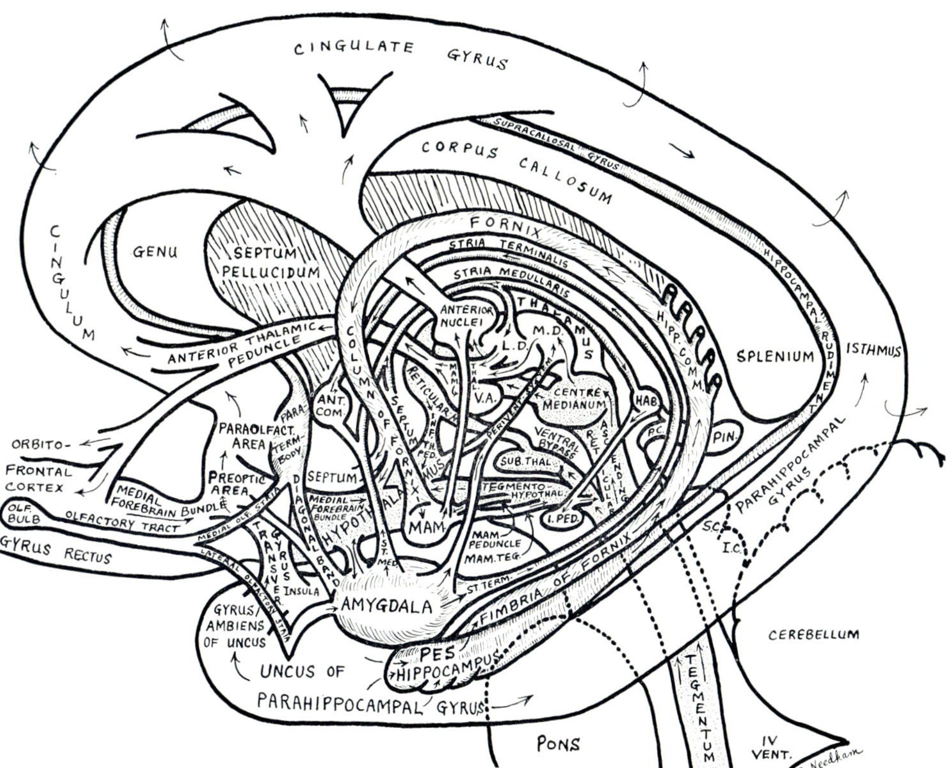

Figure 68. The central neuraxis of the brain. The brain stem reticular core establishes connections with the limbic system at many diencephalic and telecephalic levels. The limbic system is the primitive, multiple-ringed, mediobasal cerebrum, the rostral counterpart of the "isodendritic core" of the brain stem. These archaic brain structures are centralized and hidden by the process of encephalization. They may be regarded as a modulating system for neothalamic-neocortical activity.

pontine reticular core can produce coma, especially when the lesion is central or bilateral.

(2) Similar effects result from hypothalamic lesions and even with basal forebrain lesions (i.e. the anterior critical point). Rostral reticular projections terminate at hypothalamic, septal and basal forebrain levels (Fig. 69).

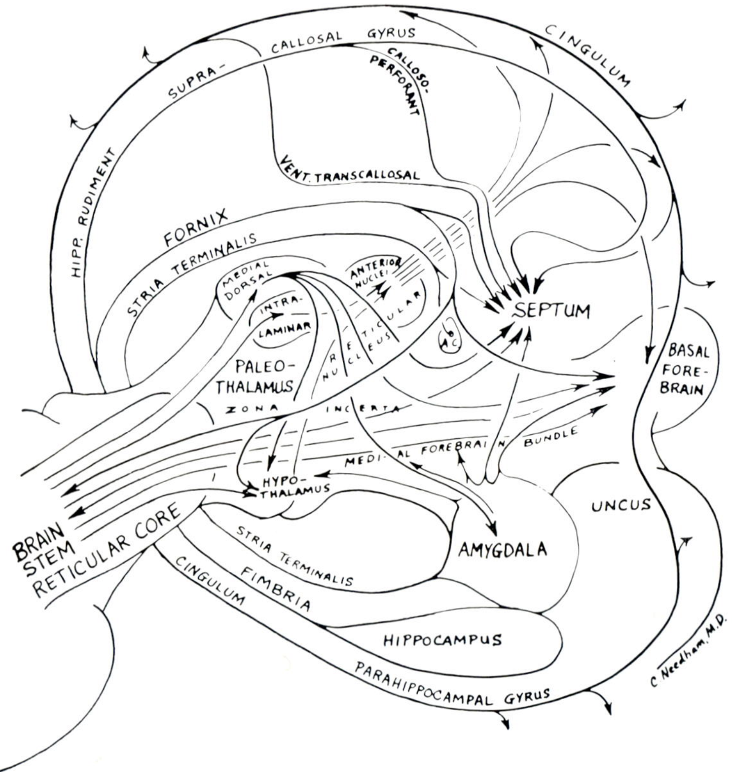

Figure 69. The old-brain. This diagram indicates the reticular, paleothalamic and limbic components of the old-brain. "Reticular activation" and "reticular suppression" can be experimentally produced from many levels, all lying within the confines of the old-brain. The old-brain is contrasted with the much larger new-brain, consisting of specific, callosal and associational bundles, neothalamus and neocortex.

(3) Coma does not necessarily follow a lesion in the medullary reticular core.

(4) The decorticate animal is not comatose if central cerebral and brain stem integrity are maintained. The rage reaction can be obtained from such preparations. Hemispherectomy similarly is compatible with the conscious state.

In summary, relatively small lesions of the phylogenetically old core systems of the upper brain stem, diencephalon and basal telencephalon specifically produce coma. The critical region lies both rostral and caudal to the third ventricle and within its lateral walls and floor (i.e. supratentorial segment). The critical region extends caudally about the aqueduct to the mouth of the fourth ventricle in the central portion (i.e. reticular tegmentum) of the midbrain and rostral pons. This centrobasal core is as vital to consciousness as the optic pathways are to vision. It is likely that in diffuse cerebral disease (e.g. anoxia, brain swelling, encephalopathy) sufficient to produce coma, deep central arousal pathways are involved as well as more superficial corticosubcortical structures.

3. Chemical physiology of the primitive projection systems.
   a. The brain amine "transmitter substances," dopamine, norepinephrine and serotonin, are largely restricted to the brain stem core, diencephalon and extrapyramidal structures.
   b. Dopamine and norepinephrine are the major catecholamines of the brain and are present in almost equal amounts.
   c. Dopamine, in addition to its independent transmitter action, is also the essential precursor of norepinephrine. The hypothalamus is one of the few brain sites where dopamine can penetrate the blood-brain barrier. It has been postulated that direct synthesis of hypothalamic norepinephrine from dopamine takes place in the hypothalamus.
   d. Regions containing the most dopamine contain the least norepinephrine and vice versa.
   e. Norepinephrine reaches its highest levels in the hypothalamus, medial thalamus and tegmental core of the brain stem.
   f. Dopamine reaches its greatest concentration in the corpus striatum and substantia nigra of the extrapyramidal system.
   g. Evidence that both catecholamines, norepinephrine and dopamine, are central transmitters is considerable. Enzymes for the synthesis and inactivation of both norepinephrine and dopamine are present in the brain.
   h. Epinephrine can drive single unit reticular neurons.
   i. Serotonin is found in significant amounts only in those structures which also contain either norepinephrine or dopamine.
   j. The distribution of serotonin most resembles that of norepinephrine.
   k. All three biogenic amines have their highest concentrations not only in primitive reticular, paleothalamic and extrapyramidal structures, but also in the ancient limbic system.

l. Within the central core of the brain stem, serotonin-containing neurons are most centrally situated (i.e. raphe system). Norepinephrine-containing neurons are more lateral (i.e. pontobulbar tegmentum) in the core. Dopamine-neurons are present in the midbrain core (i.e. ventromedial tegmentum). These are demonstrated by histofluorescence techniques.

m. Total destruction of the most central serotonin-neurons of the brain stem raphe system produces a maintained alert state (i.e. total insomnia).

n. These lines of evidence have implicated noradrenergic and serotonergic mechanisms in arousal and sleep.

B. Cerebellar physiology

The cerebellum acts like a motor computer for all phases, tonic and kinetic, of motor activity. It is a brain stem appendage which can continuously modify motor activity by direct and relay projections to all motor levels of the neuraxis (Fig. 70). Cerebellar physiology should be considered in conjunction with central motor mechanisms (see Ch. 9, "Central Cerebral Syndromes"). Cerebellar cortical neurons exhibit spontaneous fast activity in the absence of external stimulation. Neurons of the deep cerebellar nuclei exhibit tonic discharge. Modulation of recipient neurons is apparently accomplished by alterations in frequency of discharge by the deep cerebellar nuclear structures. Stimulation of the vermis directly influences static and kinetic motor activity. Stimulation of the cerebellar hemisphere appears to indirectly modulate motor activity by thalamocortical relay to the motor cortex.

Resection of a cerebellar hemisphere results in ipsilateral ataxia and hypotonia. If the resection includes the dentate nucleus, an ataxic tremor may occur. Section of the brachium conjunctivum may result in ataxia, hypotonia and tremor. Section of the restiform body leads to a less well-lateralized dysequilibrium. Resection of the vermis may result in extensor hypertonus. Midline lesions tend to result in truncal ataxia. Nystagmus may accompany cerebellar lesions and may result from damage to vestibular nuclei or imbalance of vestibular input following large cerebellar resections.

The vermis, fastigium and flocculonodular lobe influence the vestibular nuclei of the brain stem. The vestibular nuclei are innervated by the vestibular nerves from the labyrinth, utricle and saccule. Further integration with eye and head movement is carried out by connections of the medial longitudinal fasciculus with the third, fourth, sixth and eleventh motor nuclei of the brain stem and upper cervical cord. The vestibulospinal system activates the reticulospinal system. The cerebellum also has reciprocal projections to the reticular core of the brain stem. The red nucleus, a main site of cerebellar projection, lies within the tegmentum and has been considered to be a specialized reticular nucleus. Rubro-olivary fibers join the central tegmental tract to innervate the inferior olive, in turn projecting widely to the cerebellum. Rubrospinal fibers in man terminate at cervical cord levels. Reticuloreticular fibers from upper brain stem to medullary core innervate the reticulospinal tract, which is the chief vector of combined extrapyramidal influence to spinal levels. Spinal influence is returned to the anterior lobe of the cerebellum. The great bulk of input however, descends from cerebral levels for relay in the pontine nuclei and distribution to the neocerebellar hemispheres of the large posterior lobe. The bulk of the output of neocerebellar cortex is upon the dentate, in turn projecting rostrally to upper brain stem, thalamic, and—by relay—to motor cortical levels. Cerebellar output is integrated with pallidal (striate) output in the VL, the VL forming the final common pathway to motor cortex. Thus the cerebellum modulates the motor activity of both the old and new motor systems at many levels of the neuraxis.

NEUROSURGICAL SYNDROMES OF THE POSTERIOR FOSSA

Development

A. Acute brain stem contusion syndrome—traumatic contusion of the brain stem results in immediate coma, often with immediate decerebrate posturing. Decorticate posturing can occur as a result of associated central cerebral contusion, and some degree of brain swelling is commonly associated. Multiple cranial nerve palsies, hemiplegia, paraplegia and quadriplegia occur. Fluctuation in signs and autonomic instability are characteristic. "Brain stem seizures" are common. A lucid interval does not occur.

B. Acute cerebellar contusion—a relatively uncommon clinical contusion syndrome in closed head injuries. An acute ataxia ipsilateral to the contused hemisphere may be present. Acute intracerebellar or extracerebellar hematoma may be associated, and results in progressive obtundation with obstructive hydrocephalus and brain stem compression.

C. Acute posterior fossa traumatic hematoma syndrome—the traumatic posterior fossa clot is much less common than the supratentorial hematoma. The posterior fossa hematoma may be epidural, subdural or occasionally intracerebellar. Signs similar to supratentorial hematoma with progressive obtundation following trauma and signs of brain stem compression occur in posterior fossa hematomas. A lucid interval, similar to that sometimes present in the supratentorial epidural, may occur.

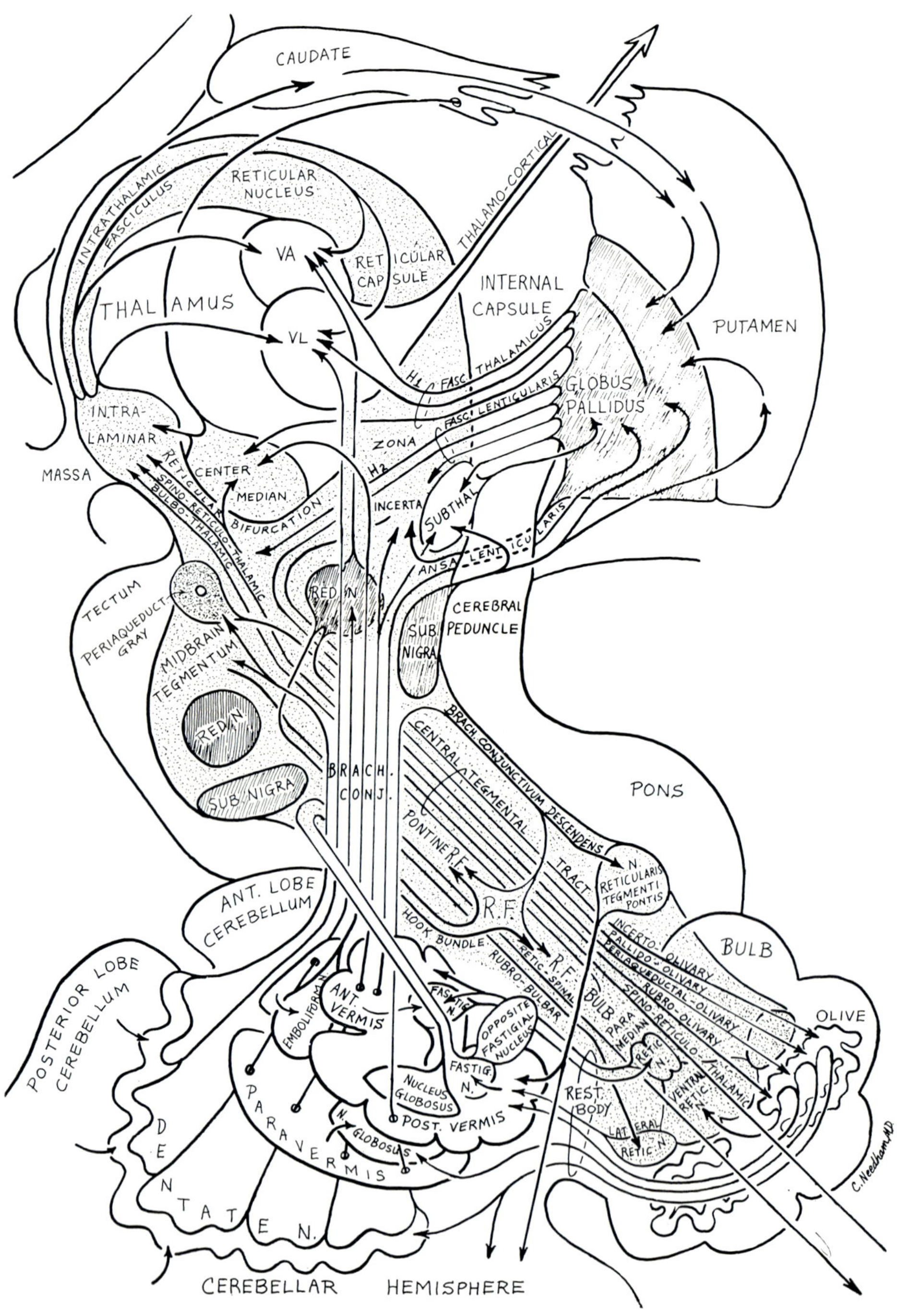
CAUDATE
INTRATHALAMIC FASCICULUS
RETICULAR NUCLEUS
THALAMO-CORTICAL
VA
RETICULAR CAPSULE
INTERNAL CAPSULE
THALAMUS
VL
PUTAMEN
H1
FASC. THALAMICUS
FASC. LENTICULARIS
GLOBUS PALLIDUS
INTRA-LAMINAR
MASSA
CENTER MEDIAN
ZONA
H2
INCERTA
SUBTHAL
RETICULAR BIFURCATION
SPINO-RETICULO-THALAMIC
BULBO-THALAMIC
ANSA LENTICULARIS
TECTUM
PERIAQUEDUCT GRAY
RED N.
CEREBRAL PEDUNCLE
SUB NIGRA
MIDBRAIN TEGMENTUM
BRACH. CONJ.
BRACH. CONJUNCTIVUM DESCENDENS
CENTRAL TEGMENTAL TRACT
PONTINE R.F.
PONS
N. RETICULARIS TEGMENTI PONTIS
ANT. LOBE CEREBELLUM
R.F.
HOOK BUNDLE
RETIC-SPINAL
RUBRO-BULBAR
BULB
INCERTO-OLIVARY
PALLIDO-OLIVARY
PERIAQUEDUCTAL-OLIVARY
RUBRO-OLIVARY
SPINO-RETICULO-THALAMIC
OLIVE
POSTERIOR LOBE CEREBELLUM
EMBOLIFORM N.
ANT. VERMIS
FASTIG. N.
OPPOSITE FASTIGIAL NUCLEUS
BULB PARA MEDIAN RETIC. N.
VENTRAL RETIC. N.
NUCLEUS GLOBOSUS
REST. BODY
LATERAL RETIC. N.
POST. VERMIS
N. GLOBOSUS
PARAVERMIS
DENTATE N.
C. Needham, M.D.
CEREBELLAR HEMISPHERE

Like supratentorial clots, there may be no lucidity, and just a course of progressive obtundation. A double lucid interval, with two phases of deterioration following initial unconsciousness, is an unusual manifestation of the posterior fossa epidural. Persistent vomiting, an occipital fracture, angiographic evidence of hydrocephalus or negative supratentorial exploratory burr holes in the traumatically comatose, deteriorating patient should suggest posterior fossa hematoma.

D. Ruptured vertebrobasilar aneurysm—often rapidly fatal. Much less common than carotid, middle cerebral and anterior communicating aneurysms. There may be total absence of localizing signs, closely simulating the much more common anterior communicating aneurysm. The presence of an asymmetrical corneal response, or negative bilateral carotid angiograms in an otherwise typical case of spontaneous subarachnoid hemorrhage should suggest an infratentorial aneurysm.

E. Spontaneous intracerebellar hematoma syndrome—the patient often has evidence of chronic arterial hypertension, but rupture of an arteriovenous malformation of the cerebellum may be responsible. There is often retention of the alert state for a number of hours. Headache is present during the alert phase in half the cases. Vomiting, vertigo, inability to stand, and progressive obtundation occur. The spinal fluid is almost always bloody.

F. Cerebellar tumor syndrome—symptoms and signs of progressive intracranial hypertension over several weeks or months, occurring most often in childhood, point to cerebellar tumor. Headache, irritability, loss of energy, vomiting, diplopia, papilledema and ataxia are characteristic. Astrocytoma (Fig. 71), medulloblastoma (Fig. 72), or ependymoma (Fig. 73) produce the same clinical picture. Recurrent episodes of meningitis or evidence of an occipital sinus tract should suggest posterior fossa dermoid. The same cerebellar and fourth ventricular tumors may also occur in adults with similar symptoms and signs. Cerebellar hemangioblastoma, subtentorial meningioma and metastatic carcinoma of the cerebellum should be included in the differential diagnosis. Choroid

Figure 70. Cerebellum, the motor computer. The cerebellum has a complex relationship with the corpus striatum. Both project to the thalamic VL, the final common path to motor cortex. Both also have an overlapping projection to the brain stem reticular core: the extrapyramidal-extralemniscal complex, depicted above. Motor integration at the spinal level is largely the composite of corticospinal and reticulospinal influence. The cerebellum effects continuous motor modification through its output, the brachium conjunctivum, containing the projections of the deep cerebellar nuclei shown above. The major input to the large posterior lobe is cerebral, via pontine nuclear projections in the brachium pontis. This input, plus the spinal input to the small anterior lobe, have been excluded.

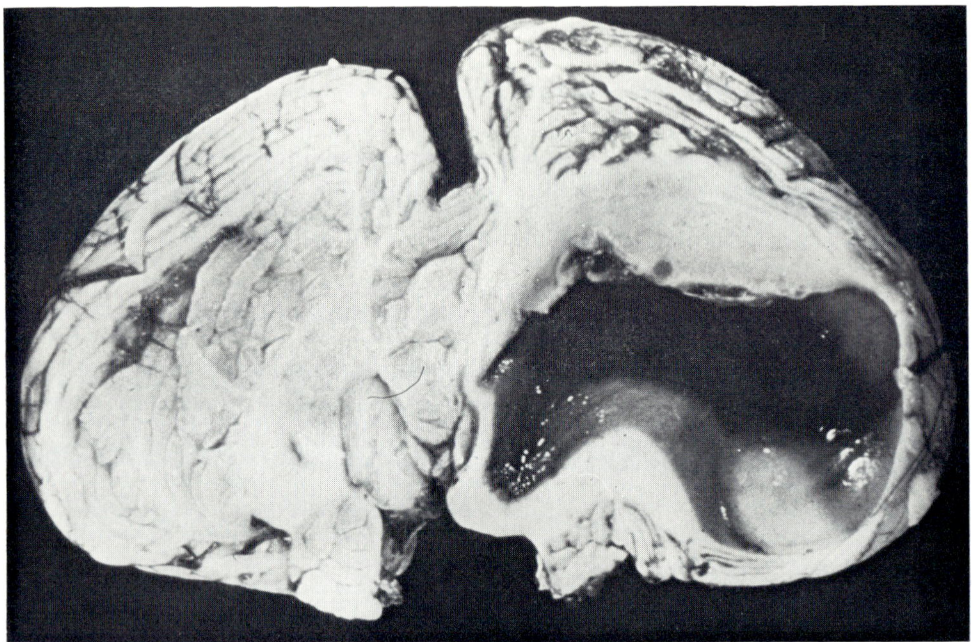

Figure 71. Cerebellar astrocytoma.

plexus papilloma of the fourth ventricle is an unusual posterior fossa tumor, but does occur in the adult. Obstructive hydrocephalus with intracranial hypertension results, just as in other cerebellar tumors.

G. Cerebellar abscess syndrome—this may present in the same manner as the cerebellar tumor, and may occur at any age. Middle ear or mastoid infection may be responsible for either cerebellar or temporal lobe abscess. Transverse sinus occlusion may be associated. Septic signs may be prominent or absent at the time of diagnosis. The abscess may be related to a posterior fossa dermoid with an occipital sinus tract and previous episodes of meningitis. Tuberculoma of the cerebellum may be responsible. The abscess may be an extension from an abscess in the cerebellopontine angle, with clinical evidence of an angle syndrome. In older age groups, an apparent cerebellar abscess may be necrotic metastatic carcinoma of pulmonary origin.

H. Infantile hydrocephalus syndrome—this is discussed at greater length in the next chapter ("Syndromes of Intracranial Hypertension"). Abnormal cranial enlargement in infancy may be the result of aqueductal stenosis, Arnold-Chiari malformation of the hindbrain, Dandy-Walker syndrome with occlusion of the outlets of the fourth ventricle (the ventricle becomes a large posterior fossa cyst), and varying forms of

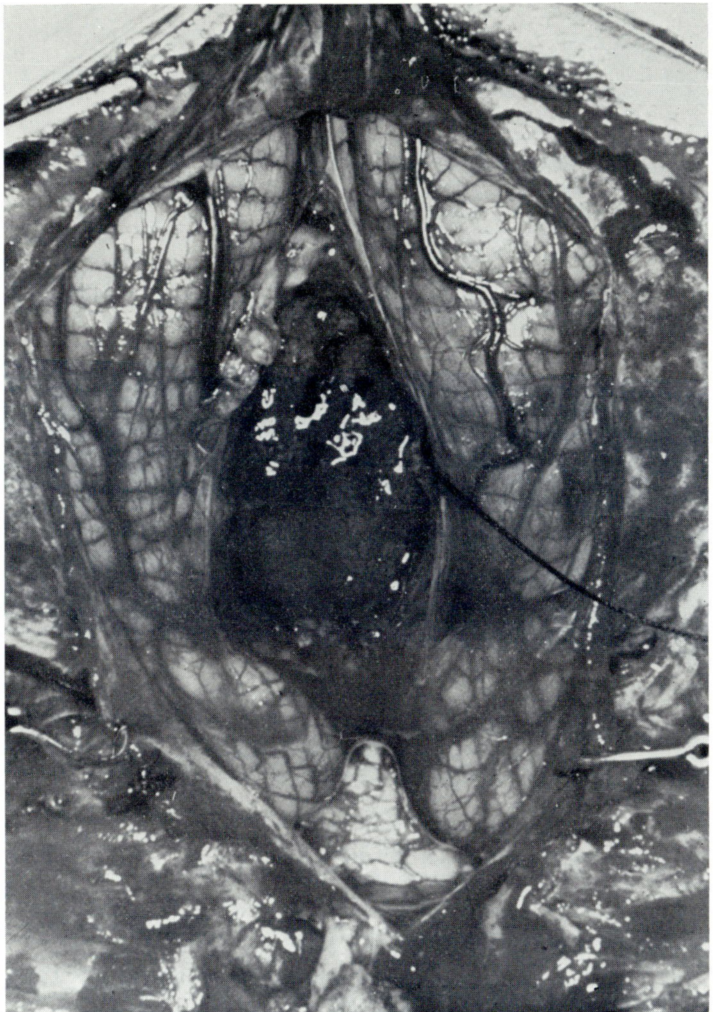

Figure 72. Medulloblastoma.

communicating hydrocephalus. The Arnold-Chiari and Dandy-Walker abnormalities resulting in hydrocephalus are infratentorial. The occlusion of the upper aqueduct in most cases of aqueductal stenosis occurs at the tentorial level. Supratentorial subdural hematomas, cerebral tumor or posterior fossa tumor may also produce cranial enlargement in infancy.

I. Brain stem glioma syndrome (Fig. 74) —less common than cerebellar tumors, but like the cerebellar tumor, the intrinsic glioma of the brain stem is most common in childhood. Progressive gait disturbance, squint,

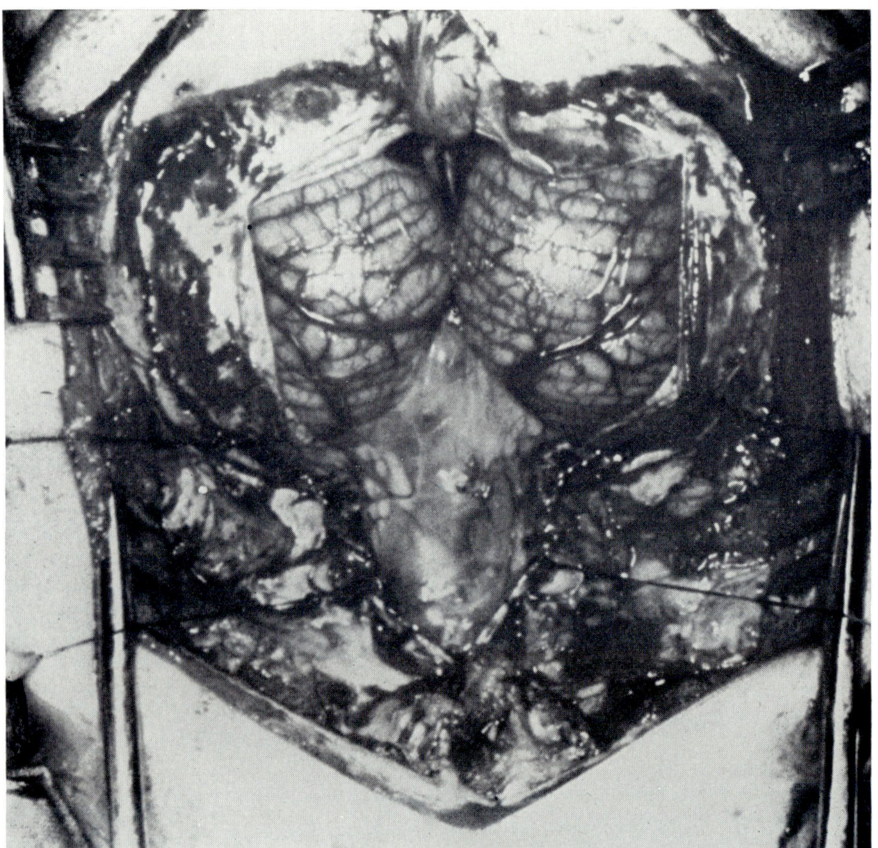

Figure 73. Ependymoma.

facial palsy or other cranial nerve signs develop over several weeks or months, without evidence of intracranial hypertension. Truncal ataxia with spasticity and pyramidal signs are common. Signs eventually become bilateral. Evidence of elevated intracranial pressure is late, in contrast to cerebellar tumor.

J. Cerebellopontine angle syndrome—this is unusual in childhood although an acoustic neuroma can present early in von Recklinghausen's disease. Most patients with angle tumors are middle-aged adults, and the most common angle tumor is the acoustic neuroma. Gradual unilateral deafness over months or years, with tinnitus, imbalance and facial asymmetry are commonly noted. Intracranial hypertension is late, in contrast to the cerebellar tumor.

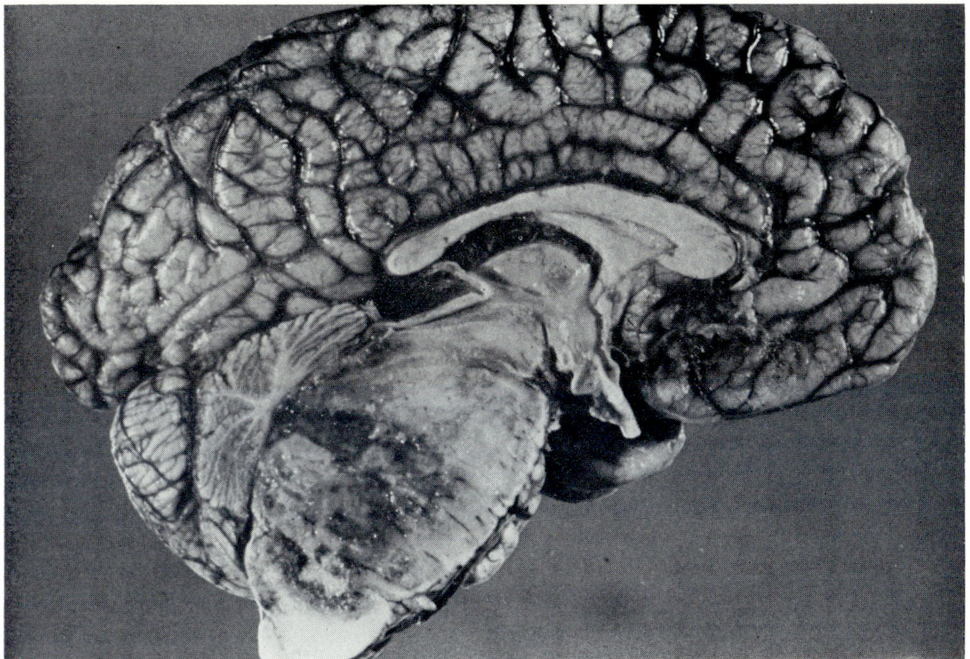

Figure 74. Brain stem glioma.

Deficits of the Posterior Fossa Syndromes

Neurosurgical syndromes of the posterior fossa are of three basic types.

1. Cerebellar.
2. Brain stem.
3. Cerebellopontine angle.

The neurosurgical cerebellar syndromes may be hemispheral or vermian. Hemiataxia is ipsilateral to the involved hemisphere, or predominantly truncal when the vermis is involved. However, with either hemispheral, vermian or fourth ventricular involvement by tumor, progressive intracranial hypertension due to obstructive hydrocephalus is the common denominator. The obstructive hydrocephalus results from tumor within the fourth ventricle, occlusion of the outlets of the ventricle and obliteration of the cisterns, or by translated compression, shift and collapse of the fourth ventricle from a hemispheral cerebellar tumor.

The posterior fossa neurosurgical syndromes of the brain stem type may be intrinsic (e.g. glioma, contusion). Alternatively, they may be extrinsic with infratentorial brain stem compression (e.g. large cerebellar or acoustic tumor, meningioma, chordoma, nasopharyngeal carcinoma, large vertebrobasilar aneurysm, infratentorial hematoma). Extrinsic upper brain stem compression by the supratentorial mass has been discussed in previous chapters.

The cerebellopontine angle syndrome of the acoustic tumor is treated separately because of its highly characteristic nature and because diagnosis can be made before significant cerebellar and brain stem compression are clinically manifest. A meningioma, epidermoid and aneurysm can simulate the acoustic tumor syndrome. The angle syndrome almost always occurs in an adult. The various other tumors extrinsic to the brain stem and cerebellum are also much more common in adult life. In contrast, intrinsic tumors of the cerebellum and brain stem are much more common in childhood.

Cerebellar tumors characteristically present early signs of elevated intracranial pressure. The pressure increase occurs more regularly and more rapidly than with tumors at other brain sites. Papilledema is almost always present, and may be chronic at the time of diagnosis; the danger of rapid visual loss is great. In contrast, the intrinsic brain stem glioma of childhood, like the extrinsic angle acoustic tumor of adult life, reveals distinctively localizing deficits early in the course, while intracranial hypertension occurs much later.

A. Cerebellar syndromes

The symptoms and signs of intracranial hypertension (e.g. headache, vomiting, papilledema) are treated in greater detail in the next chapter since they are common to a host of neurosurgical mass syndromes. While in most brain tumors the signs of elevated pressure are the last to appear, in cerebellar tumors these signs are the earliest. Headache, irritability, vomiting, diplopia, and papilledema are directly related to the elevated pressure occurring with the obstructive hydrocephalus, due in turn to fourth ventricular compression or obliteration by cerebellar tumor. Young children may not complain of headache or diplopia; loss of normal childhood energy and vomiting may be the only symptoms due to pressure. Cerebellar signs are superimposed on the clinical picture:

1. Ataxia and hypotonia.

The most important cerebellar signs are ataxia and hypotonia. The childhood cerebellar tumor most often presents a truncal ataxia, even when the bulk of the tumor is hemispheral rather than vermian. This apparent paradox is the result of the influence of hydrocephalus, which itself can produce a truncal form of ataxia. A wide-based gait with impairment of tandem walking is characteristic. Circle walking and hopping may bring out ataxic deficits which are not obvious. Cerebellar ataxia typically occurs on attempted complex movement. The ataxia persists despite visual assistance. If severe, there may be inability to stand without support. If the patient can stand unsupported, there may be persistent falling when walking is attempted or with eye closure. In hemispheral tumors with ipsilateral hypotonia, there is a marked tendency to fall to the side of the tumor. In vermian tumors or hemispheral tumors with marked hydrocephalus, the hypotonia may be most marked in both legs, with a tendency to fall in place rather than to either side. Increased tone in the extremities indicates brain stem compression or actual invasion of the brain stem by the cerebellar tumor. Truncal ataxia combined with spasticity, in the absence of intracranial hypertension, should suggest intrinsic glioma of the brain stem rather than cerebellar tumor.

When the patient is placed in bed, the ataxia of the erect position may all but disappear. The contribution of hypotonia to the patient's incoordination can be tested, in relative isolation from ataxia, with the patient supine. Heel-knee-tibia testing and toe-to-finger testing may reveal lower extremity ataxia while the patient remains supine. When the patient is prone with the knees flexed to 90°, oscillations of the ataxic leg occur when the patient is instructed to keep the legs erect. In cerebellar tumors with demonstrable lower extremity ataxia, there may be minimal upper extremity ataxia. The hemispheral tumor with ipsilateral hypotonia may produce ipsilateral impairment in finger-to-nose, finger-to-finger and rapid alternating movement testing. There may be decomposition of movement in a jerky intermittent fashion. There may be dysmetria with overshooting. An ataxic intention tremor may be noted, characteristically without tremor at rest. Pouring a glass of water, writing (i.e. ataxic macrographia), and tying shoelaces are good sample tests to reveal incoordination.

2. Nystagmus.

Evidence of nystagmus may not be present even when there is marked ataxia. When nystagmus occurs, it is usually most marked on lateral gaze, and is coarser to the side of a hemispheral tumor. When nystagmus is absent, the patient is rapidly brought to a full sitting position from the supine. Nystagmus induced by this maneuver can occur in vermian tumors of the cerebellum and in intrinsic brain stem tumors. Spontaneous vertical nystagmus can occur in anterior vermian tumors and in intrinsic brain stem tumors. Nystagmus, when present, is an important sign. Supratentorial brain tumors which produce a pseudocerebellar ataxia (e.g. frontal tumors) are not associated with nystagmus. There are some exceptions, however. The supratentorial tumor most often associated with nystagmus is temporal. The finding of nystagmus in a tumor suspect should always direct attention to the posterior fossa. This is particularly true in childhood.

3. Other signs of cerebellar tumor.
   a. Stiff neck—this may be due to herniation of a cerebellar tonsil or extension of tumor through the foramen magnum into the upper cervical canal. However, nuchal rigidity may also be present without foramen magnum impaction. There may be head tilting and suboccipital tenderness. Neck stiffness tends to increase as intracranial pressure becomes marked.
   b. Signs of brain stem compression by cerebellar tumor.
      (1) Obtundation of consciousness.
      (2) Cranial nerve signs—abducens palsy with resultant diplopia is usually the result of increased intracranial pressure rather than direct brain stem compression by the cerebellar tumor. It is usually unilateral. Compression of the dorsolateral pons can produce a facial assymmetry. Actual extension of cerebellar tumor into the brain stem can produce other cranial palsies.
      (3) Reflex signs—the usual cerebellar tumor results in hypoactive deep tendon reflexes, especially in the lower extremities. Plantar reflexes are normal. Hyperactive reflexes, a Babinski sign or evidence of spasticity points to brain stem compression by the cerebellar tumor. The same effect can be produced by invasion of the brain stem by the cerebellar tumor. However, brain stem compression by a large cerebellar mass is more common than actual brain stem invasion by tumor.
      (4) Brain stem seizures—these were once known as "cerebellar fits." Most cases of cerebellar tumor are not associated with any convulsive activity. However, severe brain stem compression, sometimes occurring during a hydrocephalic attack with an acute rise in intracranial pressure, can produce sudden and episodic extensor rigidity. The patient assumes the decerebrate posture, with autonomic instability, pupillary dilatation and deep coma. Apnea and cyanosis may occur during such an attack.*
4. Cerebellar tumor types.

The clinical picture of cerebellar tumor described above does not

---

**Note:* While brain stem seizures and hydrocephalic attacks can occur together in the large cerebellar tumor, the term "brain stem seizure" is not synonymous with the term "hydrocephalic attack." A typical brain stem seizure may occur in brain stem contusion without any evidence of hydrocephalus or even of elevated intracranial pressure. A typical hydrocephalic attack can occur in the acute obstruction of the foramen of Monro by the colloid cyst of the third ventricle. Hydrocephalic attacks are considered in greater detail in the next chapter.

allow an exact diagnosis as to tumor type in the individual case. The pathologically benign "juvenile astrocytoma" of the cerebellum and the malignant medulloblastoma both produce the same clinical picture. Both are most common in childhood, but both also occur in adult life. The juvenile astrocytoma is most common in the cerebellar hemisphere, but also occurs in the vermis. The medulloblastoma is most common in the vermis, but also occurs in the hemisphere. The medulloblastoma commonly invades the meninges and may metastasize in the CSF. The juvenile astrocytoma may locally invade the meninges, but does not spread by CSF metastasis. The juvenile astrocytoma is commonly cystic with a mural nodule; it may be solid. The ependymoma of the fourth ventricle similarly cannot be clinically differentiated. It also occurs in childhood and in adult life. It also involves the vermis and may extend into the hemisphere of the cerebellum. The ependymoma commonly extends through the foramen magnum into the upper cervical region; stiff neck, however, is common in any cerebellar tumor. The ependymoma seeds the CSF. The hemangioblastoma of the cerebellum presents the clinical picture of the cerebellar tumor in adult life. There may be polycythemia. This tumor is most common within the cerebellar hemisphere and often has the gross appearance of a cystic juvenile astrocytoma. It may have a mural nodule. The vermis may be involved. The tumor may be attached to the meninges and compress the cerebellum from without; angioblastic meningioma may be simulated. The choroid plexus papilloma is an uncommon tumor, and when it occurs it usually grows within the lateral ventricle, the typical case being a form of childhood hydrocephalus. However, when it occurs in the fourth ventricle, it produces a typical cerebellar syndrome with obstructive hydrocephalus in the adult. In the older age group, metastatic carcinoma of the cerebellum should be considered with astrocytoma and hemangioblastoma. Glioblastoma of the cerebellum is exceedingly rare. The cerebellar tumor syndrome can be simulated by cerebellar abscess, cerebellar tuberculoma and posterior fossa dermoid (which may be secondarily infected). Parasitic cysts of the posterior fossa can produce the same picture.

B. Brain stem syndromes

Neurosurgically operable mass lesions producing brain stem signs are ordinarily extrinsic to the brain stem proper. Midbrain compression is usually due to a supratentorial-transtentorial process (e.g. uncal herniation), rather than due to a posterior fossa mass. The entire brain stem can be shifted downward (e.g. central transtentorial herniation) by supratentorial mass effect. Cerebellar tonsillar herniation (e.g. foraminal impaction) through the foramen magnum can occur with either the supratentorial or subtentorial mass. Brain stem involvement by the supratentorial mass is considered in previous chapters.

Three basic brain stem syndromes of neurosurgical interest are considered in this section.

1. Brain stem glioma syndrome—a progressive intrinsic brain stem syndrome which should be contrasted with the cerebellar tumor syndrome.
2. Brain stem contusion syndrome—on acute intrinsic brain stem syndrome which should be contrasted with the traumatic supratentorial and infratentorial hematoma syndromes.
3. Syndromes of brain stem compression by posterior fossa mass—brain stem compromise by various infratentorial mass lesions extrinsic to the neuraxis.

Deficits of the brain stem syndromes include the following:

1. Syndrome of the brain stem glioma—the patient is usually a child with a history of progressive gait disturbance of several weeks or months duration. A squint and facial asymmetry may have been noted. Motor and occasionally bulbar paralysis may occur symptomatically. Headache, vomiting and mental symptoms are typically absent. Presenting signs include the following:
   a. Multiple bilateral cranial nerve signs.
      (1) Abducens palsy—this is the most common cranial nerve involved and may be unilateral or bilateral; there may be an associated horizontal conjugate gaze paralysis; nystagmus is less common. A small pupil due to Horner's syndrome may be present.
      (2) Facial palsy—this commonly presents as a peripheral facial diplegia; unilateral facial palsy may occur; if hemiparesis is also present, it tends to occur on the side opposite the unilateral facial weakness.
      (3) Trigeminal palsy—when present, a unilateral diminution of corneal sensation is most common; this decrease may be bilateral and the corneal reflexes are typically also impaired by facial weakness; hemifacial hypesthesia with crossed hemihypesthesia of the body may occur.
      (4) Palatal, pharyngeal and laryngeal paralysis may be noted with associated dysphagia and dysarthria. The gag reflex is depressed. Pseudobulbar signs may occur. Hypoglossal weakness with or without atrophy is occasionally noted. Attacks of hiccoughing sometimes occur. Palatal myoclonus is rare.

b. Pyramidal tract signs.
   (1) Hyperactive reflexes most marked in the lower extremities are common.
   (2) Unilateral or bilateral Babinski signs and ankle clonus are also common. Decreased superficial abdominal reflexes and positive Hoffmann's signs also occur.
   (3) Motor paralysis assumes one of three forms: hemiplegia, paraplegia or quadriplegia. The paralysis is spastic despite the coexistence of "cerebellar" ataxia. When hemiplegia occurs early, it tends to be of the crossed type, on the side opposite any unilateral cranial nerve signs. Even when motor paralysis is unilateral, there are usually bilateral hyperactive tendon reflexes or bilateral Babinski signs. Unilateral paralysis soon becomes bilateral, and decerebrate posturing may occur. When spastic paraplegia is initially noted, normal bladder function and the absence of a sensory level, with cranial nerve and upper motor neuron signs, point to a brain stem origin.

c. Truncal ataxia.
   (1) The disturbance of gait is a prominent sign. The patient walks on a wide base. The pelvis tends to be projected forward and the trunk backward. There is a definite tendency to fall backward, although the child may fall to either side. There may be inability to stand without support. Extremity ataxia may be minimal despite marked swaying during ambulation. When the patient is tested supine in bed, there may be no evidence of ataxia.
   (2) The other major cerebellar sign, hypotonia, is typically absent. Thus, truncal ataxia with lower extremity spasticity favors brain stem tumor, while truncal ataxia with hypotonia of the legs favors midline cerebellar tumor. Conversion of such hypotonia to spasticity may occur with brain stem extension or compression by cerebellar glioma.
   (3) Nystagmus and other cerebellar signs are much less common than truncal ataxia. Nystagmus may sometimes be induced (positional nystagmus) by rapidly lifting the child from the supine to the sitting position. Such induced nystagmus can occur with either brain stem or midline cerebellar tumors.

d. Normal fundi—this is a major sign because it separates the brain stem glioma from the majority of other posterior fossa tumors of childhood. Headache and papilledema are late signs of brain stem glioma. When they occur with brain stem signs, cerebellar tumor with brain stem compression or extension of cerebellar tumor to the pons should be ruled out. Late cases of brain stem glioma may produce obstructive hydrocephalus due to aqueductal and fourth ventricular stenosis. They are usually readily differentiated from other causes of aqueductal block by the presence of well-developed multiple cranial nerve, long tract and ataxic signs.

2. Syndrome of the brain stem contusion.

Acute brain stem injury is commonly the result of automotive trauma. The most common sign is coma from the time of injury; this is nonspecific since immediate unconsciousness which persists can occur in both supratentorial and infratentorial hematomas extrinsic to the brain stem. The spectrum of associated signs, including cranial nerve and vital signs with motor and reflex deficits, are highly variable in brain stem contusion. Many of these signs may be closely simulated by extracerebral or intracerebral hematoma with secondary brain stem compression. Angiography and exploratory burr holes are often required because of the frequently great clinical similarity between these acute primary and secondary brain stem syndromes. In the traumatically comatose patient with brain stem signs, a history of alertness for a period following injury favors secondary brain stem compression. A history of immediate decerebration at the scene of injury favors primary brain stem contusion. Usually such history is not available, the patient being comatose upon arrival in the emergency room. The signs of the primary contusion of the brain stem are as follow:

a. Coma—the patient is not arousable to conscious levels despite noxious stimulation. Such stimuli may elicit semipurposeful movement, reflex withdrawal, decerebrate posturing, or no motor response at all. Bilateral diminution or absence of corneal responses are good indicators of the level of impaired sensorium. Unequal or unilateral abnormalities of corneal response have different significance and are discussed below.

b. Cranial nerve signs.

(1) Fundi—the optic discs and retinae are usually normal. Occasionally, retinal hemorrhages accompany an associated traumatic subarachnoid hemorrhage. The early development of papilledema suggests brain swelling due to an associated cerebral contusion; hematoma must be ruled out; both edema and hematoma tend to produce a deepening level of coma; both commonly occur with entirely normal fundi. The late development of papilledema several weeks after injury suggests a post-traumatic communicating hydrocephalus. This is usually the result of traumatic subarachnoid hemorrhage.

(2) Oculomotor, trochlear and abducens paralyses—these tend to be present in various combinations bilaterally and asymmetrically in brain stem contusion. Both internal and external ophthalmoplegia are common. Fluctuating changes in pupillary size are notable. Pupillary abnormalities which defy explanation on another basis are common in brain stem contusion. Progressive oculomotor palsy with a dilating pupil beginning unilaterally must always suggest the presence of an ipsilateral supratentorial hematoma. Isolated abducens palsy has no sharp localizing significance; it commonly indicates elevated intracranial pressure. A downward shift of the brain stem secondary to supratentorial mass may result in unilateral or bilateral abducens palsies. A primary brain stem contusion may also produce unilateral or bilateral abducens paralysis. An isolated trochlear paralysis is rare.

(3) Gaze paralysis—abnormalities in conjugate ocular movement are common in brain stem contusion. Gaze may appear normal until the head is turned from side to side or flexed and extended. Such cephalic manipulation may induce disconjugate gaze, sometimes with changes in pupillary size. Alternatively, gaze may be grossly disconjugate without any manipulation. There may be conjugate ocular deviation to either side and the head may be slightly rotated. In brain stem lesions, such conjugate ocular deviation is not readily overcome by cephalic manipulation. When the normal compensatory ocular movements to head turning are diminished or absent, caloric stimulation may induce the oculovestibular reflex. If oculovestibular paralysis persists, simultaneous cold and warm water irrigation of opposite external auditory canals may induce ocular movement. In severe brain stem damage, there may be total paralysis of the oculovestibular response to all stimuli. If irrigation elicits only vertical eye movement, a pontine destructive lesion may be suspected. A brain stem nystagmus of undulatory type with slow, approximately regular to and fro movements may be noted in contusion. This nystagmus precedes total paralysis of gaze.

(4) The corneal reflex—bilateral diminution of the corneal responses may reflect the level of obtundation. Unilateral marked diminution or absence of corneal response suggests brain stem trigeminal involvement; facial paralysis must be ruled out.

(5) Facial paralysis—central facial weakness associated with hemiplegia on the same side as the facial palsy should suggest supra-

tentorial hematoma. Such paralysis is usually contralateral to the hematoma, but may be ipsilateral (Kernohan's notch). In contrast, facial paralysis on one side with hemiplegia on the opposite side occurs with brain stem lesions. Peripheral facial weakness involving the entire hemiface can be due to the brain stem contusion itself or to peripheral facial nerve involvement in an associated basilar skull fracture. Signs of fracture of the cranial base (mastoid ecchymosis, CSF or hemorrhagic otorrhea) are particularly common in association with brain stem contusion. Basilar fracture may of course be absent in the presence of marked brain stem injury. Signs of basilar skull trauma are not of good differential value, since they may also be present in supratentorial or infratentorial hematoma as well.

(6) Bulbar paralysis—decrease in gag reflex, palatal, pharyngeal and laryngeal weakness may occur in brain stem contusion.

c. Vital signs—fluctuation in vital signs is characteristic of brain stem contusion.

(1) Hyperventilation alternating with normoventilation and periodic apnea may occur. Noisy hyperventilation is also common in midbrain compression due to supratentorial mass.

(2) Fluctuations in pulse and blood pressure are also common in brain stem contusion. A persistent tendency for systemic hypertension with bradycardia or tachycardia should suggest intracranial hypertension (e.g. brain swelling or hematoma). Systemic hypotension with tachycardia may be due to brain stem contusion, but associated acute gastrointestinal bleeding should be ruled out.

(3) Hyperthermia, hypothermia, episodic diaphoresis and diabetes insipidis—these suggest a hypothalamic—high brain stem contusion.

d. Motor deficits—these are highly variable in the acute brain stem contusion, but motor signs in the extremities are virtually always present.

(1) Decerebration—hypertonic hyperextension and hyperpronation of the extremities either spontaneously or related to noxious stimulation is common. For practical purposes, this indicates a midbrain or pontine level. External compression of the midbrain may produce the same effect. Pontine contusion may be associated with typical decerebrate posturing of the upper extremities and flaccidity of the lower extremities. Bilaterally small pupils also favor a pontine level. Decerebration

is usually bilateral but may be unilateral; in the latter case, there is commonly a coexistent hemiplegia of the opposite limbs. Decerebrate attacks may occur with neck retraction and opisthotonus. Vital signs may fluctuate markedly during such tonic brain stem seizures and profound apnea may occur. Unilateral focal clonic seizures of face, arm or leg are not common and suggest associated cerebral contusion.

(2) Decortication—generalized rigidity with flexion of the upper extremities and extension of the lower extremities may be seen in association with signs of brain stem contusion. This decorticate rigidity usually indicates some degree of associated cerebral contusion of deep central cerebral type.

(3) Paralysis—in brain stem contusion, paralysis may take the form of hemiplegia, paraplegia, triplegia or tetraplegia. Isolated brachial or crural monoplegias are uncommon. Weakness may be partial or complete. Tone may be increased, normal or reduced and often fluctuates between hypertonic and hypotonic states. In pontine failure, an atonic paraplegia often associated with small pupils occurs. In medullary failure, an atonic tetraplegia, often with bilaterally dilated pupils, may occur as a terminal event.

(4) Motor restlessness—the comatose patient exhibiting almost continuous or increasing random or semipurposeful movements of restless, irritable type may present a diagnostic problem. Such activity is seen in high brain stem-subfrontal contusion. However, increasing restlessness may be due to rising intracranial pressure with impending transtentorial herniation (e.g. hematoma). Subarachnoid hemorrhage with meningeal irritation may be responsible. Bladder distension may produce a similar picture in the comatose patient.

e. Reflex signs.

Unilateral or bilateral Babinski signs are common in brain stem contusion. They are often associated with other pyramidal signs. However, a Babinski sign is also common opposite an epidural, subdural or intracerebral hematoma. At times, these supratentorial hematomas may result in an ipsilateral Babinski. This occurs with shift of the midbrain to the opposite tentorial edge, with "notching" of the cerebral peduncle on the side opposite the mass. Since the corticospinal fibers decussate in the medullary pyramids, pyramidal signs and paralysis can in this instance be ipsilateral to the supratentorial clot. In addition, an extracerebral hematoma which sufficiently compresses the midbrain via uncal herniation can produce bilateral Babinski signs. An intracerebral hematoma which extends into the ventricle, or extends into the midbrain, or compresses the midbrain similarly can produce bilateral Babinski signs. The significance of the Babinski sign is greatest when it is opposite an oculomotor palsy, for it then suggests supratentorial hematoma on the side of the dilated pupil.

3. Syndromes of brain stem compression by posterior fossa mass.

   The intracerebellar mass and cerebellopontine angle tumor which may compress the brain stem are dealt with separately because of their distinctive syndromes. An uncommon group of infratentorial spacetaking lesions remains which includes tumor, aneurysm and hematoma.

   a. Chordoma of the clivus.

      This unusual and slowly progressive tumor erodes the clivus behind the dorsum sellae and in front of the pons. The hallmark of this tumor is multiple bilateral cranial nerve palsies. Abducens palsy, unilateral or bilateral, in the absence of signs of elevated intracranial pressure, may be the earliest deficit. Intracranial hypertension is late. The chordoma dislocates the brain stem posteriorly. It erodes into the sphenoid sinus anteriorly and may protrude into the posterior nasopharynx. It extends upward into the interpenduncular cistern, compressing the oculomotor nerves and cerebral peduncles. It extends rostrally as a retrochiasmatic mass with compression of the chiasm, optic tracts and third ventricular floor. It may erode the sella. It extends caudally into the foramen magnum producing neck pain and nuchal rigidity. Lateral extension into a cerebellopontine angle may occur. Cranial nerves two through twelve may eventually be involved in association with pyramidal tract signs; cranial nerve and pyramidal signs are distributed bilaterally in various combinations. Cerebrospinal fluid leak and meningitis may occur.

   b. Tumor syndrome of multiple bilateral cranial nerve palsies with late intracranial hypertension.

      This distinctive syndrome may result from various tumors of the posterior fossa. In the child, the brain stem glioma is most common. In the young adult, glioma, chordoma and nasopharyngeal lymphoma should be considered. In the older adult, clivus chordoma, meningioma and nasopharyngeal or metastatic carcinoma of the cranial base are diagnostic possibilities.

      Multiple unilateral cranial nerve palsies in the adult suggest acoustic neuroma, meningioma, or cholesteatoma of the cerebellopontine angle. A chromophobe adenoma or meningioma of

Meckel's cave may extend into the posterior fossa and produce a multiple cranial nerve syndrome.

Such multiple cranial nerve syndromes due to slowly or moderately progressive tumors should be contrasted with the acute multiple cranial nerve syndrome associated with hydrocephalic attacks. In this instance, symptoms and signs of intracranial hypertension are present before the onset of multiple cranial nerve palsy. The cranial nerve signs in this unusual syndrome are falsely localizing, typically bilateral, often symmetrical and may fluctuate in severity. This multiple cranial nerve syndrome is considered in the next chapter.

c. Syndrome of the foramen magnum meningioma (Fig. 75).

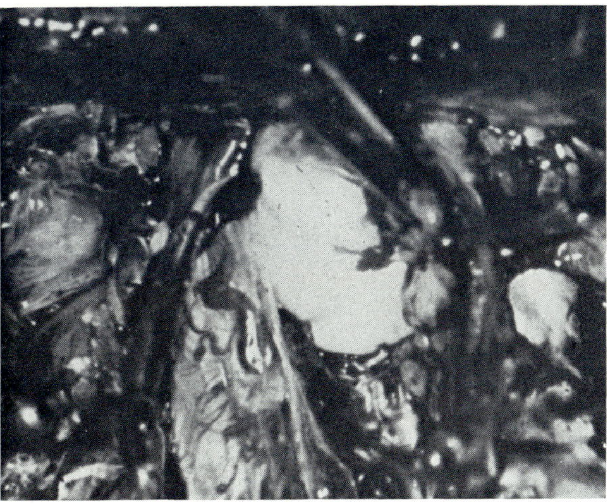

Figure 75. Foramen magnum meningioma.

These slowly growing tumors of the adult compress the lower brain stem at the medullary-cervical junction. The medulla may be compressed anteriorly, posteriorly or posterolaterally. The characteristics of this foramen magnum syndrome include the following:

(1) Suboccipital and neck pain with cervical rigidity. An abnormal posture of the head may be noted.

(2) Shoulder, arm and occasionally spinal pain and paresthesias.

(3) Progressive extremity paralysis. This may take several forms.

(a) Spinal hemiplegia—the face is characteristically spared but the tongue may be involved.

(b) Cruciate paralysis—there is brachial diplegia with weakness greater in the arms, the legs being relatively spared. Nonetheless, Babinski signs, clonus and hyperactive reflexes are often noted in the lower extremities despite their relative strength.

(c) Spastic paraplegia—the upper extremities are relatively spared. Loss of position sense in the arms with pyramidal signs in the legs is a common combination.

(d) Triplegia and tetraplegia—this may occur in a "round-the-clock" fashion from the arm to the leg of the same side, then to the opposite leg and finally to the opposite arm.

(4) Sensory deficits—hemihypesthesia or a bilateral sensory level may be detected. The sensory deficit may extend as high as C_2 and the face may also be involved. Position sense may or may not be impaired. Stereoanesthesia simulating astereognosis may be present.

(5) Sphincter and respiratory paralysis—may occur in association with the tetraplegic syndrome.

(6) Horner's syndrome—may be present.

(7) Papilledema—may occur, but uncommon at the time of clinical presentation.

(8) Lower cranial nerve signs—paralyses of cranial nerves ten, eleven and twelve are present only occasionally. Attacks of hiccoughing may occur.

(9) Ataxia—this is usually mild and overshadowed by the presence of paralysis. Occasionally, ataxia, either hemiataxia or truncal ataxia, may be prominent.

(10) The entire course is slowly progressive.

d. Syndromes of the vertebrobasilar aneurysm.

Aneurysms of the vertebrobasilar system are much less common than those of the internal carotid, anterior or middle cerebral vessels. Small aneurysms usually present clinically at the time of their rupture with subarachnoid hemorrhage. Large aneurysms may be diagnosed before rupture when brain stem-cranial nerve compression occurs due to local mass effect. Brain stem and cerebellopontine angle syndromes can be produced. The sites of such vertebrobasilar aneurysms are the following:

(1) Aneurysm of the upper bifurcation of the basilar artery.

(2) Aneurysm of the midbasilar artery.

(3) Aneurysm of the vertebral artery—just below the lower bifurcation of the basilar artery.

(4) Aneurysm of the basilar or vertebral branches, e.g. aneurysm of the anterior or posterior-inferior cerebellar arteries.

Typical syndromes are as follow:

(1) Syndrome of rupture of the aneurysm of the basilar bifurcation (Fig. 76).

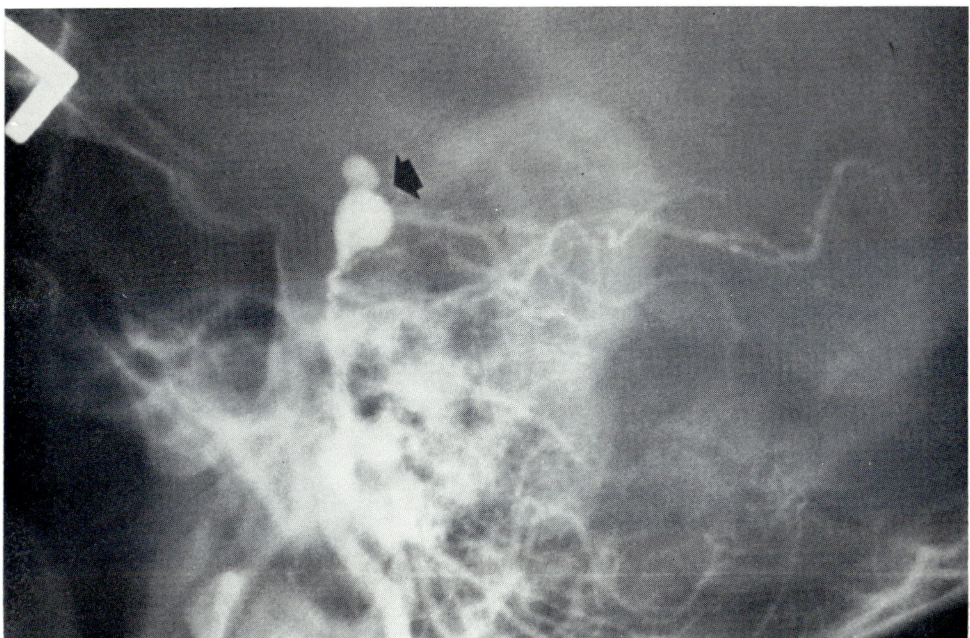

Figure 76. Aneurysm of the basilar bifurcation. A daughter aneurysm is present, along with spasm of the basilar artery.

Hemorrhage upon rupture of any vertebrobasilar aneurysm may be rapidly fatal. This may be the result of arterial spasm with brain stem ischemia, hemorrhage into the substance of the brain stem, or compression of the brain stem and cerebrospinal fluid pathways by posterior fossa hematoma. The aneurysm of the upper basilar bifurcation will be employed as an example of the hemorrhagic syndrome.

The midline aneurysm of the basilar bifurcation lies at the caudal extreme of the circle of Willis, between the cerebral peduncles. Like the midline anterior communicating aneurysm of the rostral extreme of the circle of Willis, a characteristic syndrome may result from rupture of either of these midline aneurysms.

(a) Immediate loss of consciousness.

(b) Visual symptoms just prior to collapse, or visual symptoms following the apoplexy if consciousness is regained.

(c) Absence of lateralizing signs.

(d) Presence of signs of subarachnoid hemorrhage (e.g. nuchal rigidity).

The rostral anterior communicating aneurysm is the more common site of hemorrhage in this syndrome. The visual symptoms are related to hemorrhage in the region of the optic nerves and chiasm. The hallmark initial loss of consciousness is related to ischemia or hemorrhage in the region of the anterior perforated substance and rostral hypothalamus. When bilateral carotid angiograms fail to reveal an aneurysm, the presence of this syndrome suggests an aneurysm of the basilar bifurcation and indicates the need for vertebral angiography. Visual symptoms including transient blindness in the presence of ruptured basilar aneurysm point to spasm of the posterior cerebral arteries. When the initial loss of consciousness is temporary, transient spasm of midline vessels of the posterior perforated substance in the region of the caudal hypothalamus and midbrain is suggested.

Transient deafness and transient brain stem signs may occur with the rupture of any vertebrobasilar aneurysm. Symptoms of vertebrobasilar insufficiency at the time of subtentorial subarachnoid hemorrhage are common. More enduring brain stem signs point to infarction or hemorrhage within the brain stem. In mesencephalic or pontine infarction or hemorrhage, coma tends to be deep and progressive. Bilateral cranial nerve palsies and tetraplegia occur in both the large brain stem infarct and hemorrhage. Unilateral cranial nerve palsies with crossed hemiplegia favor brain stem infarction, but can be seen in early hemorrhage into the brain stem by a laterally situated aneurysm. Generalized rigidity and decerebration with tonic brain stem seizures may occur. Coma marked by extreme autonomic lability, shivering and pupillary abnormalities with sparing of extraocular motor power may be seen with hemorrhage directly into the third ventricle. This may occur with aneurysms of the rostral or caudal extremes of the circle of Willis; it is also seen in hypertensive intracerebral hemorrhage. In the comatose patient with spontaneous subarachnoid hemorrhage, but without any motor or other obvious localizing deficit, a unilateral diminution in the corneal response may be the only clinical clue suggesting aneurysm within the vertebrobasilar circulation.

(2) Prerupture syndromes of the large vertebrobasilar aneurysm —these large aneurysms may closely mimic a slowly progressive tumor. However, variations in the clinical course with sudden

appearance of signs or with remission or fluctuation of signs should suggest the possibility of aneurysm in the adult patient. Local subtentorial compression syndromes include the following:

(a) Interpeduncular oculomotor compression by upper basilar bifurcation aneurysm—this is an uncommon source of third nerve palsy due to unruptured aneurysm. Oculomotor palsy is much more frequently due to an internal carotid-posterior communicating aneurysm.

(b) Cerebellopontine angle aneurysm—an aneurysm with unilateral compression of cranial nerves seven, eight, and five may simulate the acoustic neuroma syndrome. Aneurysm of the anterior-inferior cerebellar artery may mimic Menièrés syndrome of recurrent vertigo. Atypical facial pain or symptomatic trigeminal neuralgia may result from an angle aneurysm.

(c) Anterior vertebrobasilar aneurysm—an aneurysm at the anterolateral pontomedullary junction may involve cranial nerves five, six, seven and eight. Crossed hemiplegia or paraplegia may be associated.

(d) Posterior-inferior cerebellar artery aneurysm and intracranial vertebral aneurysm—these aneurysms may mimic the lateral, anterior or posterior medullary infarction syndromes (see "Brain stem infarction syndromes"). However, these aneurysms are quite uncommon. The lateral medullary syndrome is common and is virtually always the result of an infarct. The other two medullary syndromes are most unusual. If a medullary syndrome occurs in a young adult with evidence of subarachnoid hemorrhage, the aneurysm may be diagnosed. Nonruptured aneurysm or tumor with medullary and lower cranial nerve compression may produce a medullary syndrome. A slowly progressive bulbar palsy may result from a paramedullary aneurysm. Extramedullary compression by meningioma, large acoustic neuroma and chordoma should be considered. Progressive bulbar palsy of some neurosurgical interest may be seen in intramedullary astrocytoma and syringobulbia.

e. Infratentorial hematoma syndromes.

These are traumatic and spontaneous. They may be extracerebellar (i.e. acute posterior fossa epidural or subdural hematoma) or intracerebellar (i.e. hypertensive cerebellar apoplexy, rupture of intracerebellar AVM). These are all relatively uncommon syndromes. The supratentorial traumatic hematomas (i.e. epidural, subdural, intracerebral) are much more common than subtentorial traumatic clots. The intracerebral hypertensive hemorrhage is much more common than spontaneous intracerebellar hemorrhage. Whether traumatic or spontaneous in origin, and whether extra- or intracerebellar in location, the pressure of the hematoma is translated to the brain stem. The posterior fossa is a relatively small space which is almost completely occupied by the brain stem and its cerebellar appendage. Cisternal and fourth ventricular obliteration and cerebellar herniation do not create much additional space to compensate for active bleeding. While consciousness may be initially maintained, as is often the case in spontaneous cerebellar hemorrhage, obtundation occurs and is progressive. Most posterior fossa acute epidurals and subdurals are associated with early progressive coma just like their supratentorial counterparts. In some cases, there may be a lucid interval, and in unusual instances, double lucidity can occur in the posterior fossa epidural. The acute epidural and acute subdural of the posterior fossa cannot be reliably differentiated from one another solely on clinical grounds. This is often true of supratentorial acute epidurals and acute subdurals presenting with progressive coma consequent to head trauma. The most important factor is the early recognition of the presence of hematoma following head injury; as a corollary, the responsible hematoma will be infratentorial in a small minority of cases. The traumatic infratentorial hematoma should be suspected in the following cases:

(1) Persistent vomiting occurs.

(2) Occipital skull fracture is noted.

(3) The pineal is in normal position in a rapidly deteriorating head-injured patient. (*Note:* Most acute epidurals and acute subdurals above the tentorium will shift the pineal to the opposite side; an eccentrically located epidural or subdural may not do this; a central cerebral or temporal lobe hematoma commonly produces midline shift of the pineal; a frontal extra- or intracerebral clot eventually displaces the pineal downward and, if large, to the opposite side; bilateral subdural hematomas may not shift the midline, but tend to depress the pineal on lateral view. Brain swelling may or may not be associated with midline shift. The echo is of value if the pineal is not calcified.

(4) Continued deterioration is noted after bilaterally negative multiple supratentorial exploratory burr holes.

(5) Carotid angiograms reveal the following:
  (a) No midline shift.
  (b) No evidence of supratentorial hematoma.
  (c) Hydrocephalus—stretching of the pericallosal arteries on lateral view and flattening of the thalamostriate veins on AP view.
  (d) Separation of the transverse sinus or torcular away from the inner table of the occipital bone (i.e. posterior fossa epidural).

Spontaneous intracerebellar hemorrhage differs from the cerebellar tumor syndrome in its sudden onset and brevity of the clinical course between onset and diagnosis. In addition, cerebellar signs may be minimal. The force of hemorrhage, like the infratentorial epidural and subdural clot of traumatic origin, is directed at the brain stem. Rupture of the hematoma into the fourth ventricle, with bloody spinal fluid and obstructive hydrocephalus, occurs. The symptoms and signs combine to produce a characteristic syndrome: acute cerebellar apoplexy syndrome.

(1) Symptoms.
  (a) There is typically no initial loss of consciousness. There may be retention of the alert state for a number of hours, depending on the rate of bleeding.
  (b) Repeated vomiting is a hallmark.
  (c) Headache is present in half the cases during the alert phase. It may be mild or severe, occipital, frontal or generalized. There may be neck and intrascapular pain. Pain may be experienced across the bridge of the nose. The headache is like that in subarachnoid hemorrhage, and photophobia may be present.
  (d) Dizziness or true vertigo commonly occur.
  (e) Inability to stand or walk is common.
  (f) Dysarthria, dysphagia or deafness may occur.
  (g) The alert phase is followed by progressive obtundation and deepening coma.

(2) Signs.
  (a) There may be a paucity of, or even total absence of, cerebellar signs during the alert phase. In some cases, ataxia and hypotonia, either most marked in the legs or ipsilateral to the clot may be demonstrated.
  (b) Nystagmus often does not occur, while many other ocular signs are present. Ocular signs include small pupils with retention of light reflexes, slight pupillary inequality, con-

jugate gaze palsy to the side of the hematoma, ipsilateral abducens palsy, forced conjugate or skew deviation, bilateral conjugate gaze palsy with retention of vertical extraocular movements.

(c) The absence of crossed hemiplegia and facial palsy during the alert phase suggests that the eye signs result from pontine compression, rather than an intrapontine hemorrhage. In some cases of cerebellar hemorrhage, an ipsilateral facial palsy may be noted, again the result of pontine compression.

(d) In most cases, the onset of paraplegia, quadriplegia and spasticity is noted in the stupor-coma phase; in occasional cases, these signs may be present in the alert phase.

(e) Plantar responses are typically flexor early, and bilateral Babinski signs are noted late.

(f) Stiff neck is common, the spinal fluid being almost always bloody. Nuchal rigidity may diminish in the deeply comatose stage.

(g) Evidence for chronic arterial hypertension (e.g. left ventricular hypertrophy, hypertensive retinopathy) is common. Normotensive status should suggest ruptured cerebellar AVM. With the onset of obtundation, progressive arterial hypertension accompanying obstructive hydrocephalus is usually noted.

This is the single most important hypertensive parenchymal hemorrhage from the neurosurgical point of view. Immediate surgical intervention can reverse the entire syndrome. In contrast, hypertensive hemorrhages into the basal ganglia or pons, if not fatal, tend to leave overwhelming deficits in their wake.

If lumbar puncture (LP) is carried out as a diagnostic aid, the following criteria are important:

(1) Truly bloody CSF does not clear in the three tubes, while the epidural bleeding of a traumatic tap tends to clear as it mixes with normal CSF.

(2) Lumbar pressure is ordinarily increased in these cases.

(3) Truly bloody CSF tends not to clot.

(4) If the hemorrhage occurred more than eight hours preceding the LP, the supernatant is xanthochromic.

(5) A normal white to red cell ratio in truly bloody CSF indicates active or recent hemorrhage. The cell count must be done promptly following the LP in order to retain accuracy.

(6) 1.0 to 1.5 mg% of protein is equivalent to 1,000 red cells in

the CSF cell count. In the presence of hematoma, the expected protein value, as judged by the number of CSF red cells, is often exceeded.

C. The Cerebellopontine angle syndrome

The majority of angle tumors are acoustic neuromas. In the majority of cases, there is a characteristic clinical course.

1. The typical patient is an adult of middle age.
2. Gradually progressive ipsilateral deafness is the most common early symptom; the history may extend over many months and even over several years. The deafness may first be noted upon answering a telephone, when an impaired speech discrimination is noted on the affected side.
3. Tinnitus may or may not be present.
4. A sense of imbalance or dizziness is common, but true vertigo is not.
5. Ipsilateral suboccipital discomfort, especially upon straining or coughing, is sometimes noted in the early stages.
6. Ipsilateral facial paresthesias may occur episodically, but pain in the trigeminal distribution is relatively uncommon.
7. Facial asymmetry may be brought to the patient's attention by relatives. The patient may become unable to close his eyelid on the deaf side.
8. Clumsiness is noted and may be intermittent at first, being most marked as a gait disturbance. Eventually the ipsilateral hand becomes less capable of finely coordinated movement.

Early diagnosis of the angle tumor

By this stage of symptomatic development, most patients have been brought to the attention of an otologist, neurologist or neurosurgeon. Evidence of the triad of unilateral deafness, peripheral facial palsy and diminished corneal sensation, all on the same side in a middle-aged adult, makes the diagnosis of acoustic neuroma extremely likely. There may be no evidence of sensory loss over the face, cerebellar signs, or intracranial hypertension at this stage, and yet a firm diagnosis can be made at this point by ancillary tests. An enlarged porus acousticus is almost always present, but may be normal in some very small tumors. The CSF protein is usually elevated and may exceed 100 mg%. In very small tumors, it may be normal or elevated. The caloric responses are usually depressed or lost on the side of the tumor. In uncommon cases with minimal deafness, loss of the caloric response when combined with other signs indicates an angle tumor. Depression or absence of the caloric response also occurs with labyrinthine disease. Deafness with an absent caloric response on the same side is nerve deafness and not middle ear deafness. While tuning fork testing is helpful in differentiating middle ear conduction deafness from sensorineural hearing loss, it does not distinguish between a cochlea (receptor) defect and a retrocochlear (nerve) defect. An otological battery of tests is employed to make this differential.

1. The Bekesy audiogram.
2. The SISI (short increment sensitivity index).
3. The ABLB (alternate binaural loudness balance test of recruitment).

The results of the test battery which favor an eighth nerve lesion (i.e. an acoustic tumor) over a cochlear defect are as follow:

1. Type 3 or 4 Bekesy (*Note:* a type 1 Bekesy can be normal or compatible with middle ear deafness. A type 2 Bekesy is usually due to a cochlear lesion, but some small acoustic tumors may have a type 2).
2. A low SISI score (*Note:* patients with cochlear lesions have high scores, while patients with normal hearing, middle ear disease or eighth nerve lesions have low scores).
3. Absence of recruitment on the ABLB (*Note:* absence of recruitment also occurs in middle ear deafness, but not with cochlear lesions).

No single test taken alone is in itself diagnostic. Specialized x-ray studies are discussed in the radiology section of this chapter.

Late diagnosis of the angle tumor

As the tumor increases in size, filling the angle, sensory loss over the face and facial palsy become associated with more marked evidence of ataxia. Headaches eventually become more generalized, and diplopia, vomiting and papilledema may be noted. Lower cranial nerve palsies with dysarthria and dysphagia, hemipalatal and pharyngeal paralysis may occur in the late stage. Abducens palsy may or may not be obvious even when diplopia is marked. Facial palsy occasionally assumes a pseudocentral type with relative sparing of the brow. Paralysis of the muscles of mastication on the side of the tumor may also be noted. In very large angle tumors, paralysis may involve the sternocleidomastoid, trapezius and ipsilateral tongue, the tongue pointing to the side of the tumor. The Romberg becomes positive with falling to the side of the tumor. Unilateral hypotonia may be very prominent and nystagmus may be present. With brain stem compression, crossed hemiplegia and hemihypesthesia can occur. Pyramidal signs can be bilateral, contralateral or ipsilateral at this stage. As papilledema becomes chronic and intracranial hypertension becomes marked, headaches usually become more severe. Suboccipital tenderness and nuchal rigidity may become extreme. Unilateral deafness is often complete before this very late stage is reached. Obstructive hydrocephalus and brain stem compression by the large tumor ultimately result in obtundation with progressive coma. The majority of angle tumors, because of their distinctive symptoms and signs, reach diagnosis before this terminal phase.

Radiological Deformities in Posterior Fossa Syndromes

Air studies are usually employed in the diagnosis of most posterior fossa tumors. Ventriculography is employed particularly for cerebellar tumors with elevated intracranial pressure and obstructive hydrocephalus. Lumbar pneumoencephalography is utilized in the diagnosis of intrinsic brain stem gliomas. The lumbar route is also commonly employed for the introduction of air or Pantopaque® in the diagnosis of cerebellopontine angle tumors. In the late stages of brain stem glioma or large angle tumor, when obstructive hydrocephalus is present, ventriculography may be utilized. Angiography is particularly indicated whenever an infratentorial aneurysm, arteriovenous malformation, meningioma or cerebellar hemangioblastoma is suspected. Angiograms are also employed when air studies are inconclusive.

A. Angiographic findings

The angiographic signs of a posterior fossa mass may be present in either or both the carotid and vertebral study.

1. The carotid angiogram and the posterior fossa mass lesion—the cerebellar tumor, abscess or hematoma, and the posterior fossa epidural or subdural clot, often present signs of obstructive hydrocephalus clearly evident on carotid angiography.
    a. Lateral displacement of the thalamostriate vein (frontal view)—this is the single best angiographic sign of ventricular dilatation. The thalamostriate vein crosses the floor of the lateral ventricle between the thalamus and caudate head. As the ventricle enlarges, this vein is displaced laterally and its curve is increased.
    b. Stretching and rounding of the pericallosal artery (lateral view)—this artery loses its normal undulations when the ventricles become moderately enlarged. Lesser degrees of hydrocephalus may be noted by thalamostriate venous displacement when the pericallosal artery appears normal. Filling of only the callosomarginal artery on the injected side, both pericallosal arteries filling as a normal variant from the opposite side, may give the erroneous impression of marked ventricular dilatation.
    c. Other carotid angiographic signs of hydrocephalus—when ventricular enlargement is marked, middle cerebral vessels may be elevated (lateral view) due to temporal horn dilatation. Lateral ventricular enlargement of great degree can also laterally displace the angiographic sylvian point (frontal view). Generalized straightening of vessels with loss of normal undulation accompanies high degrees of intracranial hypertension.
    d. The hydrocephalus produced by the posterior fossa mass lesion is

a generally symmetrical enlargement of the supratentorial ventricular system. A similar hydrocephalus may result from third ventricular or incisural tumors or aqueductal stenosis.

2. The vertebral angiogram and the posterior fossa mass lesion.
   a. Cerebellar tumors.
      (1) The vertebral angiogram may be considered normal even when supratentorial ventricular enlargement due to cerebellar tumor is obvious.
      (2) The common cerebellar tumors of childhood, the astrocytoma, medulloblastoma and ependymoma do not ordinarily produce a tumor blush. They are characterized by stretching of cerebellar vessels around a relatively avascular mass within the hemisphere (Fig. 77) or vermis.
      (3) The posterior-inferior cerebellar artery.
         (a) Tonsillar herniation—this is commonly present in cerebellar tumors. The hernia is angiographically shown by downward dislocation of the posterior-inferior cerebellar artery below the foramen magnum. However, this artery

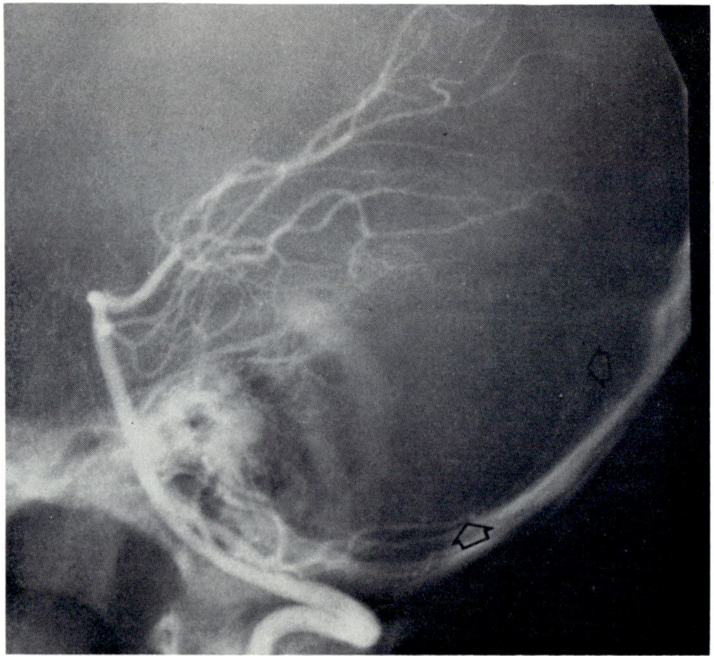

Figure 77. Cystic cerebellar astrocytoma on vertebral angiogram. The superior cerebellar artery is displaced upward and stretched over the dome of the tumor. The posterior-inferior cerebellar artery is displaced caudally and stretched over the posterior pole of the tumor (arrows).

may at times wander below the foramen magnum as a normal variant. In tonsillar herniation, the downward dislocation of this vessel may be extreme. The artery is stretched and may reach the arch of the atlas or axis. In tumors of the cerebellar hemisphere, the tonsil on the side of the tumor is herniated to greater degree, so that the posterior-inferior cerebellar artery is lower on the tumor side. If the vertebral opposite the hemispheral tumor is injected, the maximal tonsillar herniation may be missed, since the posterior-inferior cerebellar artery on the tumor side may not fill. In vermian tumors, or hemispheral tumors with vermian extension, the tonsils may be equally herniated. It is important to note that tonsillar herniation does not necessarily indicate a posterior fossa mass. The supratentorial mass with advanced intracranial hypertension and downward transtentorial herniation may produce cerebellar tonsillar herniation as well. When the impaction of tonsils at the foramen magnum is extreme, an acute hydrocephalic attack may result from occlusion of the fourth ventricular outlets (i.e. foraminal impaction). The hydrocephalus and tonsillar herniation of the cerebellar tumor should not be confused with the hydrocephalus due to Arnold-Chiari malformation of the hindbrain. In this instance, cerebellar tissue including the tonsils and posterior-inferior cerebellar artery are located in the upper cervical canal. A portion of the medulla, which may be angulated, and the fourth ventricle, may also be situated in the upper cervical canal; meningomyelocele may be associated.

(b) Vermian branch of the posterior-inferior cerebellar artery—this paramedial branch supplies the caudal vermis. A tumor of the vermis shifts this branch laterally; a tumor of the cerebellar hemisphere shifts it medially.

(4) The superior cerebellar artery.

(a) This vessel may be displaced upward (lateral view) by a hemispheral tumor, the opposite vessel remaining in normal position.

(b) The vermian branch to the rostral vermis is laterally shifted by a vermian tumor and medially shifted by a hemispheral tumor (AP view).

(c) Upward transtentorial herniation of the superior cerebellar vermis—both the superior cerebellar and posterior cerebral arteries may be dislocated upward by this tentorial herniation due to posterior fossa mass. The superior cerebellar artery may even rise higher than the posterior cerebral artery for a portion of its course. On the venous phase, the vein of Galen is dislocated upward; the basilar vein is pushed up and forward. The middle cerebral vein fills in retrograde fashion from the basilar vein when the latter is obstructed in its course around the brain stem (i.e. whether transtentorial herniation occurs from above or below). In cerebellar tumors, the tendency for foramen magnum herniation is greater than for tentorial herniation. The rigidity of the tentorium and the presence of supratentorial enlargement of the ventricular system tend to minimize the degree of upward cerebellar herniation.

(5) The basilar artery may be pushed forward against the clivus by cerebellar and brain stem tumors. If hydrocephalus and tonsillar herniation are associated, the forward basilar dislocation is likely due to cerebellar rather than brain stem tumor. Forward dislocation of the basilar artery is not as good a sign as downward posterior-inferior cerebellar or upward superior cerebellar arterial displacement.

(6) The precentral cerebellar veins are close to the midline in the region of the superior vermis. A cerebellar hemispheral tumor shifts these veins medially, rostrally and superiorly; vermian tumors shift these veins laterally and rostrally.

(7) While the common cerebellar tumors of childhood tend to appear as a relatively hypovascular mass without tumor stain, the posterior fossa tumors of high angiographic vascularity are more common in adult life.

(a) Meningioma—subtentorial meningiomas are much less common than supratentorial varieties. They have a tendency to be angioblastic. They rarely occur in childhood, but may in association with von Recklinghausen's disease; under these circumstances they may be malignant. The posterior fossa meningioma may be encased by cerebellum and may resemble the hemangioblastoma. The meningioma may be the subtentorial component of a tentorial tumor, growing through the tentorium itself, or through the incisura. It may be the subtentorial portion of a meningioma arising from Meckel's cave of the middle fossa. It may arise from the clivus, the anterior or posterior lip of the foramen magnum, or from the cerebellopontine angle. Occlusion of a major venous sinus (i.e. transverse) may be associated with growth of this tumor.

(b) Hemangioblastoma (Fig. 78)—this tumor may present a highly vascular or a mixed vascular-avascular appearance,

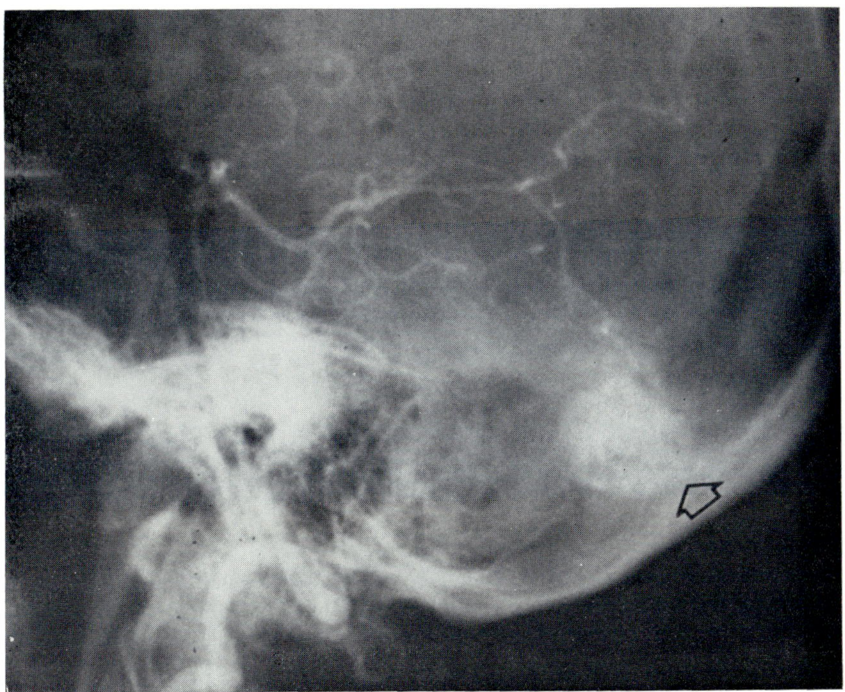

Figure 78. Cerebellar hemangioblastoma on vertebral angiogram. The highly vascular tumor stain is subtentorial.

the solid portions of the tumor showing hypervascularity. If a large cyst is present (i.e. like a juvenile astrocytoma) with a small mural nodule, the tumor may appear as a predominantly avascular mass.

(c) Metastatic carcinoma of the cerebellum—like metastases to the cerebrum, these deposits may present as either a hypovascular or hypervascular mass. Multiplicity is the best angiographic sign suggesting metastatic disease, but the cerebellar metastasis often presents as a single mass.

(d) Glioblastoma of the cerebellum—high-grade astrocytomas of the cerebellum are quite rare; when they occur they may involve both cerebellum and brain stem in continuity. The vast majority of cerebellar astrocytomas are of low grade (i.e. "juvenile" astrocytomas) and are hypovascular.

(e) Arteriovenous malformation of the cerebellum—these are usually angiographically visible and may be extremely prominent; arteriovenous shunts, with tortuous abnormal vessels and rapid circulation through early filling of veins are notable. This hypervascularity may be associated with a hypovascular mass effect if hematoma is also present. They may present at any age and are a source of acute cerebellar hemorrhage in the normotensive patient. Hematoma may obscure the presence of a small malformation. "Telangiectasia" which are not angiographically visible may result in significant hemorrhage. Cerebellar and pontine malformations (Fig. 79) are much less common than supratentorial AVM's.

b. Brain stem tumors.

(1) As in the cerebellar tumor, the vertebral angiogram may be normal in the intrinsic brain stem glioma.

(2) Pontine gliomas usually do not reveal a tumor blush. Marked vascularity may be due to arteriovenous malformation of the pons rather than glioma.

(3) Forward dislocation of the basilar artery against the clivus may be due to brain stem or cerebellar tumor. It is not a reliable sign. Pontine tumors may expand the brain stem and even grow forward into the prepontine cistern without great dislocation of the basilar artery. The vermian branch of the posterior-inferior cerebellar artery may be displaced posteriorly with the fourth ventricle by the pontine mass. Mesencephalic enlargement may widen the angular arch of the superior cerebellar arteries and displace the precentral cerebellar veins posteriorly. Prepontine and peduncular veins may be displaced forward. Despite these vascular changes, pneumoencephalography usually provides much more definitive evidence of pontine enlargement.

(4) Prepontine tumors of the clivus (e.g. chordoma or meningioma) produce backward dislocation of the basilar artery. A large cerebellopontine angle tumor may produce lateral basilar artery displacement as it displaces the pons to the opposite side. These extra-axial tumors tend to occur in older age groups than the intrinsic pontine glioma. The normal course of the basilar artery is subject to greater variability with the passage of time; it can be highly tortuous in the arteriosclerotic age group. "Ectasia" of the basilar artery may result in an unusual-

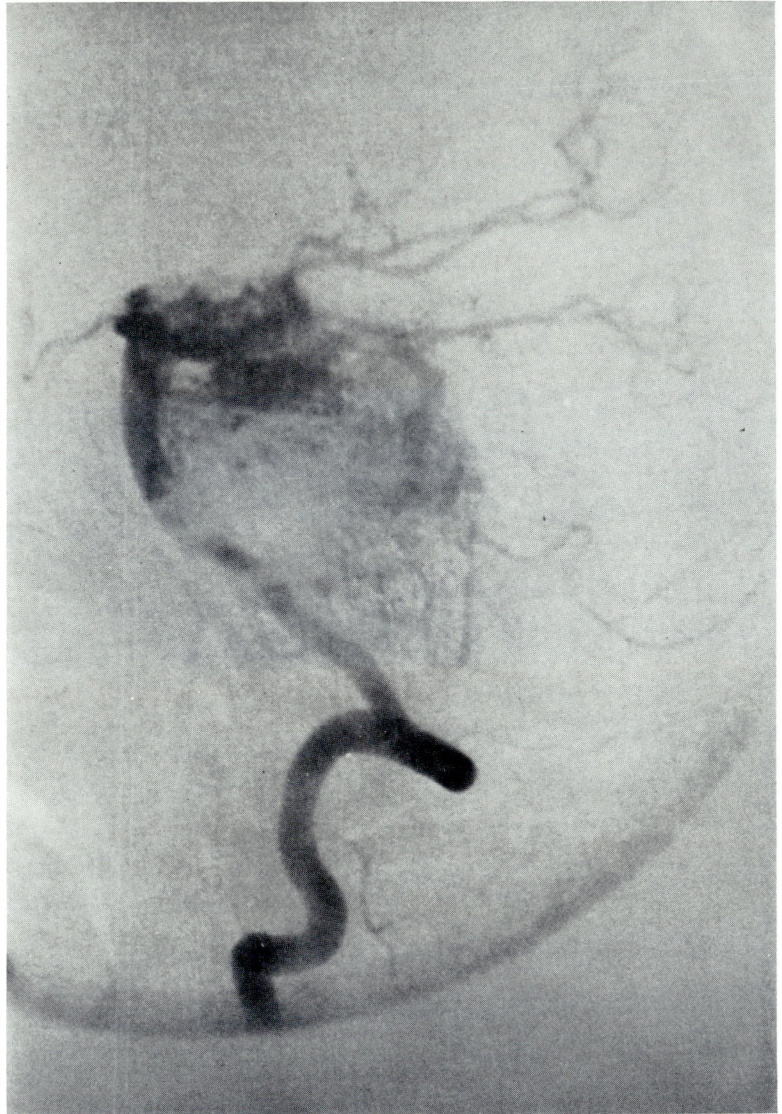

Figure 79. Pontine arteriovenous malformation.

ly large vessel which takes a circuitous course rostrally and laterally to the brain stem.

(5) Intrinsic tumors of the brain stem, prepontine tumors and cerebellopontine angle tumors produce intracranial hypertension relatively late in the clinical course. When these tumors reach early diagnosis because of their characteristic neurological deficits, the evidence for tonsillar or transtentorial

herniation and hydrocephalus is absent or minimal. This contrasts sharply with cerebellar tumors in which hydrocephalus, tonsillar herniation and intracranial hypertension are common early in the course.

c. Cerebellopontine angle tumors.

(1) The acoustic neuroma accounts for the great majority of cerebellopontine angle tumors. While tumor blush and vascular displacement occur with many of these tumors, vertebral angiography may be considered negative while other radiological techniques show unequivocal evidence of this angle tumor. Subtraction studies and special views may be required to clearly demonstrate the vascular abnormalities. Meningioma (Fig. 80), glomus tumor, aneurysm or basilar ectasia may produce an angle syndrome requiring vertebral angiography for accurate diagnosis. Epidermoid tumor of the angle is ordinarily hypovascular by comparison.

(2) The tumor stain of an acoustic tumor may be due to pathological vessels arising from the anterior-inferior cerebellar artery or its internal auditory branch. The anterior-inferior

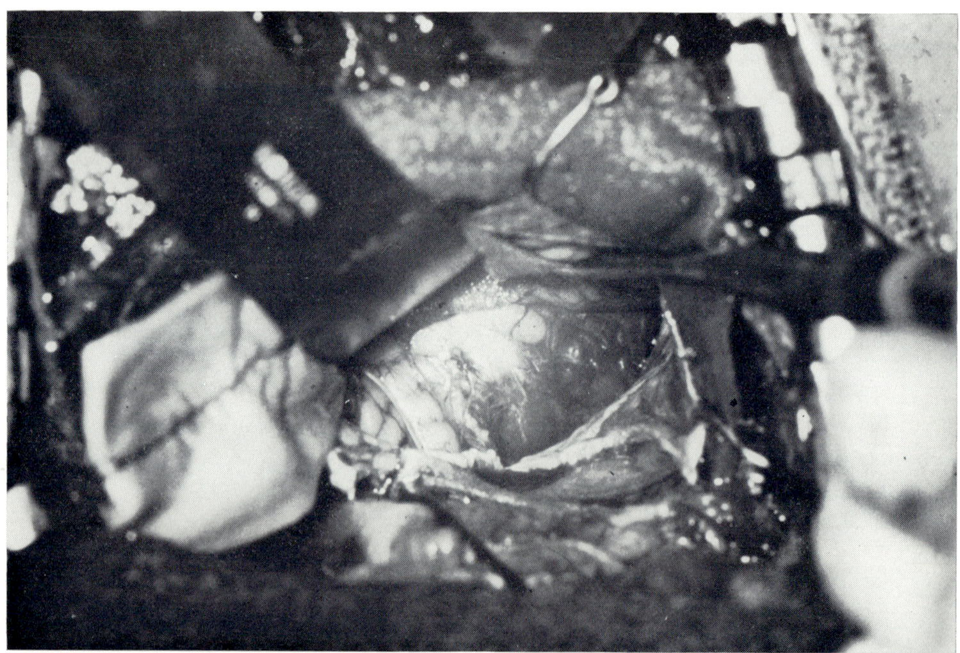

Figure 80. Angle meningioma. The posterior surface of a large meningioma is exposed, filling the right cerebello-pontine angle. This can be compared with the empty angle exposed in Figure 81 for retrogasserian neurectomy by the posterior fossa approach.

cerebellar artery normally courses in the cerebellopontine angle and may enter the internal auditory canal under normal conditions. The internal auditory artery may not be visible. When present, it arises as an anterior-inferior branch and less often as a basilar branch.

(3) When the anterior-inferior cerebellar supply is normally reduced on one side, the posterior-inferior cerebellar supply is excessive. This form of vascular supplementation is common. As a consequence, an angle tumor may obtain most or all of its pathological vascular supply from the posterior-inferior cerebellar artery. If the vertebral on the tumor side is not injected, this pathological vascular supply may not be visualized. Occasionally, tumor vessels will be derived from the superior cerebellar artery.

(4) In addition to tumor vessels, an angle tumor may produce the following vascular displacements:

(a) Anterior-inferior cerebellar artery—this may be elevated, depressed or straightened by an angle tumor.

(b) Superior cerebellar artery—this is shifted rostrally by a large angle mass.

(c) Posterior-inferior cerebellar artery—this is shifted caudally by a large angle mass; when sufficiently large, tonsillar herniation on the tumor side may be noted.

(d) Basilar artery—this tends to shift laterally with dislocation of the pons to the opposite side by a large angle mass.

(e) Petrosal vein (half-axial view)—this passes from the region of the flocculus to the superior petrosal sinus, where it lies adjacent to the internal auditory meatus. The petrosal vein and its tributaries are deformed by an angle tumor; when the tumor is large, the vein may not fill. The petrosal vein lies beneath the fifth nerve, while the anterior-inferior cerebellar and internal auditory arteries accompany the seventh and eighth nerves in the angle between the pons and cerebellum.

B. Pneumographic findings

1. Cerebellar tumors.

The hypertensive, obstructive hydrocephalus secondary to the cerebellar mass renders ventriculography the air study of choice. Lumbar pneumoencephalography may precipitate acute foraminal impaction with increasing intracranial hypertension; it may also fail to produce ventricular filling. The characteristics of the air study in the cerebellar mass include the following:

a. Lateral ventricles.
   (1) Virtually always enlarged to some degree.
   (2) May be extremely enlarged.
   (3) Relatively symmetrical dilatation in most cases.
   (4) Ventricular fluid is under increased pressure at the time of ventricular puncture.
   (5) The occipital horn and atrium may be elevated on the side of a cerebellar hemispheral tumor.
   (6) Subarachnoid air is not visualized over the cerebral hemispheres in most instances.
b. Third ventricle.
   (1) Usually enlarged to some degree, but may be normal.
   (2) The posterior third ventricle may be narrowed, while the anterior third may be dilated, in the presence of upward cerebellar herniation.
   (3) No intra-third ventricular mass is present.
c. Aqueduct.
   (1) The upper aqueduct (above the incisura) is dilated or normal, while the lower aqueduct is deformed or obliterated.
   (2) "Hockey-stick aqueduct"—angulation of the aqueduct at the incisural level; the entire aqueduct normally has a smooth curve.
   (3) Vermian tumor—displaces the aqueduct forward; the minimal normal distance from aqueduct to dorsum sella is 30 mm.
   (4) Hemispheral tumor—displaces the lower aqueduct to the opposite side.
d. Fourth ventricle, vallecula, cisterna magna.
   (1) Like the lower aqueduct, the fourth ventricle and basal cisterns may be entirely obliterated.
   (2) The fourth ventricle may be completely obliterated by either vermian or hemispheral cerebellar tumors.
   (3) The fourth ventricle may fill and reveal characteristic deformities in either vermian or hemispheral tumors.
      (a) Vermian tumor—may deform the apex of the ventricle. The superior vermian tumor displaces the ventricle downward and deforms its anterior wall, while pushing the aqueduct forward. The inferior vermian tumor displaces the ventricle upward and buckles the lower aqueduct.
      (b) Hemispheral tumor—may deform the lateral recess of the ventricle and shifts the ventricle to the opposite side. The hemispheral tumor is apt to only partially occlude the outlets of the ventricle, so that the vallecula fills. The valle-

cula is shifted away from the hemispheral mass. The cisterna magna, if visualized at all, is narrowed beneath the cerebellar mass.

2. Brain stem tumors.

   Lumbar pneumoencephalography is the procedure of choice.

   a. The fourth ventricle and aqueduct are displaced backward, in an arch concave anteriorly (lateral view).
   b. The prepontine cistern is usually narrowed, the greatest expansion of the brain stem usually noted at the pontine level (lateral view).
   c. The fourth ventricle usually remains in the midline (frontal view).
   d. The ventricular system is usually patent and the lateral ventricles commonly appear at the upper limits of normal in size, or slightly dilated.
   e. Expansion of the upper brain stem is associated with backward dislocation of the upper aqueduct as well, and elevation of the posterior floor of the third ventricle. Complete aqueductal obstruction occurs late, and is typically not present at the time of diagnosis.
   f. Prepontine tumors may also shift the fourth ventricle and aqueduct backward; the curvature of the arch is not as smooth. The prepontine cistern is usually widened, rather than narrowed, by tumor anterior to the brain stem; the cistern may be filled by tumor.
   g. Cerebellar tumors may narrow the prepontine cistern just as brain stem gliomas. However, the aqueduct and fourth ventricle are deformed (or obliterated) in characteristic ways by the cerebellar mass; the aqueduct and fourth ventricle are not pushed backward as they are in pontine glioma. Cerebellar tumors characteristically have greater evidence of hydrocephalus at the time of diagnosis than do brain stem gliomas.
   h. Cerebellopontine angle tumors in the vast majority of cases occur in middle or late adult life, while brain stem gliomas, like cerebellar tumors, are most common in childhood. The angle tumor does not ordinarily require differentiation from the intrinsic glioma of the brain stem because of this age difference. A large angle tumor laterally dislocates the brain stem and may deform the fourth ventricle in a manner differing from the intrinsic brain stem tumor. Occasionally, a pontine glioma will eccentrically enlarge into the cerebellopontine angle, filling the lateral cistern; even under these circumstances, diffuse pontine enlargement due to the intrinsic glioma is apparent on pneumography.

3. Cerebellopontine angle tumors.

Air or Pantopaque study of the posterior fossa by the lumbar route are the procedures of choice in the diagnosis of angle tumor. Ventriculography is usually not adequate for diagnosis. Vertebral angiography is helpful for selected cases but is usually not required.

a. Pneumoencephalographic findings.

(1) The earliest abnormality is usually elevation of the cerebellopontine recess on the tumor side (PA half-axial) with a normal recess on the opposite side. This elevation may be mimicked by the shadow of a normal crural cistern passing around the cerebral peduncle.

(2) The angle tumor may be seen within the angle cistern (Fig. 81), or the cistern may be obliterated by the tumor; the latter must be differentiated from nonfilling of this cerebellopontine cistern due to inadequate injection of air or inadequate head positioning.

(3) If the angle cistern is obliterated by tumor, widening of the medullary cistern on the tumor side is an indirect sign of an

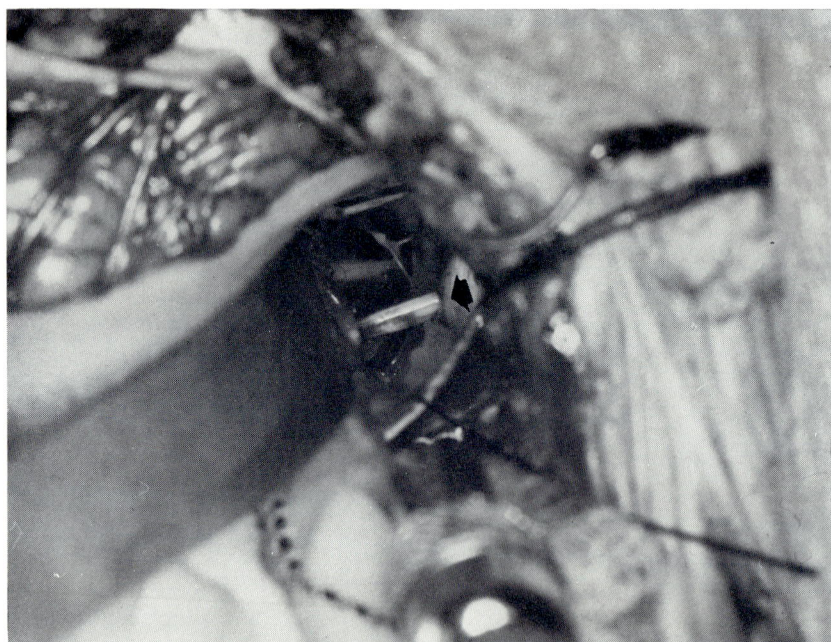

Figure 81. Cerebellopontine angle. The seventh and eighth cranial nerves cross the angle to enter the internal auditory canal at the meatus (arrow). The trigeminal root lies deeper, in the forward reaches of the angle. The anterior-inferior cerebellar artery can be seen crossing the seventh and eighth nerves medially in the angle. This artery supplies the pontine tegmentum as well as cerebellum.

angle mass. Widening of the ambient cistern on the tumor side may also be noted. The prepontine cistern may be normal or reduced depending on the size of the angle tumor and the direction of its growth.

(4) A small angle tumor may not affect the fourth ventricle and aqueduct. Larger tumors distort the position of the fourth ventricle and lower aqueduct. The displacement of the fourth ventricle characteristically exceeds that of the aqueduct.

(a) The fourth ventricle and lower aqueduct are usually displaced posteriorly and laterally to the opposite side.

(b) Depending on the direction of tumor growth in the angle, degree of posterior displacement of the ventricle and lower aqueduct may exceed or be less than the lateral shift of these structures.

(c) "Banana-shaped ventricle" (frontal view)—the fourth ventricle is commonly deformed by large angle tumors and may be deformed out of proportion to the degree of midline shift. The concavity is on the tumor side. As the tumor compresses the pons, the brain stem and ventricle rotate as well as shift. The fourth ventricle is narrower than normal (frontal view) even if it retains a close to midline position.

(d) Growth of a large angle tumor toward the cerebellar hemisphere may superimpose the findings of cerebellar mass upon the lateral aspect of the ventricle, and tonsillar herniation on the tumor side may be noted. Large angle tumors growing rostrally may elevate the posterior third ventricle and deform the upper aqueduct. In such cases, the cisternal changes and lower aqueductal-fourth ventricular deformities are also present. In late cases with very large angle tumors, hydrocephalus may be prominent as a result of fourth ventricular and cisternal block; the fourth ventricle may be markedly compressed and shifted. Occasionally, the fourth ventricle itself participates in the hydrocephalus, enlarging while its lateral wall on the tumor side is flattened. In such late cases with advanced intracranial hypertension and obstructive hydrocephalus, ventriculography may be required as the initial air study; fourth ventricular deformity suggesting a large angle tumor may be noted.

b. Posterior fossa myelographic findings.

While the lumbar pneumogram has the advantage of a higher rate of fourth ventricular filling, the introduction of Pantopaque by the lumbar route may be employed as the preferred test. It is easier to fill and visualize an internal auditory canal with positive contrast than with air. Such filling of a canal with Pantopaque can effectively rule out a small intracanalicular acoustic tumor. The positive contrast effectively outlines an extracanalicular angle tumor as well. The findings on posterior fossa myelography include the following:

(1) Nonfilling of the internal auditory canal on the suspect side, with a normal angle and filling of the opposite canal: compatible with intracanalicular tumor.
(2) Nonfilling of the canal on the suspect side with a small filling defect bulging into the angle.
(3) An obvious filling defect in the angle due to tumor mass.
(4) Evidence of brain stem shift and tonsillar herniation in large angle tumors. Fourth ventricular deformity may be noted in those cases in which ventricular filling occurs.
(5) Filling defects closely adjacent to major arterial shadows indicate the need for vertebral angiography to rule out aneurysm or vascular anomaly in the angle.

C. Plain x-ray findings

1. Cerebellar tumors.

Since cerebellar tumors commonly present with intracranial hypertension in childhood, the most common abnormality on plain skull x-rays is suture separation. Suture separation greater than 2 mm is abnormal after age three. Most patients with suture separation due to elevated pressure are prepubertal, but it can also occur later in adolescence. Widening of the coronal suture is usually most marked even in posterior fossa tumors. Suture separation may be limited to the coronal, or it may include the sagittal and lambdoid sutures as well. Some degree of obvious cranial enlargement may be present in the cerebellar tumor of childhood. Thinning or bulging of the suboccipital bone may be present. Occasionally, a cerebellar tumor presents in infancy; progressive cranial enlargement is typical. An inion in high position and lambdoidal sutural enlargement out of proportion to the separation of other sutures should suggest a Dandy-Walker posterior fossa cyst in such infants. Cerebellar tumors presenting in adult life most often produce pressure atrophy of the dorsum sella and posterior clinoids as a result of chronic intracranial hypertension. Increased convolutional markings on the inner table of the vault constitute a late sign of elevated pressure. The plain skull x-rays are commonly abnormal in the suspected cerebellar tumor. However, the findings are those of intracranial hypertension and are generally non-pathognomonic as to actual tumor site in the individual case.

2. Brain stem tumors.

   Plain skull x-rays in the usual intrinsic pontine glioma of childhood are quite normal. This normality contrasts with the suture separation due to childhood cerebellar tumor.

3. Cerebellopontine angle tumor.

   In contrast to brain stem tumors, plain x-ray studies are of great positive diagnostic value in angle tumors. In contrast to cerebellar tumors, plain x-ray studies in angle tumors present local bone erosive changes pointing to the site of the lesion; only in late cases of angle tumor is pressure atrophy of the sella demonstrable. Plain x-ray studies including PA, half-axial, Stenver's views and laminography may be virtually pathognomonic of the presence of an angle tumor. Some plain x-ray abnormality is present in the majority of cases (Fig. 82). However, negative plain films do not rule out an angle tumor in the individual case. Positive plain x-ray changes in angle tumors include the following:

   a. Erosion is usually first noted at the roof of the meatus of the internal auditory canal. The angle tumor is most commonly an acoustic neuroma attached to the superior vestibular nerve in the region of the meatus. The meatus is eroded as the tumor grows out of the canal into the angle. The totally intracanalicular neuroma is much less common at the time of diagnosis than the tumor which extends to some degree into the cerebellopontine recess. Such totally intracanalicular tumors may erode only the roof of the canal leaving the meatus relatively intact until later expansion occurs. Another relatively uncommon neuroma is the one which is attached to the eighth nerve as it crosses the angle without any tumor extension into the meatus or canal. Thus, most acoustic tumors at the time of diagnosis involve the canal, the meatus and the angle.
   b. As the meatus is eroded, it changes from a diameter smaller than the canal to one larger than the canal diameter: there is a progressive opening of the porus acousticus.
   c. Following meatal erosion, demineralization of the petrous apex may become prominent.
   d. Such erosions are not absolutely pathognomonic of acoustic neuroma, since they can also occur with other angle tumors (i.e. meningioma, epidermoid, glomus tumor, glioma extending into the angle, aneurysm). Hyperostosis in the region should suggest

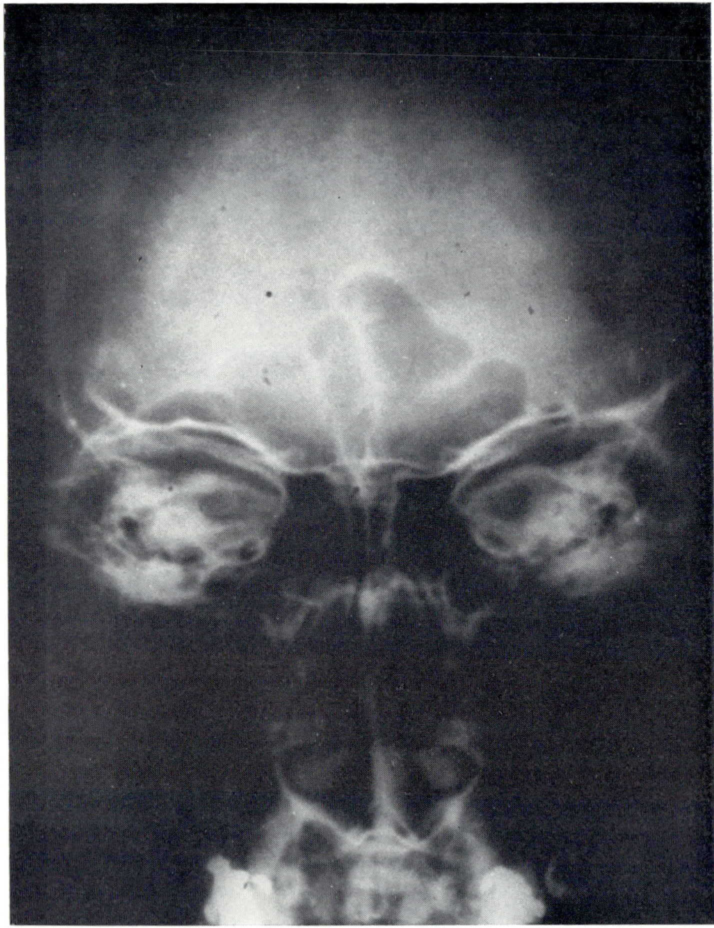

Figure 82. Abnormal internal auditory canal on plain x-ray study. The canals are projected through the orbits. The left canal is enlarged due to an acoustic neuroma. The right canal is normal.

meningioma. Epidermoids commonly erode the petrous apex. Glomus tumor should be suspected if erosion involves the region of the jugular bulb. Tumor calcification in the angle should suggest the possibility of an epidermoid or meningioma. Calcification in the wall of an aneurysm must be kept in mind. Evidence of increased vascular markings may point to meningioma, glomus tumor or arteriovenous malformation. Petrositis may result in erosive or hyperostotic bony change in the petrous apex. The findings on plain x-rays that suggest that the angle tumor may *not* be an acoustic neuroma may be summarized as follow:

(1) Whenever an angle syndrome occurs with entirely normal plain x-rays and laminograms, another tumor type may be responsible; an acoustic neuroma is not ruled out, however.
(2) Preservation of the internal auditory canal and meatus in the presence of an erosive lesion of the petrous bone.
(3) Erosion of the cranial base (Fig. 83).
(4) Hyperostosis or tumor calcification.
(5) Abnormal vascular markings.

These assorted angle tumors may also produce the characteristic plain x-ray findings of an acoustic neuroma. If a *nonacoustic* tumor is suspected because of an unusual clinical syndrome (e.g. an angle syndrome combined with trigeminal neuralgia), or be-

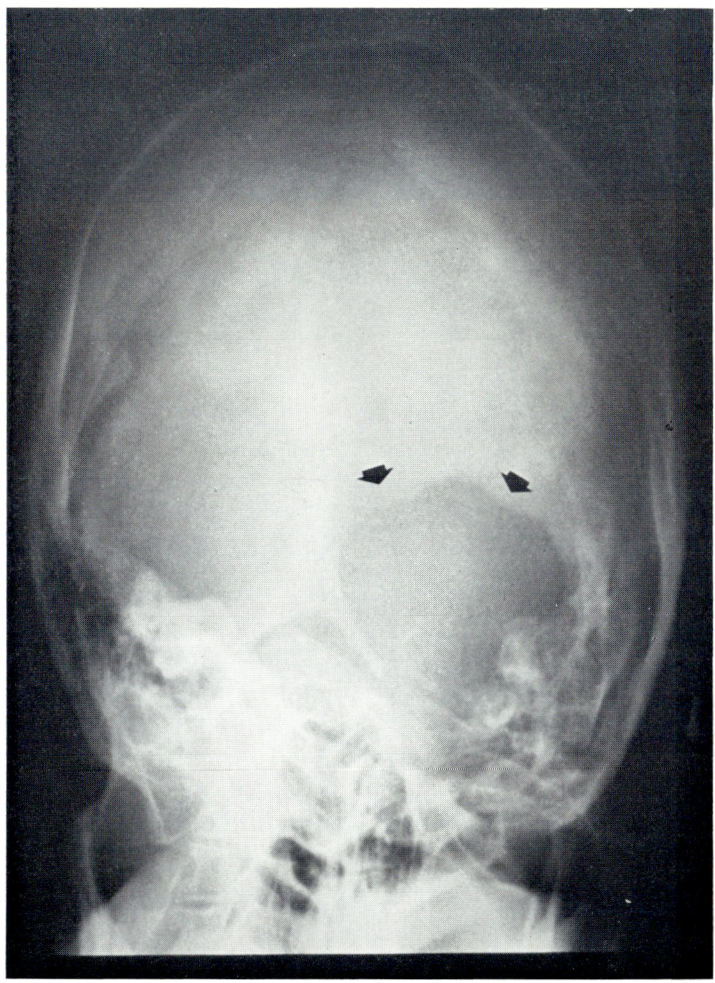

Figure 83. Erosion of the cranial base due to glomus jugulare tumor.

cause of unusual plain x-ray findings, the differential diagnosis can be supplemented by the following:

(1) Lumbar pneumoencephalography—the assorted *nonacoustic* tumors tend *not* to elevate the cerebellopontine recess.

(2) Vertebral angiography—tumor vessels will be noted in meningiomas and glomus tumors (and in many acoustic neuromas as well) while aneurysm or arteriovenous malformation can be ruled out.

EEG

1. Cerebellar tumors commonly result in an abnormal EEG reflecting elevated intracranial pressure.
2. However, elevated intracranial pressure can result in either a normal or abnormal EEG. A normal EEG in a child with papilledema is a point in favor of a cerebellar rather than cerebral tumor.
3. The abnormal EEG reflecting elevated intracranial pressure usually reveals generalized slowing and increased amplitudes. The abnormally slow rhythms are often most marked occipitally, but may be most prominent frontally in cerebellar tumor. Occipital delta activity occurs in cerebellar and posterior third ventricular tumors. Bilateral alpha slowing is seen in states of reduced alertness and is nonspecific as far as tumor localization is concerned. Bilateral frontal slowing not of frontal origin can result from central cerebral, brain stem or cerebellar tumors.
4. When EEG abnormalities are asymmetrical, the side of greatest abnormality does not reliably reflect the side of the cerebellar tumor.
5. A normal EEG is common in the intrinsic brain stem tumor and in the cerebellopontine angle tumor. A normal EEG does not rule out a cerebellar tumor. A normal EEG does not rule out the presence of elevated intracranial pressure. A normal EEG is particularly common in cases of "benign" hydrocephalus, the EEG more often being abnormal when hydrocephalus results from neoplastic obstruction.

CHAPTER 12

SYNDROMES OF INTRACRANIAL HYPERTENSION

Clinical Correlates

THIS FINAL CHAPTER is devoted to the common final event produced by the progressive intracranial mass: elevated intracranial pressure. These neurosurgical syndromes transcend a strictly regional approach, and by virtue of their production of intracranial hypertension, can be considered together. The chief clinical manifestations of intracranial hypertension are headache, vomiting, papilledema and stupor. These are essentially nonlocalizing features. Various cranial nerve abnormalities commonly accompany elevated intracranial pressure. Some of these are also nonlocalizing, reflecting only the existence of a pressure syndrome. Others have localizing value. It is most important to avoid lumbar puncture when an intracranial mass lesion is suspected on clinical grounds. The hazard of brain herniation is increased by lumbar puncture. After the spinal needle is removed, there is continued escape of CSF through the lumbar theca into the epidural space in the presence of an intracranial mass. Furthermore, lumbar puncture pressure may not accurately reflect intracranial and intraventricular pressure. The clinical symptoms and signs of intracranial hypertension therefore assume great importance.

A. Headache

Headache is the most common symptom of intracranial hypertension. It is usually of insidious onset with a progressive tendency to increase in severity, duration and frequency. The majority of brain tumors are ultimately associated with headache of this character. Similarly, the chronic subdural hematoma or brain abscess may produce headache of this type. Headache of more acute onset should always suggest intracranial hemorrhage. Such sudden headache may indicate arterial hypertension with intracerebral hemorrhage. Subarachnoid hemorrhage from a ruptured aneurysm or acute extradural hematoma following cranial trauma may be accompanied by severe acute headache. Headache is, of course, a prominent symptom of intracranial hemorrhage only if the patient remains alert enough to complain. The acute onset of headache may occur in certain brain tumors with ventricular obstruction and "hydrocephalic attacks." If consciousness is lost at the peak of such an attack, the severity of the headache may be totally forgotten by the patient. Hemorrhage within the substance of a brain tumor may also present with headache of sudden onset. In contrast, certain slowly growing tumors may be associated with headaches of insidious onset and an apparently nonprogressive character. The low-grade cerebral astrocytoma or meningioma may be accompanied by such chronic stable headaches for months or years. Focal or generalized recurrent epileptic seizures without headaches may be the only indicator of such a tumor during this period of time. The presence of intracranial hypertension should always be suspected when headaches, despite their mode of onset, assume a progressive, worsening character.

The headache of intracranial hypertension is typically a morning headache at the outset. The headache may awaken the patient or it may appear shortly after arising from bed. The headache is sometimes associated with vomiting. If vomiting occurs, the headache may be relieved. The patient may not experience nausea or anorexia. Eventually, with increasing frequency, the headaches appear later in the day and are unrelieved by analgesics. The headache is variously described as dull, throbbing or bursting; it is always painful and not lightly considered by the patient. The headache is aggravated by coughing, sneezing and straining. It may also be worsened by extension of the neck or by any sudden movement. The headache is usually bilateral and typically bifrontal. It may be generalized. It may be suboccipital and associated with neck pain. Both the supratentorial and the infratentorial mass can produce bifrontal, suboccipital and nuchal pain. Unilateral headaches or unilateral predominance of pain can occur. Such headaches may historically precede the more typical bifrontal headaches of elevated intracranial pressure. Unifrontal headaches may indicate trigeminal involvement. Unitemporal headaches may occur on either side of a supratentorial tumor. Hemicrania suggesting migraine is an unusual manifestation of brain tumor. Unilateral postauricular and suboccipital pain is common on the side of the cerebellopontine angle tumor. All such unilateral forms of headache have no sure localizing value unless supported by localizing neurological deficits. Headache as the first symptom of brain tumor occurs typically in cerebellar-fourth ventricular neoplasm. These tumors are more common in childhood, a time of life when recurrent headache is an unusual symptom. The child may not clearly indicate the site of cranial discomfort. Headache may assume the form of irritability, subtle personality change or loss of normal childhood energy. Headache as the first symptom of brain tumor in the adult often occurs with the temporal lobe mass. The frontal lobe tumor is apt to announce itself clinically with seizures, personality change or motor deficit before recurrent headaches bring the patient to medical attention. Mental disturbance and apathy are particularly severe with tumor extension to the corpus callosum. Such patients may not complain of headache despite intracranial hypertension. The colloid cyst of the third ventricle may present only with headaches which suddenly appear and even resolve with changes in cephalic position. These headaches may be severe and may be associated with impairment of consciousness or transient blindness at the peak of the attack. Recurrent episodes of severe headaches with syncope should suggest acute ventricular obstruction. The headaches of intracranial hypertension are often associated with nonspecific symptoms such as light-headedness, a sense of imbalance and tinnitus. True vertigo suggests an infratentorial lesion. Transient deafness, like transient blindness, can occur with the headaches of advanced intracranial pressure.

Symptomatic relief from the headache of intracranial hypertension does not necessarily imply relief from the intracranial pressure itself. In children with cerebellar tumors, early headaches may be less intense following "springing" of cranial sutures, while vomiting continues and papilledema worsens. The patient with intracranial hypertension due to brain tumor still has elevated pressure between attacks of headache during symptom-free intervals. The individual episode of headache in the tumor patient does not necessarily indicate a rise in intracranial pressure over previous levels. It may result from traction upon pain-sensitive basal dura or arterial channels with or without an accompanying pressure elevation. In the adult with subarachnoid hemorrhage due to ruptured aneurysm, the patient may complain bitterly of headache often associated with photophobia and neck pain due to meningeal irritation. Relief of such headache can occur with diminished bleeding. However, such headaches may also appear to be relieved as consciousness is slightly clouded by progressive brain swelling associated with the arterial spasm of subarachnoid hemorrhage.

B. Vomiting.

Vomiting is not as common a symptom of intracranial hypertension as headache. Vomiting more commonly occurs in children than in adults with elevated pressure. Vomiting is usually associated with morning headache. Vomiting may be the only symptom of elevated intracranial pressure, especially in those too young to complain of headache. Vomiting may symptomatically reflect the intracranial hypertension of infantile hydrocephalus or infantile subdural hematomas. The usual symptoms and signs of elevated pressure may be delayed by the expansile capacity of the infantile skull. Vomiting in children old enough to complain of headache may still appear as an isolated symptom of elevated pressure in the fourth ventricular tumor. Such vomiting may be sudden and projectile and unassociated with nausea. However, the vomiting of intracranial hypertension may also be nonprojectile, effortless and accompanied by definite nausea and anorexia. Vomiting can occur on a periodic basis with symptom-free intervals. Such "cyclic vomiting" can occur with hydrocephalic attacks and intermittent ventricular obstruction. Vomiting may also be intractable and associated with progressive dehydration and weight loss.

C. Papilledema (Fig. 84)

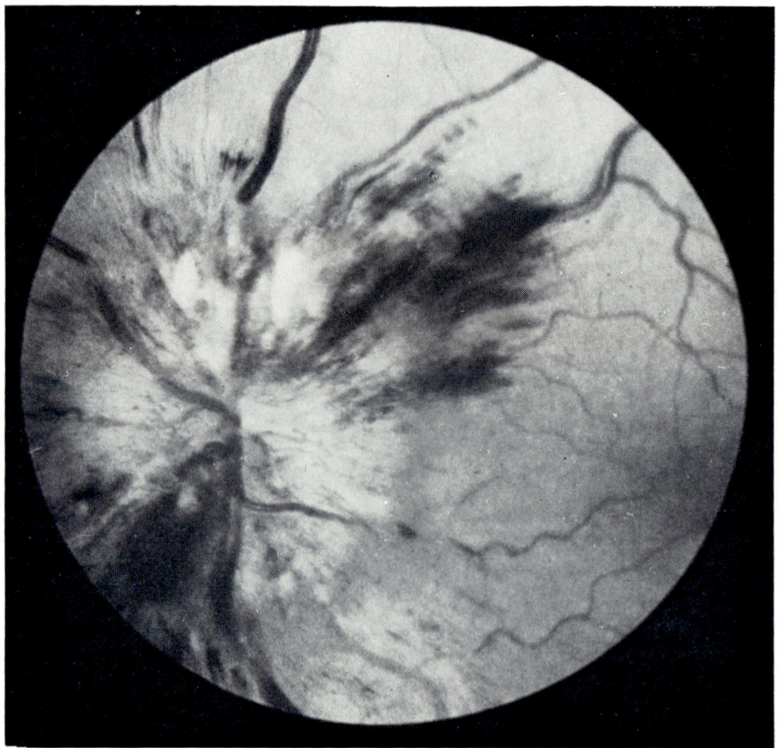

Figure 84. Papilledema.

Papilledema is the classical sign of intracranial hypertension. Early papilledema may be limited to blurring of the nasal margin of the disc, pink discoloration of the disc, congestion and tortuosity of retinal veins and loss of venous pulsations. Venous pulsations can be induced in certain normal individuals, in which they are difficult to visualize, by employing gentle ocular pressure during ophthalmoscopy. Such venous pulsation cannot be induced when papilledema is present. The width of veins increases so that the normal vein:artery ratio of 3:2 is exceeded. Blurring of the disc margin eventually makes the entire disc edge indistinct; the disc appears wider, and reddening of the disc makes it resemble the surrounding retina. Edema of the papilla obliterates the detail of the physiologic cup and elevates the disc. The retinal vessels are deflected over the edge of the prominently elevated disc onto the surrounding retina. The difference in strength between the two lenses employed to sharply place in focus a prominent vessel on the disc surface and a prominent retinal vessel at the disc edge is the measure of disc elevation in diopters. Most cases of papilledema reveal 2 to 4 diopters elevation, but higher grades of 8 to 9 diopters can occur. Radial retinal hemorrhages around the disc or on the disc itself are common in papilledema. They tend to be flame-shaped and lie adjacent to retinal veins. They may be punctate. The hemorrhages of papilledema do not usually extend out into the periphery of the retina. The hemorrhages may appear early in an acute papilledema. At other times, hemorrhages may be absent even with advanced papilledema. White or grayish-white spots may be seen on the disc and surrounding retina especially in later stages. Equally characteristic of papilledema is functionally preserved vision in the early stages. There may be a striking disparity between the absence of visual symptoms and the funduscopic picture of choked discs. Papilledema is almost always bilateral, although it may be asymmetrical. Unilateral papilledema points to an orbital rather than intracranial source. The Foster Kennedy syndrome with papilledema opposite the side of a frontal tumor producing ipsilateral optic atrophy is exceptional. Visual fields in papilledema reveal enlargement of the blind spot which is asymptomatic.

Papilledema can be readily differentiated from "papillitis" (i.e. optic neuritis) . Both conditions may resemble one another on funduscopic examination. Papillitis is an inflammatory swelling of the disc which does not indicate intracranial hypertension. Papillitis may produce blurred margins, increased disc diameter, disc elevation and retinal hemorrhages upon and around the disc. The differential points are as follow: Papillitis is almost always unilateral. When bilateral, papillitis tends to be sequential rather than simultaneous. Ocular pain is common in early papillitis and is aggravated by movement of the eye. Rapid central visual failure is common in papillitis. The patient may have visual symptoms even before the onset of funduscopic evidence of disc swelling. Visual acuity is reduced. Visual fields reveal not only enlargement of the blind spot, but also central and paracentral scotomas. Peripheral quadrant and sector-shaped field cuts also occur.

Papilledema may at times be mistaken for "hypertensive retinopathy." The patient presenting with either process may have systemic hypertension, neurological deficit, bilateral disc swelling and retinal hemorrhage. The differentiation is based upon the narrowing of retinal arteries with localized irregularities, "silver-wire" effect, and "A-V nicking" in hypertensive retinopathy. Retinal hemorrhages extend into the peripheral retina instead of being merely upon and about the region of the disc as in papilledema. "Cotton wool" exudates of grayish-white appearance also extend into the peripheral retina, unlike the white spots of papilledema which lie on or about the disc. A "macular star" may be present with yellowish-white bright dots of lipoid material about the macula. Evident of chronic renal disease and chronic hypertensive cardiomegaly is confirmatory. "Central retinal vein thrombosis" may cause some confusion because of venous distension, edema of the disc and retinal hemorrhage. However, this process is unilateral, the hemorrhages are massive and peripheral in the fundus as well as in the disc and central fundal regions. Retinal veins are extremely tortuous and macular hemorrhages are promient. Visual deterioration is immediate and marked. "Drusen" (i.e. hyaline bodies) of the optic disc can cause disc swelling bilaterally and can therefore be mistaken for papilledema. However, drusen of the disc is associated with a yellow rather than a pink disc, and there is no venous dilatation and no retinal hemorrhage. The drusen itself may or may not be seen. If it lies on the disc surface, it appears as a glassy, yellowish-white, nodular mass. "Pseudopapilledema" is a congenital glial overgrowth which produces an enlarged, blurred disc which may be associated with tortuosity of both retinal arteries and veins. The tortuosity of vessels is greater than the degree of disc elevation. There are no hemorrhages. The process is usually bilateral and may be associated with hyperopia or myopia.

Although papilledema with well-developed funduscopic changes is ordinarily asymptomatic, transient visual symptoms can occur. The transient episodes consist of blurring of vision, the appearance of a cloud or veil, distortion of color vision or total blindness. These transient episodes are characteristically brief, lasting only a few seconds, but occasionally will last as much as thirty seconds. The brevity of these attacks and the fact that visual acuity remains normal between attacks is characteristic of papilledema. "Amblyopic attacks" due to papilledema represent a late sign of intracranial hypertension. They may occur at the peak of headache or they may occur without other symptoms. The majority of patients with papilledema do not give the history of such transient episodes of blindness. Increasing frequency of such attacks indicates progressively increasing intracranial hypertension and heralds the danger of permanent blindness.

In papilledema, the swelling of the optic disc exceeds the edema of the retina about the disc. Such edema will ultimately extend to the region of the macula if intracranial hypertension is unrelieved. At this point, central visual acuity fails and an enlarging central scotoma appears. Hemorrhages may similarly extend to the macular region and damage central vision. With the onset of early signs of secondary optic atrophy, peripheral constriction of visual fields becomes prominent and progressive (Fig. 85). This is usually most noted in the nasal fields, but

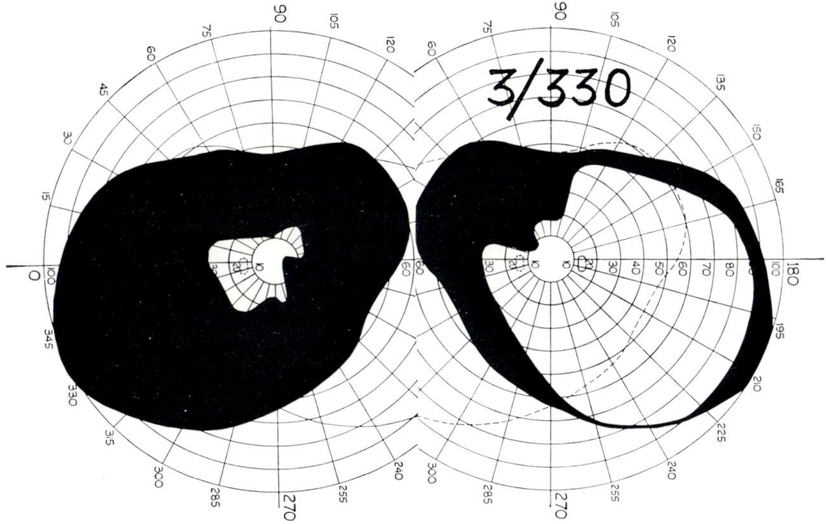

Figure 85. Visual fields in advanced papilledema. Marked peripheral field constriction is present on one side and early constriction is evident on the opposite side. The patient had a large right sphenoid ridge meningioma with chronic papilledema (Fig. 51).

is essentially concentric. The earliest sign of secondary optic atrophy occurring in papilledema is a grayish-white discoloration at the peripheral border of the edematous disc. As the atrophy proceeds, the disc becomes less elevated and less pink, and eventually the entire disc becomes pale. Retinal veins becomes less distended and retinal arteries become narrow and surrounded by white sheaths of glial proliferation. Secondary atrophy proceeds despite the fact that intracranial hypertension remains high. Secondary optic atrophy can be differentiated from primary atrophy because the secondarily atrophic disc remains increased in width, its margins remain blurred and remnants of previous hemorrhages are present. As the atrophy proceeds, peripheral and central field defects unite. Spared paracentral tubular vision may persist. Total blindness may result. Blindness may become permanent after one of a series of amblyopic attacks. The ultimate visual failure of papilledema may be compounded by the localizing visual defects of tumors involving the intracranial optic pathways. For example, hemianopia may be added to the visual field defects of papilledema in glioblastoma invading the optic radiation.

Papilledema can occur with intracranial hypertension of any etiology. Its presence indicates a brain tumor until proven otherwise. Papilledema may be absent in certain brain tumor cases even with advanced intracranial pressure. Brain tumors presenting with papilledema may be supratentorial or infratentorial, intracerebral or extracerebral. At one extreme is the cerebellar-fourth ventricular tumor with a high incidence of papilledema, usually in the absence of visual symptoms. At the opposite extreme is the pituitary tumor with a low incidence of papilledema, often in the presence of visual failure. Papilledema in a general way reflects the incidence of brain tumors. It is more commonly due to infratentorial tumor in the child, and more often due to supratentorial tumor in the adult. Tumors which are critically located with regard to the ventricular system (i.e. those which produce obstructive hydrocephalus) are particularly apt to produce high-grade papilledema. Larger tumors located at a distance from the ventricular system (e.g. tumors of the frontal pole) may never produce papilledema, despite intracranial hypertension due to the mass of the tumor itself. Slowly growing extracerebral tumors (e.g. meningioma of the middle sphenoid ridge) may reveal themselves clinically at a late stage when the tumor is huge. Papilledema present at that time is usually chronic with secondary atrophy and pallor of the optic disc. Rapidly growing intracerebral tumors (e.g. glioblastoma) associated with cerebral edema may present with more acutely swollen optic discs. However, the presence of papilledema does not necessarily correlate with the pathological malignancy of the tumor. The low-grade cerebellar astrocytoma typically produces high-grade papilledema due to fourth ventricular obstruction and hydrocephalus. The high-grade glioblastoma does not necessarily produce papilledema at the time of its clinical presentation. Asymmetry of papilledema can be misleading. Such asymmetry can be due to cerebellar tumor. Papilledema is not necessarily worse on the side of a supratentorial tumor. When papilledema is much greater on the side opposite a tumor, partial or complete obstruction of the foramen of Monro should be suspected. The lateral ventricle on the tumor side may be compressed, while the opposite lateral ventricle may be obstructed and hydrocephalic. Large tumors in the sylvian and parasylvian regions are apt to present in this manner. Papilledema may be totally contralateral in the presence of ipsilateral optic atrophy. The usual source of this Foster Kennedy syndrome is olfactory meningioma or frontal glioma.

Intracranial hypertension of sudden onset may be quite severe without the development of papilledema. For example, the acute epidural hematoma usually produces progressive coma, brain stem compression and intracranial hypertension without swelling of the optic discs. Acute intracranial hemorrhage of any etiology may result in sudden intracranial hypertension without papilledema. When evidence of chronic papilledema is present in intracranial bleeding, sudden hemorrhage into a brain tumor (e.g. glioblastoma, oligodendroglioma) should be suspected. This does not deny the fact that an acute papilledema can occasionally occur within several hours of a sudden and severe episode of intracranial hypertension. Rapid swelling of the discs with acute hemorrhage can occur. Acute subarachnoid hemorrhage due to ruptured aneurysm can result in both retinal and preretinal hemorrhages. The optic discs may be surrounded or obscured by such hemorrhages. The optic discs themselves are usually not elevated in the presence of preretinal hemorrhage following acute subarachnoid hemorrhage. While this is not a true papilledema, the preretinal hemorrhage reflects the presence of subarachnoid bleeding and the likelihood of intracranial hypertension. Preretinal hemorrhages include the subhyaloid boat-shaped type and hemorrhages into the vitreous.

In head trauma cases, extracerebral or intracerebral hematomas, cerebral contusion with brain swelling, or communicating hydrocephalus resulting from subarachnoid hemorrhage are all sources of intracranial hypertension. Posterior fossa hematomas should be included. All these complications of head injury commonly occur without papilledema and early diagnosis must be made on other grounds. However, the development of papilledema in the head trauma case has significance. It means that intracranial pressure has become elevated, if not already so. It may thereby indicate the presence of a previously unsuspected hematoma. Most cases of intracerebral or extracerebral hematoma of acute onset reveal a general tendency toward progressive deterioration. The "lucid interval" occurring in a minority of acute epidural hematomas may be misleading if the patient is seen early in the postconcussive recovery phase following trauma. Rapid deterioration usually occurs quickly, however, making expanding extradural clot the leading diagnosis. Under certain circumstances, patients with eccentrically located epidural or subdural hematomas may appear to be improving following the initial trauma.

Development of papilledema in such circumstances may be the only indicator of such an eccentric clot. Traumatic brain swelling reaches its peak three to four days following a cerebral injury. When brain swelling is generalized, the patient is somnolent; he may be comatose depending on the severity of brain swelling and brain stem compromise. Papilledema may or may not accompany such generalized brain swelling. Still later development of papilledema in the head-injured patient should suggest communicating hydrocephalus due to traumatic subarachnoid hemorrhage. At the time papilledema is noted, the patient may have made an apparently good recovery from the head injury and may even be totally asymptomatic.

The age of the patient at the onset of intracranial hypertension is an important factor. The presence or absence of papilledema in the pediatric age group has special significance. The expansile nature of the infantile cranial vault provides a measure of safety. The abnormal head growth associated with congenital hydrocephalus, subdural hematomas and tumors occurring in infancy is usually not accompanied by papilledema. Fullness and tension of the anterior fontanelle, dilated scalp veins, irritability and vomiting support the impression of intracranial hypertension despite the "safety valve" of unfused sutures. Papilledema in infancy should suggest the diagnosis of sagittal sinus thrombosis. Dilated scalp veins forming a "caput medusa" about the anterior fontanelle and evidence for intracranial hemorrhage favor the diagnosis. A tympanitic "cracked-pot note" on cranial percussion, positive transillumination and "sunset eyes" favor hydrocephalus. Subhyaloid hemorrhages favor infantile subdurals. The latter diagnosis is confirmed by subdural taps. Meningitis is not usually associated with papilledema. Failure of clinical response to adequate antibiotic therapy or the development of papilledema in a case of meningitis should suggest intracranial hypertension due to one of four possibilities: subdural effusion, brain abscess, venous sinus thrombosis or postmeningitic hydrocephalus. While visual failure due to papilledema can occur at any age, rapid visual deterioration is particularly prominent in the cerebellar-fourth ventricular tumor of childhood. This occurs despite the presence of "springing" of the cranial sutures.

D. Stupor

Impairment of consciousness to some degree is common in intracranial hypertension. It is common enough to constitute a major manifestation of elevated intracranial pressure. However, just as headache, vomiting and papilledema are not present in all instances of intracranial hypertension, so too the patient with elevated pressure is apt to be fully alert. This is particularly true if the onset of the pressure syndrome is gradual. In fact, the patient with elevated pressure may be quite irritable and may have difficulty sleeping. All graduations on the spectrum of consciousness to deep coma are encountered in the neurosurgical syndromes associated with intracranial hypertension. A certain mental torpor, a loss of mental acuity, is common in elevated intracranial pressure. Mental agility may vary. Confusional episodes occur. Episodic somnolence may be present. Such impairments may be present only at the apex of an attack of severe headache. "Stupor" implies that the obtunded patient remains arousable, although his verbal and motor responses may be somewhat delayed. "Coma" implies that the patient is no longer arousable to conscious levels, despite the intensity of noxious stimulation. This phase is divisible into "semicoma" in which purposeful movements still persist, and "deep coma" in which motor responses are primitive and nonpurposeful. Noxious stimulation at the deep coma level may produce reflex withdrawal, stereotyped rigid decorticate or decerebrate responses, or no motor response at all. Progressive intracranial pressure of gradual onset ultimately propels the patient into a state of reduced consciousness or coma if neurosurgical attention is not obtained in the early phase. Intracranial pressure of sudden onset may immediately result in progressive coma, and may totally bypass the traditional triad of headache, vomiting and papilledema.

Obtundation does not necessarily imply that intracranial hypertension exists. The hypothalamic tumor and the brain stem contusion provide clinical examples of depressed consciousness which may exist without intracranial hypertension. However, progressive impairment of consciousness in the neurosurgical setting must always be regarded as evidence for intracranial hypertension and intracranial mass until proven otherwise. Stupor progressing to coma is the cardinal sign of brain stem compression. Such compression occurs as a result of uncal transtentorial herniation, central transtentorial herniation, tentorial packing, or foraminal impaction at the level of the foramen magnum. Any supratentorial mass can produce both transtentorial and foraminal impaction. The infratentorial mass usually produces foraminal impaction. Herniation of the cerebellar tonsils with compression of the lower brain stem and outlets of the fourth ventricle with obstructive hydrocephalus occurs. The acute hydrocephalus causes further impaction and further depression of consciousness. The supratentorial mass producing midbrain compression at the incisura of the tentorium impairs consciousness by compromise of reticular function in the midbrain tegmentum. There may be midbrain compression, distortion, displacement, ischemia and central stem hemorrhage. The supratentorial mass can be relatively localized as in a tumor, hematoma or abscess. A more generalized supratentorial mass effect can occur in massive diffuse cerebral edema and in acute hydrocephalus. The responsible supratentorial mass may be intra- or extracerebral. Compression of the midbrain is associated with compromise of the critical CSF and deep venous pathways surrounding the midbrain at the tentorial opening. These factors contribute to the intracranial hypertension already present due to the bulk of the supratentorial mass. Midbrain compression at the tentorial level can occur anterolaterally, posteriorly and centrally. These are accounted for by uncal herniation, posterior hippocampal herniation and central transtentorial herniations, respectively (Fig. 86). Preceding transtentorial herniation, other brain herniations (e.g. subfalcial) which were clinically silent may have occurred without reduction of consciousness until eventual midbrain compression. A lateral or rostral intra-or extracerebral mass is most apt to produce subfalcial herniation. Slowly growing lateral tumors, such as outer sphenoidal meningiomas of globose type, may produce marked subfalcial herniation over a long period before diagnosis or ultimate transtentorial herniation. Frontopolar tumors readily produce herniation under the relatively narrow border of the anterior falx. Frontopolar tumors may also shift the entire hemisphere toward the occipital pole, and the base of the frontal lobe may herniate into the middle fossa. If these hernias occur slowly enough, they may be evident on angiography but not on clinical evaluation. In contrast, transtentorial herniation is almost always clinically detectable. Diagnosis and treatment must be carried out promptly before irreversible compromise of the brain stem occurs. All three forms of transtentorial herniation clinically present essentially the same pattern.

1. Progressive impairment of consciousness is constant.
2. Generalized mild increase in tone is common and often is most marked in the neck and the legs ("nuchocrural rigidity").
3. Early irritability is common, but not always present.
4. Oculomotor palsy.

This begins with pupillary dilatation. It is almost always on the side of the mass. The patient may still be alert when the pupil is beginning to dilate. He may already be stuporous. The slightly dilated pupil may still react to light. With further dilatation, the pupil becomes sluggish. The pupil eventually becomes fixed and fully dilated, and extrinsic oculomotor palsy is noted. The fixed dilated pupil with divergent gaze is seen during the comatose stage. Further midbrain compromise is associated with bilateral dilatation of the pupils and loss

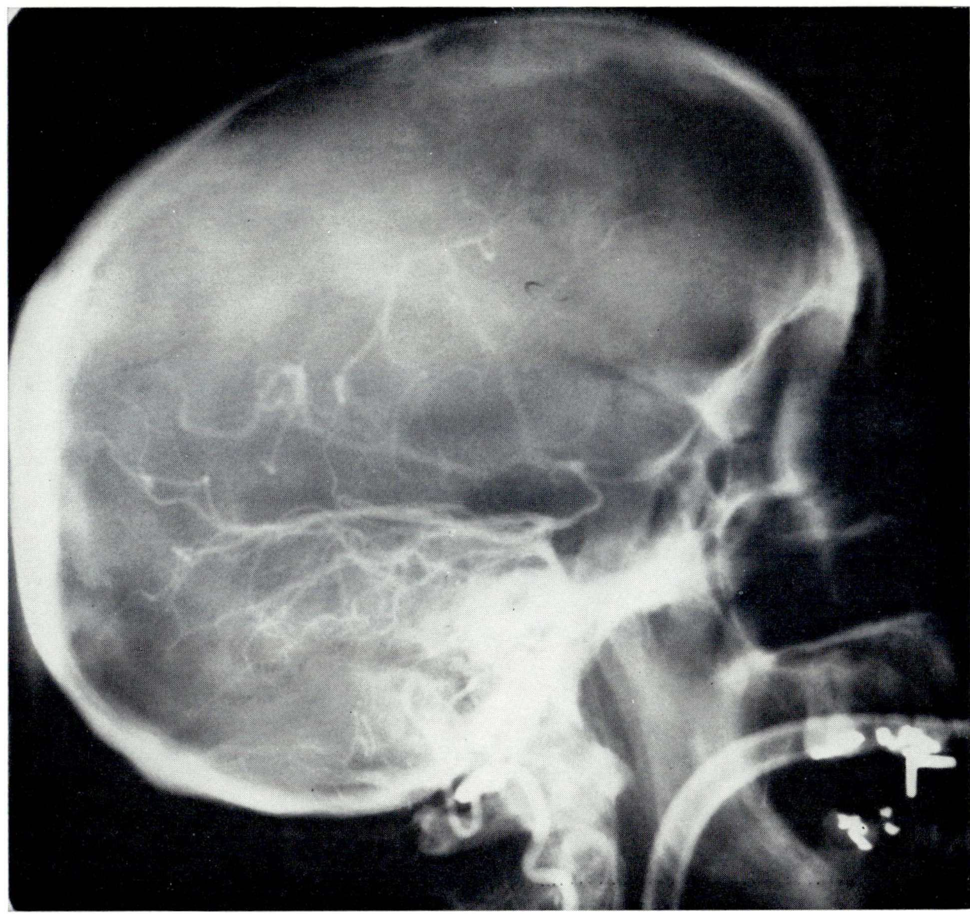

Figure 86. Combined transtentorial and tonsillar herniation. Multiple bilateral cranial nerve palsies, including the bulbar cranial nerves, in a forty-two-year-old woman with advanced papilledema, led to this vertebral angiogram. There is downward dislocation of the brain stem, posterior-inferior cerebellar, superior cerebellar and posterior cerebral arteries. Note the elevation of the right middle cerebral artery, filling via the right posterior communicating artery, over a supratentorial mass. A right carotid angiogram revealed the tumor to be a large right sphenoid ridge meningioma (Fig. 51).

of light reflexes bilaterally. Before the pupils are fully dilated, in some cases of transtentorial herniation, pupillary dilatation can be induced by neck flexion. Loss of upward gaze on neck flexion is a sign of "tentorial packing" in which the posterior hippocampal gyri are bilaterally herniated with compression of the midbrain tectum and tegmentum. Further midbrain compromise leads to disconjugate gaze and ultimate loss of oculovestibular response. The oculomotor palsy itself is most often the result of uncal herniation against the medially adjacent third nerve. Temporal lobe tumor and the middle fossa extradural hematoma produce typical examples. However, subdural hematoma over the convexity, or a sylvian, presylvian or suprasylvian mass can also result in an uncal hernia. More medial masses or diencephalic tumors can produce oculomotor palsy by central transtentorial herniation. The brain stem is dislocated downward and the oculomotor nerve is stretched over the petroclinoid ligament.

5. Hemiparesis.

Contralateral motor weakness may already be present as a localizing sign of the supratentorial mass. Such weakness becomes more profound with compression of the ipsilateral cerebral peduncle by a herniated uncus. If no preexistent motor deficit is present, the hemiparesis results entirely from compression of the peduncle. While the patient is alert or drowsy, only a slight drift may be detected. Facial weakness or arm weakness, or faciobrachial weakness occurring alone are not due to uncal herniation, but rather are localizing signs of the mass lesion. This is due to the fact that the corticospinal fibers to the leg are outermost in the peduncle and are affected early. The weakness always includes the leg and is usually a hemiplegia in uncal herniation. The face may or may not be spared. Facial fibers are more medial in the peduncle. Hemiplegia is most often contralateral to the mass, but Kernohan's notch can occur. If the midbrain is shifted sufficiently to the opposite side and the tentorial incisura is sufficiently narrow, the opposite cerebral peduncle can be compressed by the tentorial edge on that side. This produces an ipsilateral hemiplegia. Hemiplegia is therefore not as good a lateralizing sign as oculomotor palsy in uncal herniation. A Babinski and hyperactive deep tendon reflexes are common on the hemiparetic side. Hemiparesis, usually contralateral to the main bulk of the mass, is common in central transtentorial and posterior hippocampal herniations as well. Quadriparesis should suggest foraminal impaction, but it can occur terminally in transtentorial herniation.

6. Vital sign changes.

As intracranial tension rapidly rises during transtentorial herniation, the vital signs show characteristic changes. Alteration in vital signs is always a late manifestation of intracranial hypertension. The characteristic alterations of a rising blood pressure, falling pulse, and change in respiratory pattern with diminishing consciousness may not all be present in the individual case. Variations in the usual vital sign picture are especially common in children with intracranial hypertension. The child with an acute supratentorial epidural hematoma and transtentorial herniation may develop bradycardia without rise in blood pressure. The child with cerebellar tumor with acute obstructive hydrocephalus and foraminal impaction also may present bradycardia without systemic hypertension. However, progressive arterial hypertension combined with bradycardia is the usual combination in children and adults with rapidly progressive intracranial pressure. There is usually a tendency toward widening of the pulse pressure. Occasionally, the arterial hypertension is accompanied by a tachycardia rather than a bradycardia. The constellation of vital signs combined with frequent evaluations of the level of consciousness is critical to early diagnosis of impending herniation.

Change in respiratory pattern in the obtunded patient is always suspect. In midbrain compression due to transtentorial herniation, respirations often become noisy and excessive tracheobronchial secretions with rhonchi may be noted. Respirations may become slow and deep. "Cheyne-Stokes respiration" may occur with hyperpnea alternating with periods of apnea. The hyperventilation phase in Cheyne-Stokes breathing reaches a peak and then declines. The hypoventilation phase is shorter than the more prominent hyperventilation phase. Cheyne-Stokes respiration also occurs in a variety of cerebral disorders without transtentorial herniation. When it appears with progressive systemic hypertension, bradycardia or diminishing consciousness, it should be regarded as evidence of transtentorial herniation until proven otherwise. "Central neurogenic hyperventilation" is a rapid, deep, sustained form of hyperpnea. No hypoventilatory interruptions occur. No crescendo effect occurs. This respiratory pattern can occur with severe midbrain compression. Central neurogenic hyperventilation is prominent when transtentorial herniation occurs as a result of intracerebral and intraventricular hemorrhage. Marked hyperthermia or shivering, early spasticity of the hemiparetic limbs or early decerebrate rigidity occur with massive intraventricular hemorrhage. An important sign in either transtentorial or foraminal hernias is change in respiratory pattern on neck flexion. Nuchal rigidity is common in both transtentorial and foraminal impaction. Attempts at neck flexion may also produce changes in blood pressure and pulse when herniation is occurring. Pronounced bradycardia or apnea can occur. In the terminal phase of transtentorial herniation, cardiorespiratory collapse occurs with hypotension, thready tachycardia and marked hypoventilation. Resistant hypothermia occurs in this phase.

When foraminal impaction with cerebellar tonsillar herniation is responsible for rapidly rising intracranial pressure, the respiratory changes differ from those of the transtentorial level. The circulatory changes, in contrast, may be identical at either level of herniation; systemic hypertension and bradycardia can occur in either case. However, when foraminal impaction with primary medullary compression occurs, respiratory failure and hypoventilation are prominent. Respiratory failure occurs much before circulatory collapse. When prolonged apnea accompanies systemic hypertension and/or bradycardia, foraminal impaction should be suspected. Ataxic respiration which is totally irregular in depth and rhythm sometimes occurs. The regular alternating rhythm of Cheyne-Stokes respiration does not occur with primary medullary compression. Other respiratory patterns do occur with medullary compression, including gasping or clusterlike breathing. These are marked by irregularity with intervals of hypoventilation and apnea. Respiration is apt to be very quiet and unlike the noisy hyperpnea of midbrain compression. Foraminal impaction with primary compression of the medulla oblongata usually results from a posterior fossa mass. Occasionally, a supratentorial mass can also produce foraminal impaction with medullary compression. If intracranial hypertension is not relieved, prolonged apnea and respiratory failure occur. Ultimately, cardiovascular collapse occurs and the apnea, hypotension, thready tachycardia and hypothermia of terminal coma appear.

The posterior fossa mass occasionally results in an upward transtentorial herniation of the superior cerebellar vermis. This is less common than foraminal impaction. It is much less common than the usual forms of downward transtentorial herniation produced by the supratentorial mass. Upward transtentorial herniation of the cerebellum with midbrain compression is often a clinically indistinguishable form of brain stem compression. The patient typically reveals progressive coma and signs of progressive intracranial hypertension. Coexistent foraminal impaction may produce apnea. Cheyne-Stokes respiration in the presence of a posterior fossa mass points to midbrain compression and is indirect evidence of upward herniation of the cerebellar vermis.

7. Decerebration.

Severe midbrain compression due to transtentorial herniation can result in this stereotyped posture of extensor rigidity. The extremities are hyperpronated, hyperextended and hypertonic. The neck is rigid. Opisthotonus with hyperextension of the neck and spine in addition to extensor rigidity of the extremities may occur. Decerebrate posturing may occur spontaneously. It may be present only with noxious stimulation. It may occur intermittently in association with marked changes in vital signs including prolonged apnea. These decerebrate attacks are tonic "brain stem seizures." They were once referred to as "cerebellar fits." Attacks of decerebration can occur as a result of a posterior fossa mass with foraminal impaction, as well as with severe compression of the upper brain stem by the supratentorial mass. They can also occur during the acute hydrocephalic attack. Decerebration is bilateral in most instances. It may appear unilaterally opposite a flaccid hemiplegia. When present bilaterally, it may prevent detection of a previously lateralizing hemiparesis of mild degree. In pontine failure consequent to upper brain stem compression, the characteristic midbrain decerebrate posture may change to a pontine form. The arms remain hyperextended, hyperpronated and hypertonic, while the legs become flaccid and paraplegia occurs. In eventual medullary failure, a flaccid quadriplegia is noted. There is total loss of reflexes in addition to cardiorespiratory collapse.

E. Cranial nerve palsies.

1. First.

Bilateral anosmia may occur in intracranial hypertension. High pressure hydrocephalus with distended frontal horns may compress the olfactory tracts and even depress the roof of the orbit on each side. This accounts for bilateral anosmia, spontaneous CSF rhinorrhea, exophthalmos and the appearance of sunset eyes seen in certain hydrocephalics. Unilateral anosmia is an important localizing sign of a frontobasal tumor.

2. Second.

Papilledema and optic atrophy are frequently present in intracranial hypertension and have been discussed separately. Transient episodes of blindness occur in some cases with papilledema. Acute hydrocephalic attacks can also produce transient visual disturbances which are often associated with the presence of papilledema. Falsely localizing field defects can occasionally occur as a result of intracranial hypertension. Bitemporal hemianopia may result from chiasmatic compression by a hydrocephalic third ventricle. Third ventricular, aqueductal or fourth ventricular obstruction may be responsible. A distended third ventricle can also herniate between the optic nerves, separating them and exposing them to lateral compression by the carotid arteries. This produces the rare binasal hemianopia. Homonymous hemianopia can result from upward compression of an occipital pole by an expanding cerebellar tumor. The pressure is exerted through the tentorium. Homonymous hemianopia can also result from transtentorial stretching of the posterior cerebral artery or transtentorial compression of the optic tract. The presence of coma due to midbrain compression masks the hemianopia. The latter may become apparent only following recovery of the patient after neurosurgical intervention.

3. Third.

Oculomotor palsy occurring with intracranial hypertension indicates impending or actual transtentorial herniation until proven otherwise. The unilaterally dilated, eventually sluggish pupil is an important danger signal indicating supratentorial mass. In the obtunded patient with a spontaneous subarachnoid hemorrhage and unilateral oculomotor palsy, both a posterior communicating aneurysm and impending transtentorial herniation must be considered. The posterior communicating aneurysm can produce third nerve palsy without transtentorial herniation, and even without rupture due to proximity of the nerve to the fundus of the aneurysm. However, intracerebral hematoma, commonly the result of middle cerebral aneurysm rupture, can result in transtentorial oculomotor paralysis. Hematoma must be ruled out, especially when obtundation is progressive. Arterial spasm with cerebral edema accompanying subarachnoid hemorrhage can produce the same clinical picture. Oculomotor palsy similarly indicates the presence of supratentorial hematoma, extracerebral or intracerebral, in head trauma cases until proven otherwise. The importance of the dilating pupil as an indicator of incipient transtentorial herniation in any supratentorial brain tumor cannot be overemphasized. The patient is often too obtunded to complain of diplopia when the latter is due to transtentorial oculomotor paralysis. Bilateral oculomotor palsy also occurs with marked upper brain stem compression and also with downward shift of the brain stem due to central supratentorial mass effect.

4. Fourth.

Isolated trochlear paralysis is rare. There is partial inability to rotate the eye down and out. There may be diplopia on downward gaze as in descending a stair. It is not ordinarily seen in cases with intracranial hypertension. It is a rare sign of superior cerebellar vermian herniation with dorsal midbrain compression, in which other ocular signs are more prominent. It may be seen with associated third, fifth and sixth nerve palsies in tumors invading the medial middle fossa, carvernous sinus or orbit, or in cavernous aneurysm. Such lesions are not ordinarily associated with the syndrome of intracranial hypertension at the time of their clinical presentation.

5. Fifth.

Loss of corneal sensation commonly accompanies deepening coma and is equal bilaterally. The corneal reflexes become sluggish and are finally lost. The noncomatose aphasic, mute, anarthric or hysterical patient who fails to respond verbally retains brisk corneal reflexes. Asymmetrical corneal reflexes suggest unilateral facial palsy or involvement of the trigeminal within the brain stem, posterior or middle fossa, cavernous sinus or orbit. Unilateral paralysis of cranial nerves five, seven, eight and possibly of lower cranial nerves on the same side in an adult can be associated with intracranial hypertension. Acoustic neuroma of the cerebello pontine angle is most likely. Meningioma of the angle may be responsible. Elevated intracranial pressure is, however, a late sign of an angle tumor. Meningioma or neuroma in the vicinity of the gasserian ganglion may produce trigeminal pain, sensory and motor loss. Oculomotor palsy and compression of the ipsilateral cerebral peduncle are associated. The tumor extends from the mesial middle fossa into the posterior fossa, and may ultimately present evidence of intracranial hypertension as it blocks the tentorial opening.

6. Sixth.

Abducens palsy is a very common accompaniment of intracranial hypertension. It is usually unilateral, but may be bilateral. It does not ordinarily indicate the presence of brain herniation, and it may occur long before other signs of intracranial hypertension. Diplopia of intracranial origin is usually due to abducens palsy, and should always raise the possibility of elevated intracranial pressure with or without an associated squint. Squint is commonly seen in infantile hydrocephalus, where there may be little to suggest intracranial hypertension other than abnormal head size and a tense fontanelle. Children with obvious lateral rectus paralysis may not complain of double vision. In contrast, adults may complain of diplopia before obvious extraocular motor weakness is evident. The symptom of double vision, even in the absence of signs, has the same serious significance as do the symptoms of progressive headache and vomiting. Intracranial hypertension must be considered. Even if lateral rectus weakness is not obvious, the two images become most widely separated in the direction of pull of the paretic muscle. Diplopia may be episodic. It may occur with attacks of headache or without other symptoms. It may occur and persist and worsen. It may occur and persist, then diminish. The progressive effects of brain tumor may render the patient unaware of the second image. The image may appear to be suppressed. At times, diplopia is described in vague terms such as "blurring" or "cloudy vision" and must be separated from sensory visual failure. Lateral rectus palsy has no localizing value when symptoms and signs of intracranial hypertension are present. In the absence of elevated intracranial pressure, abducens palsy can have definite localizing value. Brain stem glioma and chordoma of the clivus are good examples of the localizing value of abducens palsy in the absence of intracranial hypertension. Elevated pressure occurs late in both tumors, while abducens palsy may be the earliest sign. In certain instances of acutely developing intracranial hypertension with downward shift of the brain stem, stretching of the abducens nerves can lead to an acute bilateral sixth nerve palsy. This is associated with oculomotor palsy and rapid impairment of consciousness.

7. Seventh through twelfth.

Unilateral peripheral facial paralysis occurring with evidence of intracranial hypertension suggests a cerebellopontine angle tumor in the adult. Since elevated pressure is a late sign of an angle tumor, the facial palsy is usually associated with other cranial nerve and cerebellar signs at this stage. In childhood, unilateral or bilateral facial palsy is common in the brain stem glioma. The cranial nerve palsy, like that of the angle tumor, precedes evidence of intracranial hypertension which occurs late. In craniocerebral injury with basilar skull fracture, peripheral facial palsy may complicate the picture of cerebral contusion or hematoma. Unilateral central facial palsy with sparing of the brow and without hemiplegia suggests a frontal or temporal mass. Facial palsy in association with intracranial hypertension almost always has localizing significance. This is also true for the remaining lower cranial nerves which may be involved by tumors within the posterior fossa. Acoustic neuroma, meningioma, cholesteatoma, metastatic tumor and carcinoma of the base of the skull may be responsible.

An unusual multiple cranial nerve syndrome can occur with advanced intracranial hypertension. When it occurs, it is associated with foraminal impaction and acute obstructive hydrocephalus resulting from fourth ventricular outlet block. The cranial nerve palsies are bilateral, symmetrical and transient. The lower cranial nerves are most commonly involved and may reveal multiple palsies. Transient tinnitus and deafness, along with transient blindness, can occur in hydrocephalic attacks. The degree of fourth ventricular outlet block appears to be intermittent. The lower cranial nerves are subjected to intermittent elevations of intracranial pressure, stretching and compression. The patient may exhibit hoarseness, dysphagia and dysarthria. Examination may reveal bilateral facial diplegia of peripheral type. Bilateral bulbar paralysis with weakness of the palate, pharynx and larynx may occur. Oropharyngeal secretions are excessive due to inability to swallow. The patient may remain alert during the attack, or obtundation may be present. Upper cranial nerves may occasionally be involved with bilateral internal and external ophthalmoplegia, and diminished corneal sensation despite preservation of an alert state. The palsies may become permanent if intracranial hypertension is unrelieved. In a singular case of sphenoid meningioma with hydrocephalus, foraminal impaction and advanced papilledema, all true cranial nerves from oculomotor to hypoglossal were involved bilaterally, symmetrically and reversibly upon reduction of intracranial hypertension (Needham et al., 1970) .

Any relatively localized intracranial mass which is not detected until the onset of symptoms or signs of elevated pressure presents in one of three ways.

1. Signs of intracranial hypertension alone are present.
2. Signs of intracranial hypertension plus signs which localize the mass are present.
3. Signs of intracranial hypertension plus falsely localizing signs are present.

The site of the mass may remain totally silent, while headaches, vomiting and papilledema indicate only the presence of elevated pressure. The colloid cyst of the third ventricle resulting in obstruction of the foramen of Monro typically presents in this way. Frequently, a chronic subdural hematoma may present only with evidence of headaches and choked discs without a previous history of trauma, so that brain tumor is suspected. The emphasis in previous chapters has been placed upon the localizing value of regional signs. However, when a patient presents with the headaches, vomiting or somnolence of intracranial hypertension, it may be difficult to elicit a definite history pointing to regional localization of a mass. The onset of the pressure syndrome may obscure the localizing value of earlier deficits. For example, stupor may prevent detection of a preexistent hemianopia or discriminatory sensory loss. Truly localizing signs which indicate the site of the responsible mass must always be distinguished from falsely localizing signs which result from intracranial hypertension. For example, when abducens palsy appears in a brain tumor suspect with evidence of intracranial hypertension, the responsible tumor may be on either side of the falx or above or below the tentorium. In the presence of brain shift, brain swelling, herniation or hydrocephalus, other focal signs may appear which are misleading with regard to the actual location of the responsible mass. The brain abscess with surrounding cerebral edema provides an example of the manner in which focal signs are valuable when intracranial hypertension exists. If a dilated pupil appears in this case, impending transtentorial herniation should be suspected. The oculomotor paresis is a highly significant sign because it indicates the hernia, reflects great mass effect, and also because it has lateralizing significance. The third nerve palsy is on the side of the abscess. However, the dilated pupil does not indicate in which cerebral lobe the abscess lies. A contralateral central facial palsy in this patient would point to either the frontal or temporal lobe, both being common sites for brain abscess. An expressive dysphasia would favor a dominant frontal location, but could occur with temporal abscess producing frontolateral transsylvian compression and edema. A contralateral superior quadrantanopia or hemianopia would heavily favor the temporal abscess, but might be absent or missed due to stupor. Clinical evidence of frontal sinusitis or middle ear infection may be extremely helpful in the differentiation, but may be absent.

In contrast to the localized intracranial mass, a more generalized mass effect may also result in intracranial hypertension. Pressure syndromes of this generalized character include the following types:

1. Ventricular—high pressure hydrocephalus.
2. Intracerebral—diffuse bilateral cerebral edema.
3. Extracerebral—bilateral subdural hematomas.
4. Cranial—premature fusion of cranial sutures.

The generalized syndrome may produce markedly elevated pressure. Examples include transtentorial herniation due to massive cerebral edema or to bilateral convexity subdurals, and the foraminal impaction of the hydrocephalic attack. At the other end of the clinical spectrum, intracranial hypertension may not be a feature of certain cases of hydrocephalus, subdural hematoma and limited cerebral edema. Similarly, limited forms of premature closure of cranial sutures are commonly compatible with normal intracranial tension. In more generalized forms of craniosynostosis, the rapidly growing brain of infancy is confined in a chamber too small for its projected growth. Optic atrophy, convulsions and mental retardation can result from the pressure of such cranial restriction. The generalized syndromes include a number of distinguishable varieties.

A. Hydrocephalus

The common feature of the various forms of hydrocephalus is ventricular enlargement (Figs. 87 and 88). The pressure within enlarged

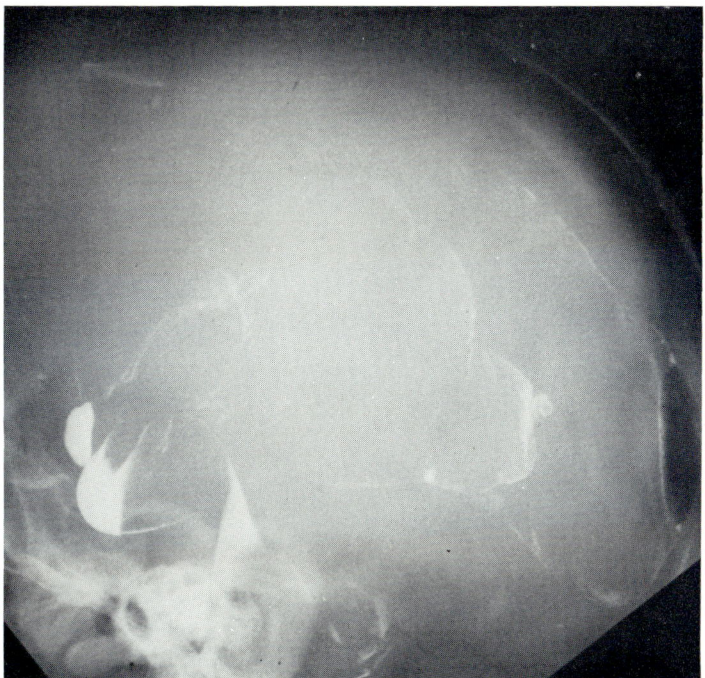

Figure 87. Hydrocephalus. Pantopaque study reveals asymmetrical dilatation of the lateral ventricular system.

ventricles may or may not be elevated. Hydrocephalus may make its clinical appearance at any age. The diagnosis may be made in utero (Fig. 89) or not until late adult life. While hydrocephalus of congenital origin may be apparent at birth or in early infancy, in certain cases congenital hydrocephalus may be undetected until adult life. Infantile hydrocephalus does not always indicate congenital abnormality. For example, hydrocephalus may result from an early meningitis or birth trauma. Hydrocephalus only results in abnormal cranial enlargement when the cranial sutures are not fused or not entirely fused. In infancy, the cranial vault is expansile due to lack of sutural fusion. Abnormal head growth may postpone other signs of intracranial hypertension. Such cranial enlargement may indicate hydrocephalus, but it may also result from infantile subdural hematomas or brain tumor. Enormous cranial enlargement or cranial enlargement noted at the time of birth heavily favor hy-

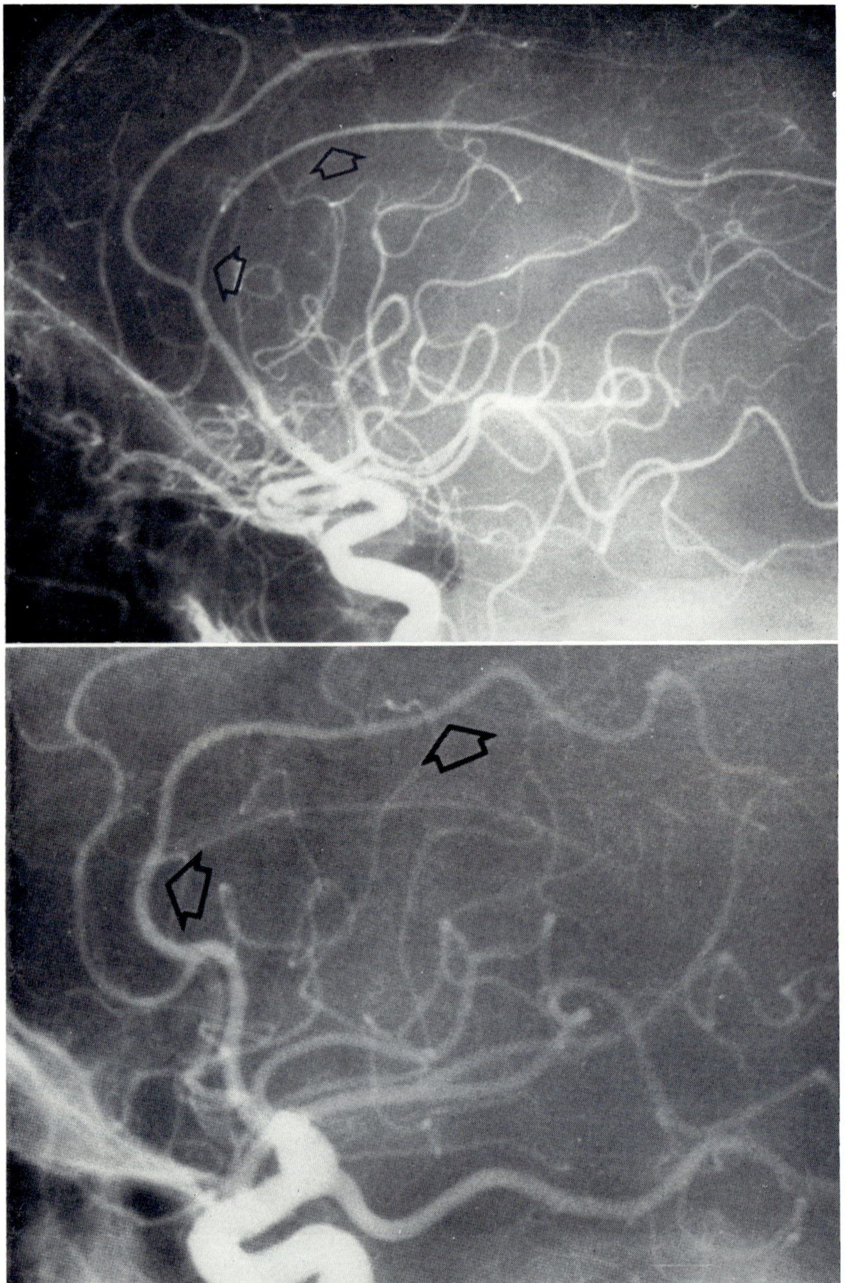

Figure 88. Hydrocephalus and the arterial phase of the carotid angiogram. The first film (*top*) reveals moderate hydrocephalus, with enough elevation of the callosal roof of the lateral ventricle to stretch and round the midline pericallosal artery. The second film (*bottom*) shows the normal undulating course of the pericallosal artery. Ventricular size can be estimated by the position of the thalamostriate vein as it crosses the lateral ventricular floor on an AP venous phase. Early hydrocephalus may be apparent on the venous phase and missed on the arterial phase.

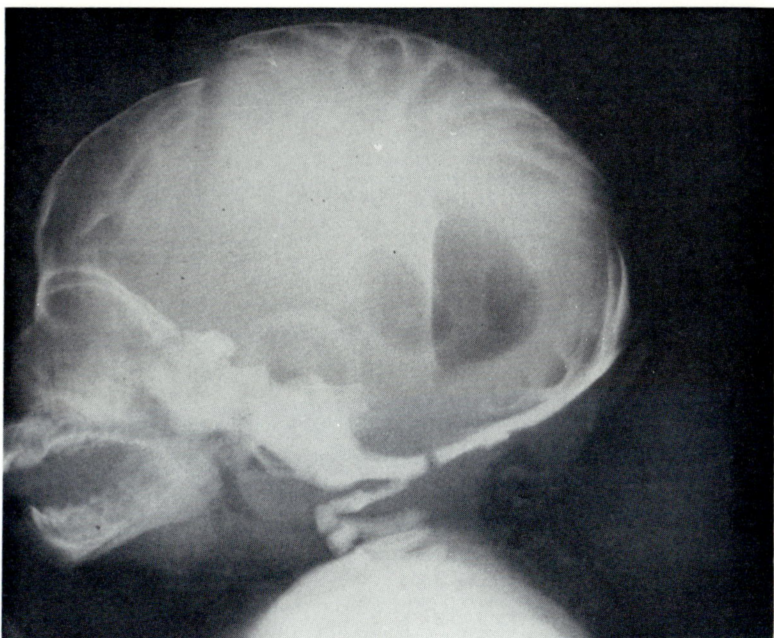

Figure 89. Hydrocephalus with craniolacunar skull. Craniolacunia of the skull may be associated with the intrauterine development of hydrocephalus and intracranial hypertension. Meningocele and encephalocele are often associated.

drocephalus rather than another intracranial mass. In childhood, springing of partially fused cranial sutures may occur with hydrocephalus or other intracranial mass. A degree of abnormal cranial growth may be recognized, but the other signs of intracranial hypertension are usually not delayed. Papilledema, headaches and vomiting often precede such late cranial enlargement. Springing of cranial sutures in childhood may of course not lead to any noticeable head growth. The fused skull of the adult prevents cranial enlargement despite the degree of intracranial hypertension. Hydrocephalus is not synonymous with an enlarged head; either may occur without the other. Many descriptive terms are employed in the various forms of hydrocephalus.

1. High pressure hydrocephalus (i.e. hypertensive hydrocephalus).

The symptoms and signs are those of intracranial hypertension. Abnormal cranial growth occurs if the cranial sutures are not fused. High pressure hydrocephalus appearing in infancy includes the following symptoms and signs:

a. Cranial enlargement.

This may be gross or difficult to detect without repeated measurements with a centimeter rule. The greatest anteroposterior circumference should increase by less than 1 cm per week in the first ten weeks of life. The average lies in the range of 0.5 cm per week. Frequent measurements should be carried out. A weekly increase of 1 cm or more is abnormal. Cranial enlargement at an abnormal rate during this initial ten-week period of life is more likely due to hydrocephalus than to subdural hematomas or other intracranial mass. The cranial vault enlargement renders the face small in appearance.

b. Enlargement and tension of the anterior fontanelle.

When the normal infant is held in the upright position and is not crying, the fontanelle should be relaxed and normal pulsations can be seen. When intracranial pressure is elevated, the fontanelle is tense and normal brain pulsations are diminished or absent. Sutural separation may be palpable.

c. Scalp vein distension.

Tortuous scalp veins with shiny scalp skin are common signs of intracranial tension in infancy.

d. "Cracked-pot" percussion note.

A hollow tympanitic sound on cranial percussion is abnormal, the normal note being flat.

e. Transillumination.

Hydrocephalic ventricles in infancy transmit light readily, while subdural hematomas do not transilluminate well. Transillumination is only a valuable sign when the ventricles are considerably enlarged.

f. Eye signs.

A squint is common. This is usually a unilateral abducens palsy, but may be a bilateral abducens or other external oculomotor paralysis. Random disconjugate eye movements and various forms of nystagmus occur. An alternating nystagmus may occur with intracranial hypertension, and may reflect blindness due to optic atrophy. Papilledema is unusual in infantile hydrocephalus. Optic atrophy is late. Slight exophthalmos is common. "Sunset" eyes with the upper portion of the iris and superior sclera of the globe being apparent is associated with downward displacement of the orbital roof on each side.

g. Spasticity.

Spasticity may be absent, but when it occurs it is most marked in the lower extremities. It is associated with hyperactive deep tendon reflexes and ankle clonus. Spastic paraparesis may occur.

h. Irritability, refusal of feedings, vomiting, and general malnutrition may occur.

i. Delayed developmental milestones and general mental retardation provide late evidence of infantile hydrocephalus.

j. Lethargy, stupor or coma appearing with marked tension of the anterior fontanelle indicates extremely elevated intracranial pressure and can occur in certain cases of infantile hydrocephalus. Changes in vital signs may be highly variable. A plethora with a flushed appearance of the face and upper thorax may appear. Persistent vomiting is common in this phase.

High pressure hydrocephalus (H.P.H.) appearing in childhood presents the symptoms and signs of intracranial hypertension with headaches, vomiting, papilledema and eventual stupor. Children may not complain of headache or diplopia. Ataxia is often a prominent feature, since H.P.H. in childhood is commonly due to cerebellar-fourth ventricular tumor. High pressure hydrocephalus in adults commonly presents the cardinal features of intracranial hypertension.

"Hydrocephalic attacks" only occur in high pressure hydrocephalus and may occur at any age. The features of hydrocephalic attack include the following:

a. Sudden bifrontal headache—suboccipital and neck pain may be associated. Vomiting may or may not occur.

b. Sudden syncope—these episodes of collapse may simulate the "drop-attacks" seen in epilepsy.

c. Tinnitus, transient deafness or transient blindness may occur.

d. Confusion, stupor or coma may follow the apex of the headache. Decerebrate—opisthotonic attacks may follow.

e. Abrupt changes in vital signs with bradycardia and apnea may occur.

f. Multiple, bilateral, transient cranial nerve palsies are quite unusual, but may accompany the attack.

g. Other evidence of advanced intracranial hypertension (e.g. papilledema) is commonly present.

2. Normal pressure hydrocephalus (i.e. low pressure hydrocephalus).

The cardinal features of this syndrome are as follow:

a. Apathetic—amnesic dementia.

b. Incontinence.

c. Ataxia or other gait disturbance.

d. Absence of signs of intracranial hypertension.

It should be noted that the above clinical features are quite compatible with the clinical diagnosis of cerebral atrophy. It should also be noted that apathy and memory loss, urinary incontinence and ataxia can result from intracranial hypertension due to obstructive hydrocephalus or to brain tumor. Therefore, the absence of signs of intracranial hypertension is critical to the diagnosis of normal pressure hydrocephalus (N.P.H.). Patients with N.P.H. are usually adults. Mental abnormalities are prominent and include memory loss, apathy and progressive sometimes fluctuating, dementia. There may be double incontinence or only urinary incontinence. Other neurosurgical syndromes such as frontal tumor, corpus callosum tumor, chronic subdural hematoma or high pressure hydrocephalus can produce a similar mental picture with incontinence. Ataxia is most marked in the lower extremities in N.P.H., but again it is nonpathognomonic. Ataxia can occur in H.P.H. due to cerebellar-fourth ventricular tumor, but this is most often a syndrome of childhood. Ataxia can also be a prominent sign in adult H.P.H. and in frontal and parasagittal tumor. The ataxia of N.P.H. can be spastic with bilateral Babinski signs; it can be truncal on a wide base; there may be parkinsonian-like features with bradykinesia and shuffling gait. There may be an inability to stand.

Most cases of N.P.H. result from communicating hydrocephalus. In contrast, H.P.H. results from noncommunicating or communicating forms.

3. Noncommunicating and communicating hydrocephalus.

Obstruction of CSF passage at the ventricular, cisternal or subarachnoid level is the usual source of hydrocephalus. Obstruction of a major venous sinus, as in otitic hydrocephalus, is an unusual cause of ventricular enlargement. Excessive production of CSF by a choroid plexus papilloma of the lateral ventricle is another unusual source of hydrocephalus.

Obstruction anywhere within the ventricular system, with ventricular enlargement proximal to the obstruction, is regarded as obstructive or noncommunicating hydrocephalus. This includes obstruction within a lateral ventricle with sequestration and enlargement of a ventricular horn, unilateral or bilateral obstruction at the foramen of Monro, obstruction at the posterior third ventricle, aqueductal stenosis, and obstruction of the fourth ventricle and its outlets. The cause of the ventricular obstruction may be intrinsic or extrinsic to the ventricular system. Thus, a medulloblastoma within the fourth ventricle itself and a cystic astrocytoma of the cerebellar hemisphere both typically produce obstructive hydrocephalus due to block of the fourth ventricle and its outlets. Shift of ventricular structures without ventricular enlargement does not constitute hydrocephalus. Obstructive hydrocephalus may be symmetrical or asymmetrical depending on the level of the block. Ventricular block is regarded as noncommunicating hydrocephalus because spinal subarachnoid pressure measured by lumbar manometrics does not reflect intraventricular pressure when the ventricles are obstructed. Lumbar puncture is quite hazardous in this situation as a result of the intracranial hypertension. Complete ventricular obstruction with H.P.H. is often present. However, depending on etiology, ventricles may be only partially or intermittently obstructed. Intraventricular pressure may be normal in the intervals between obstruction, when the latter is intermittent. Even in these cases, the general clinical picture is usually that of H.P.H. rather than N.P.H. For example, papilledema may be present in a case of colloid cyst of the third ventricle and detectable during the symptom-free intervals between attacks of foramen of Monro block. Some degree of ventricular enlargement is commonly present despite the absence of acute obstruction. Obstructive hydrocephalus may appear at any age. It is most often congenital or neoplastic in origin. Traumatic or infectious inflammatory processes with ventriculitis, ependymitis or periaqueductal gliosis are occasionally responsible for the ventricular block.

In contrast, communicating hydrocephalus may result in either H.P.H. or N.P.H. Communicating hydrocephalus is usually due to obstruction at the cisterns or cerebral subarachnoid passages. Thrombosis of the sagittal, transverse and sigmoid sinuses is an unlikely source of ventricular enlargement. Cisternal, subarachnoid and venous sinus block are "distal occlusions" which result in free communication between ventricular and spinal subarachnoid fluid. Spinal pressure tends to reflect intracranial pressure in the absence of ventricular block. Communicating hydrocephalus exists when the distal occlusion is sufficient to produce ventricular enlargement. This form of hydrocephalus is only nonobstructive in the sense of open ventricular pathways. There may be a congenital failure of development of surface subarachnoid pathways. Communicating hydrocephalus is commonly a result of meningitis or meningoencephalitis with subarachnoid adhesive scarring and occlusion. Tuberculous and other forms of basal meningitis may occlude the cisterns. The cisterns are merely basal expansions of the subarachnoid space. They must remain patent enough to permit passage of CSF around the brain stem, through the tentorial door to the cerebral convexities. Meningitis with subdural effusions may be ultimately complicated by communicating hydrocephalus. Subarachnoid hemorrhage due to birth trauma, later cranial trauma, ruptured aneurysm or arteriovenous malformation or other vascular accident may similarly occlude CSF passages. The initial trauma responsible for infantile subdural hematomas may be accompanied by subarachnoid hemorrhage. Evacuation of such subdurals may later be associated with ventricular enlargement which can result from either communicating hydrocephalus or compressive brain atrophy. When communicating hydrocephalus results in H.P.H., the same pressure signs develop as in the noncommunicating form. Communicating hydrocephalus is also encountered as the major source of N.P.H.

4. Hydrocephalus ex vacuo (i.e. central cerebral atrophy).

   This term describes ventricular enlargement resulting from cerebral atrophy rather than from obstruction to CSF pathways. There is total freedom of passage of CSF at all levels. Lumbar manometric pressure reflects the reduced or normal intracranial pressure. It may therefore be regarded as a totally nonobstructive form of communicating hydrocephalus as long as the essentially atrophic nature of the process is kept in mind. Unlike true communicating hydrocephalus with subarachnoid—cisternal block, H.P.H. never results from hydrocephalus ex vacuo. However, like true communicating hydrocephalus, the clinical picture of N.P.H. can be closely duplicated. The central cerebral atrophy with enlarged ventricles may be accompanied by variable degrees of cortical atrophy. Diffuse parenchymal disease of almost any etiology may be responsible for the ultimate atrophic process. When ventricular dilatation results from central cerebral atrophy, the "callosal angle" on the AP supine air study commonly exceeds 140°. When ventricular enlargement results from communicating hydrocephalus due to subarachnoid or cisternal block, the callosal angle is often less than 120°, and the subarachnoid passages commonly fail to fill upon lumbar pneumoencephalography.

5. Occult hydrocephalus.

   This refers to any late onset hydrocephalus previously undetected. Aqueductal stenosis occurring in the adolescent or young adult is an example of the noncommunicating form of occult hydrocephalus. Communicating types commonly occur on an occult basis. Occult hydrocephalus may take the form of either N.P.H. or H.P.H.

6. Arrested hydrocephalus.

   Any form of hydrocephalus proven to be nonprogressive can be termed "arrested." Great caution must be employed, since the natural course of both noncommunicating and communicating forms is toward progressive worsening with continued ventricular enlargement. Clinical signs can sometimes be misleading in that they may appear stable during the phase of progressive ventricular expansion.

7. Specific hydrocephalic syndromes.

   a. Aqueductal stenosis.

      Congenital stenosis, forking or septa resulting in aqueductal occlusion is a common source of infantile hydrocephalus. Cranial enlargement may be noted in utero, at birth or in early infancy. The symptoms and signs of H.P.H. are characteristic. The lateral and third ventricle are enlarged. Distention of the lateral ventricles may be relatively symmetrical or moderately asymmetrical. The aqueduct is usually stenotic in its rostral portion. Severe obstruction may be associated with ventricular diverticulae, secondary transseptal communication and marked cortical thinning. Secondary forms of aqueductal occlusion can mimic infantile aqueductal stenosis. This occurs in aneurysm of the great vein of Galen, teratoma in the region of the pineal and in posterior third ventricular cyst. When hydrocephalus due to aqueductal occlusion occurs in childhood or adult life, periaqueductal gliosis may be responsible, but cerebellar, fourth ventricular and pineal tumors must be ruled out. Aqueductal occlusion sufficient to produce hydrocephalus is a late sign of brain stem glioma.

b. Dandy-Walker syndrome.

Occlusion of the outlets of the fourth ventricle usually presents as infantile H.P.H. In unusual cases, it may present later in childhood or in the young adult. The usual features with expansion of the infantile cranium and bulging fontanelle are present. A prominent occiput is characteristic. The inion may be palpably elevated and lambdoidal suture separation palpable. In this syndrome, the posterior fossa transilluminates as well as the supratentorial region, due to the presence of the greatly dilated fourth ventricle which expands the entire posterior fossa and compresses surrounding structures. A deficient cerebellum is present and does not prevent such transillumination. The distended fourth ventricle may extend into the upper cervical canal. It displaces the brain stem forward and the tentorium upward. The lateral and third ventricles are also enlarged. A prominent occiput may occur in normal infants, but cranial growth and development is otherwise normal. An occipital encephalocele is sometimes associated with hydrocephalus and should be differentiated. Most cases of aqueductal stenosis are not associated with a prominent occiput.

c. Arnold-Chiari malformation.

This hindbrain malformation is commonly associated with infantile hydrocephalus and myelomeningocele. The abnormal cerebellum projects into the cervical canal along with a distorted medulla oblongata. The elongated fourth ventricle may be totally or partially within the upper cervical canal. Both the outlets of the fourth ventricle and the basal cisterns may be occluded. Cranial enlargement with H.P.H. may not occur until repair of the myelomeningocele, following which hydrocephalus may rapidly become apparent. Other spinal defects may occur. Myelomeningocele is sometimes associated with aqueductal stenosis. The Arnold-Chiari malformation may present in later life as a form of occult hydrocephalus without obvious spinal abnormality. Cerebellar signs may be present at that time.

d. Arachnoiditis and hydrocephalus.

Inflammatory adhesive arachnoiditis may result in infantile hydrocephalus. Hemorrhage or infection related to trauma or meningitis may be responsible. The symptoms of H.P.H. usually appear weeks or months after the acute inflammatory episode. Congenital failure of development of surface subarachnoid pathways may present the same picture in early infancy. Arachnoiditis with communicating hydrocephalus may present at any age in an occult form with either H.P.H. or N.P.H. In communicating hydrocephalus, there is enlargement of the entire ventricular system, which may or may not include the fourth ventricle. There is free communication between the fourth ventricle and cisterna magna. Absence of filling of surface subarachnoid pathways is characteristic. Basal cisterns may or may not be obstructed.

e. Intraventricular tumors and hydrocephalus.

A number of features are typical of the hydrocephalus resulting from intraventricular tumor.

(1) The majority of intraventricular tumors are associated with hydrocephalus.
(2) The hydrocephalus is almost always of the obstructive, noncommunicating type.
(3) Intracranial hypertension may be due to the local bulk of the tumor plus the generalized mass effect of the hydrocephalic ventricles.
(4) Intracranial hypertension of marked degree may reflect the obstructive hydrocephalus with critically located tumors of minimal bulk.
(5) Intracranial hypertension due to hydrocephalus may be the only clinical indicator of the presence of a brain tumor.
(6) Intracranial hypertension and ventricular obstruction can be partial, intermittent or complete.
(7) The obstructive hydrocephalus due to tumor can be symmetrical or asymmetrical.
(8) Tumors which obstruct at the third ventricular, aqueductal or

fourth ventricular level commonly produce relatively symmetrical hydrocephalus. Cerebral tumors commonly produce asymmetrical hydrocephalus. Exceptions occur: anterior third ventricular tumors may produce asymmetrical hydrocephalus, while certain lateral ventricular tumors may produce relatively symmetrical hydrocephalus.

(9) Tumors resulting in obstructive hydrocephalus may lie entirely within the ventricle or may involve both the ventricle and surrounding cerebrum or cerebellum. Tumors may be totally extraventricular and achieve hydrocephalus by ventricular compression without actual invasion. Large "metaventricular tumors" at a distance from the ventricular channels may result in translated compression of the foramen of Monro and hydrocephalus. Such tumors can be intracerebral or extracerebral. Compression of the ipsilateral ventricular system with dilatation of the opposite lateral ventricle is common. Compression of basal and incisural cisterns may contribute. A supratentorial tumor can also produce hydrocephalus by inducing downward shift of the brain stem with foraminal impaction of the outlets of the fourth ventricle and tonsillar herniation.

(10) The intraventricular tumor can produce ventricular enlargement before actual ventricular obstruction occurs.

(11) Ventricular enlargement may be present between episodes of ventricular obstruction, when the latter is intermittent.

(12) The intraventricular tumor may dilate the ipsilateral ventricle and compress the opposite lateral ventricle; this is the reverse of the ipsilateral compression and contralateral dilatation commonly seen with extraventricular cerebral tumors.

(13) Brain tumors affect the ventricular system in characteristic ways, and specific sites of ventricular obstruction often suggest specific tumor types.

(14) Multiple ventricular tumors can arise from CSF spread. Medulloblastoma, ependymoma, glioblastoma and pinealoma can metastasize via CSF pathways. Multiple ventricular nodules occur in tuberous sclerosis, and astrocytomas may be associated.

f. Specific ventricular tumors.

(1) Fourth ventricle.

The most common tumors in childhood which produce hydrocephalus are the cerebellar-fourth ventricular tumors. They are discussed in greater detail with the syndromes of the posterior fossa. Cerebellar astrocytoma, medulloblastoma and ependymoma produce H.P.H. in childhood. Dermoid cyst in the posterior fossa can be suspected by previous episodes of meningitis or evidence of an occipital sinus tract. Dermoid cyst and choroid plexus papilloma of the fourth ventricle may present the same picture of H.P.H. as the other posterior fossa tumors. Truly intraventricular tumors of the fourth ventricle such as medulloblastoma, ependymoma and choroid plexus papilloma, cannot be clinically differentiated from tumors which may be entirely extraventricular such as cystic cerebellar astrocytoma with fourth ventricular compression. Parasitic cysts are more common in the fourth ventricle than at other ventricular sites.

(2) Posterior third ventricle.

(a) Pinealoma (Fig. 90).

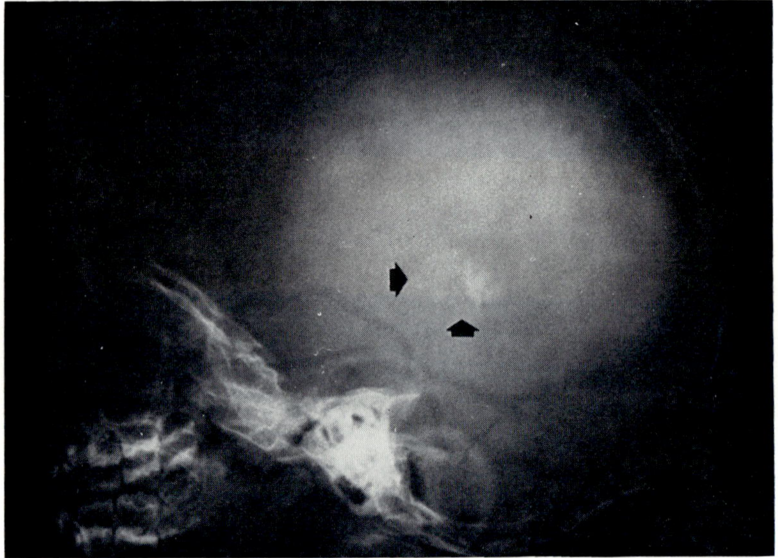

Figure 90. Pinealoma. Tumor calcification is noted in the region of the pineal. The cranial sutures are separated due to obstructive hydrocephalus with intracranial hypertension. The differential includes teratoma.

This tumor presents in childhood or in early adult life primarily as a third ventricular mass with symptoms of H.P.H. Posterior third ventricular and aqueductal occlusion produce intracranial hypertension. Characteristically, there is distention of the rostral third and lateral ventricles, and compression of the suprapineal recess and quadrigeminal cistern. The tumor is usually relatively rounded, but may vary in outline. Abnormal tumor calcification is frequently visible on plain x-rays. Prominent pineal calcification in childhood or adolescence, associated with symptoms of intracranial pressure, suggests pinealoma. Associated signs include precocious puberty in males or hypogonadism in either males or females. Sexual infantilism or precocious puberty can sometimes occur with "benign" hydrocephalus without pineal or other tumor. Eye signs also indicate the presence of a pineal tumor. These include vertical gaze palsy, pupillary dilatation with loss of light reflexes but preserved accommodation, and bilateral ptosis. A similar syndrome is produced by teratoma in the pineal region.

(b) Other posterior third ventricular masses.

A minority of posterior third ventricular tumors prove to be of nonpineal and nonteratomatous origin. In infancy, aneurysm of the great vein of Galen may present with obstructive hydrocephalus and cardiac failure. In childhood, hydrocephalic signs dominate the clinical picture in this malformation. In unusual cases, aneurysm of the vein of Galen may present with intracranial hemorrhage in the adult (Fig. 91A,B). As in other vascular malformations, spontaneous venous occlusion may occur; occlusive involvement of the vein of Galen leads to bithalamic hemorrhage and brain edema.

In childhood, the astrocytoma, ependymoma (Fig. 92) or metastatic deposit from medulloblastoma may be responsible for a third ventricular mass. In adult life, a glioma or tentorial meningioma may present as a posterior third ventricular mass. Large aneurysms of the basilar bifurcation have in unusual cases been responsible for posterior-inferior third ventricular occlusion and hydrocephalus.

(3) Anterior third ventricle.

(a) Craniopharyngioma.

This is the most common anterior third ventricular tumor presenting with intracranial hypertension in childhood. It usually presents as an anterior midline mass, elevating the rostral floor of the ventricle. It is relatively smooth, and suprasellar calcification is usually visible. The sella may or may not be expanded. The foramen of Monro

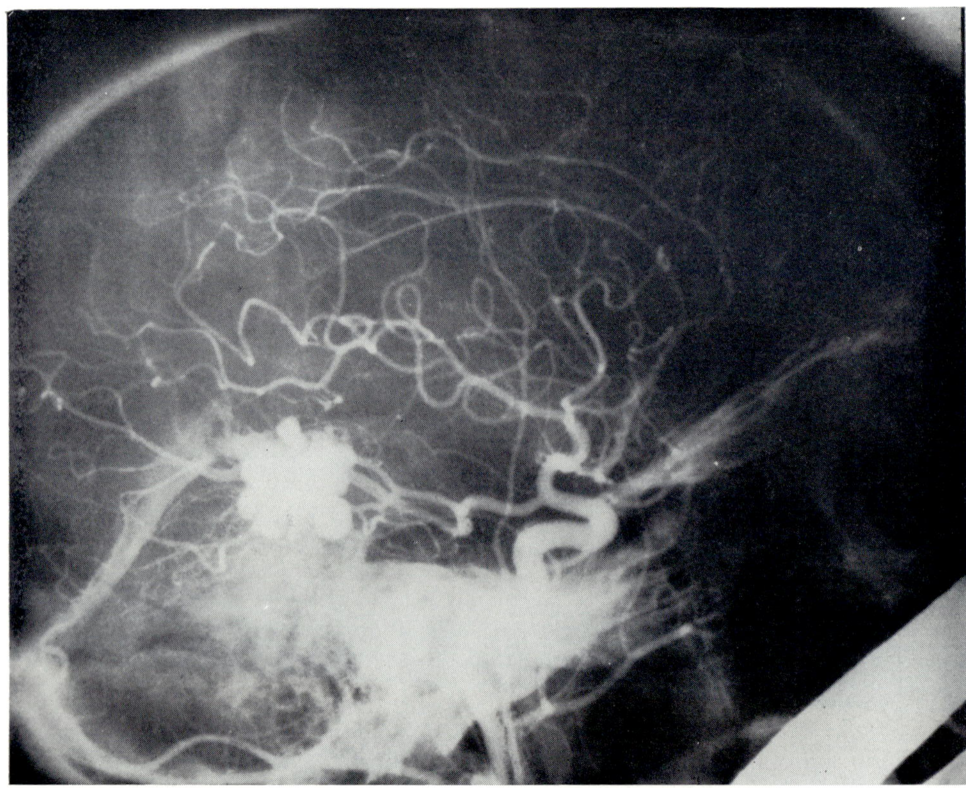

Figure 91. Arteriovenous malformation of Galen. The lateral arteriogram *(A)* shows and arteriovenous malformation attached to the vein of Galen, with early filling of the straight sinus. Stretching of the pericallosal artery indicates obstructive hydrocephalus. Posterior cerebral arterial supply to the malformation is evident in both the lateral and AP view *(B)*.

may be obstructed with dilatation of the lateral ventricles. The tumor may be present at any age, but intracranial hypertension is most common in childhood. Bitemporal or homonymous hemianopia, optic atrophy and hypothalamic-pituitary disturbances are commonly associated.

(b) Colloid cyst (Fig. 93 A-C).

This anterior third ventricular cyst most often presents in adult life. Intermittent symptoms of H.P.H. without other accompaniments are typical. Sudden bifrontal headache brought on and sometimes relieved by change of position of the head is characteristic. Headache may be unilateral and one or both foramina of Monro may be obstructed. Hydrocephalic attacks may be accompanied by

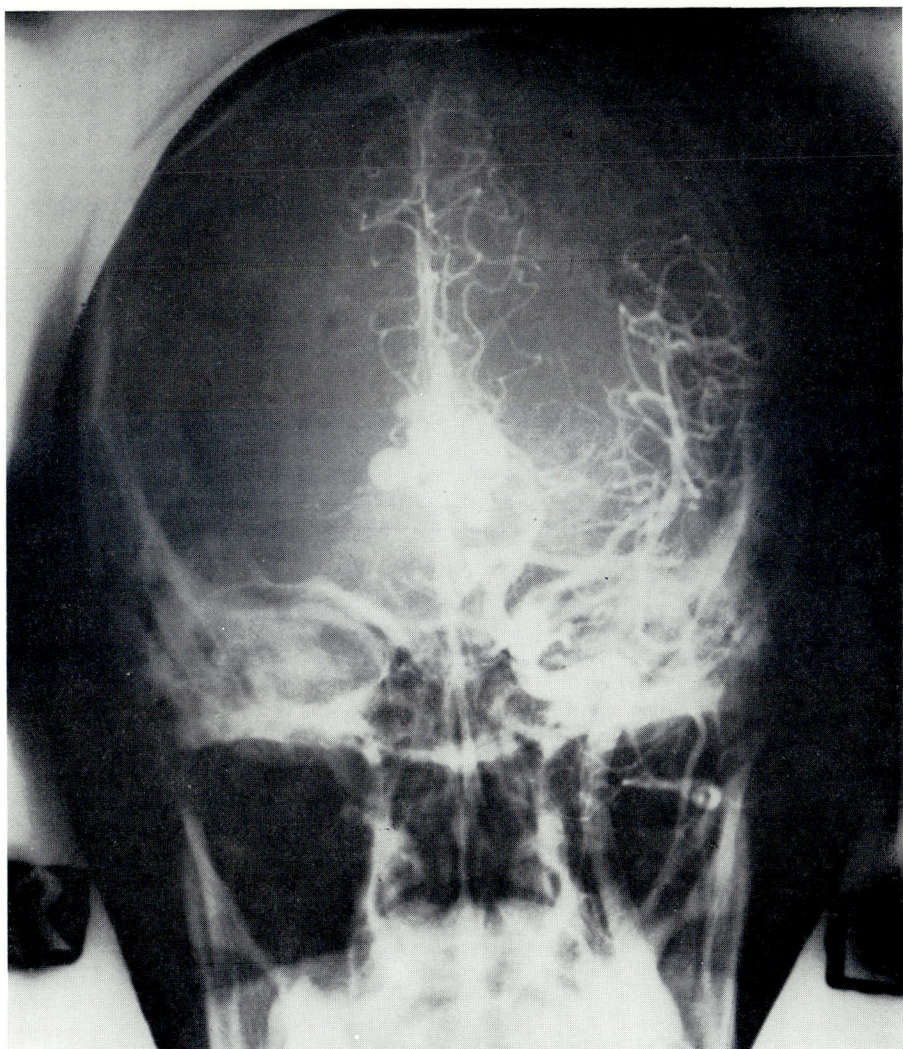

Figure 91 B.

stupor or syncope. "Drop attacks" may be simulated. Alternating hemiparesis is an unusual sign, but can occur in midline tumors with hydrocephalus. The hemiparesis is transient and subsequently appears in transient fashion on the opposite side.

Note: Alternating hemiparesis without hydrocephalus may be due to a parasagittal meningioma. In the adult, the source of alternating hemiparesis is usually vascular and may be related to migraine, carotid or embolic disease.

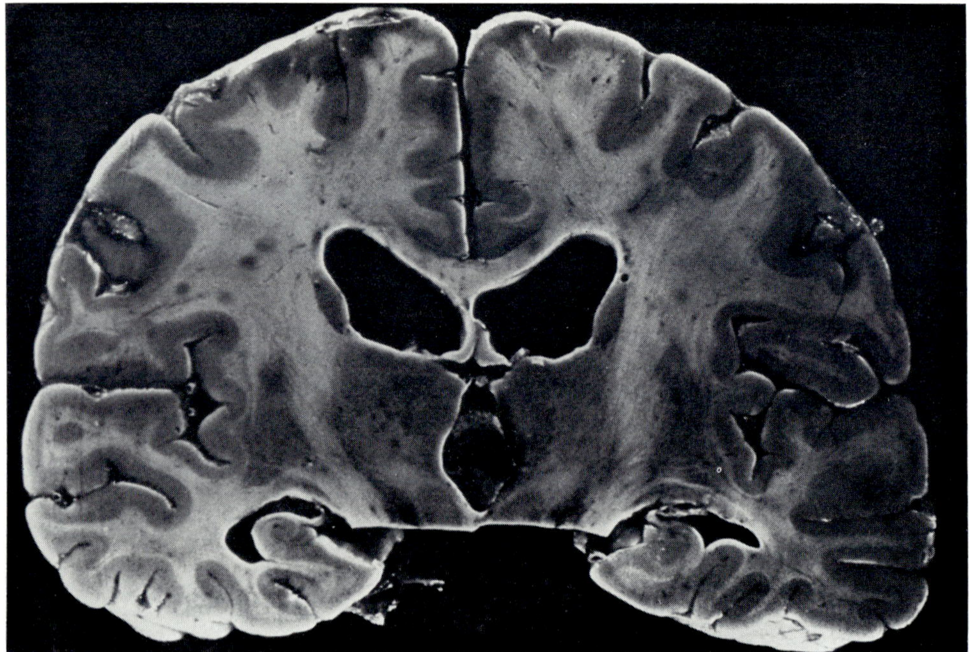

Figure 92. Third ventricular ependymoma with hydrocephalus. Ependymoma may involve any segment of the ventricular system. It most often involves the fourth ventricle (Fig. 73). It may also occur as an intracerebral tumor of the cerebral hemisphere with lateral ventricular tumor as well.

Colloid cysts are uncommon in childhood. An anterior third "ependymal cyst" is a rare source of infantile hydrocephalus. The usual colloid cyst is smooth, oval or round in outline and is attached to the anterior third ventricular roof. It is not calcified and is usually less than 2 cm in diameter. Moderate to marked distention of the lateral ventricles is often present, which is usually roughly symmetrical. The cyst may bulge through the foramen of the larger ventricle when asymmetry is prominent.

(c) Other anterior third ventricular masses.

Cerebral gliomas may obstruct the foramen of Monro and grow within the third ventricle. The hypothalamic astrocytoma may present as an irregular third ventricular mass. It may be associated with the optic glioma of childhood, with extension from the hypothalamus into the subhemispheric optic pathway. The astrocytoma may appear in childhood or adult life as an extension from a septal or thalamic glioma. An irregular anterior third ventricular mass tends to be malignant, in contrast to the smoother outlines of the craniopharyngioma and colloid cyst. Calcification is not ordinarily present in such gliomas.

"Ectopic" pinealoma or teratoma can also present as an anterior third ventricular mass which is either smooth or irregular. Visible calcification may be present. The tumor may occur in infancy or childhood. Teratoma also presents within the cerebral hemisphere in early life or in the region of the pineal.

Extraventricular tumors of large size can result in compression of the foramen of Monro without actual ventricular extension of the tumor. The pressure effects are translated by such "metaventricular" tumors to the foramen. Distention of one or both lateral ventricles with H.P.H. results. This effect can occur with deep cerebral gliomas and with large basal meningiomas. The frontobasal meningioma may foreshorten, amputate or separate the anterior horns while occluding the foramen of Monro.

(4) Lateral ventricle.

(a) Choroid plexus papilloma.

This is an unusual tumor which most commonly occurs in the trigone of the lateral ventricle in infancy or early childhood. The characteristic picture is H.P.H. with cranial enlargement in the absence of focal signs. The tumor rarely presents as an occult H.P.H. in adult life. The hydrocephalus is usually considered to be the result of excessive production of CSF by the papilloma. High CSF protein and papilledema may suggest the diagnosis in an otherwise typical case in infantile hydrocephalus. The severe communicating hydrocephalus results in enlargement of the entire ventricular system. The lateral ventricular enlargement is relatively symmetrical, despite unilaterality of the papilloma. The somewhat larger ventricle is on the side of the papilloma. The tumor is not usually calcified on x-ray. It should be noted that normal choroid plexus may be visibly calcified and may be asymmetrical. The papilloma also may occur in the third or fourth ventricle, although less often than in the lateral ventricle. Under these circumstances, the hydrocephalus is apt to be obstructive rather than communicating.

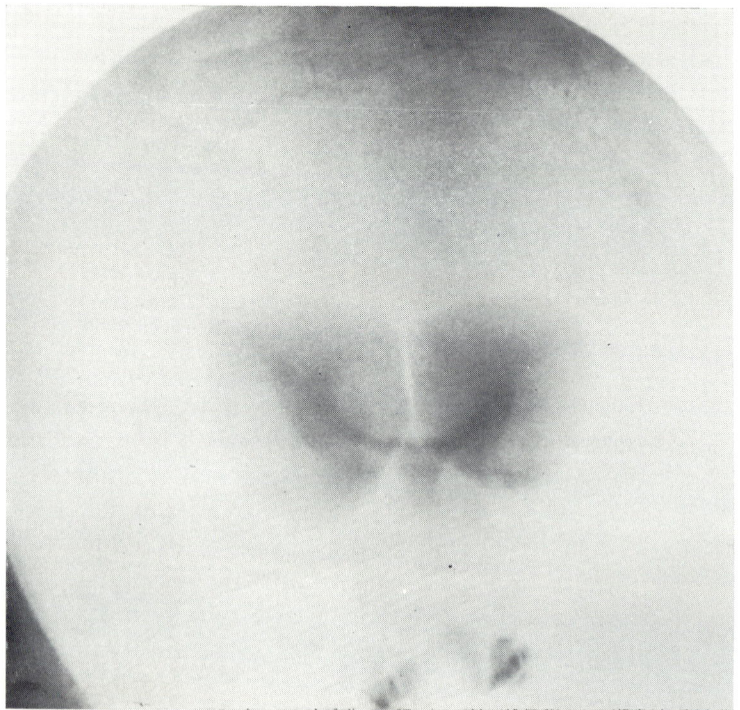

Figure 93. Colloid cyst of the third ventricle. The AP ventriculogram (A) shows a round midline mass in the roof of the third ventricle with compression of the foramen of Monro on each side. The anterior horns of the lateral ventricles are dilated. The lateral ventriculogram (B) shows a smooth round mass projecting upward through the foramen of Monro into the floor of a dilated lateral ventricle. A lateral automogram (C) allows clearer definition of the mass in the anterior roof of the third ventricle.

(b) Intraventricular cholesteatoma.

Epidermoid tumors occur in the lateral, third and fourth ventricles, in the cerebellopontine angle, and within the bones of the vault and base of the skull. Ventricular enlargement is common, especially in the region of the trigone, where the grossly irregular intraventricular cholesteatoma is most common. As with other intraventricular tumors, ventricular enlargement can occur well before actual ventricular obstruction. Because of its slow growth, most patients are adults.

(c) Intraventricular meningioma.

The primary intraventricular meningioma without dural attachment is an unusual tumor which occurs in the trigone. Hydrocephalus most marked in the region of the

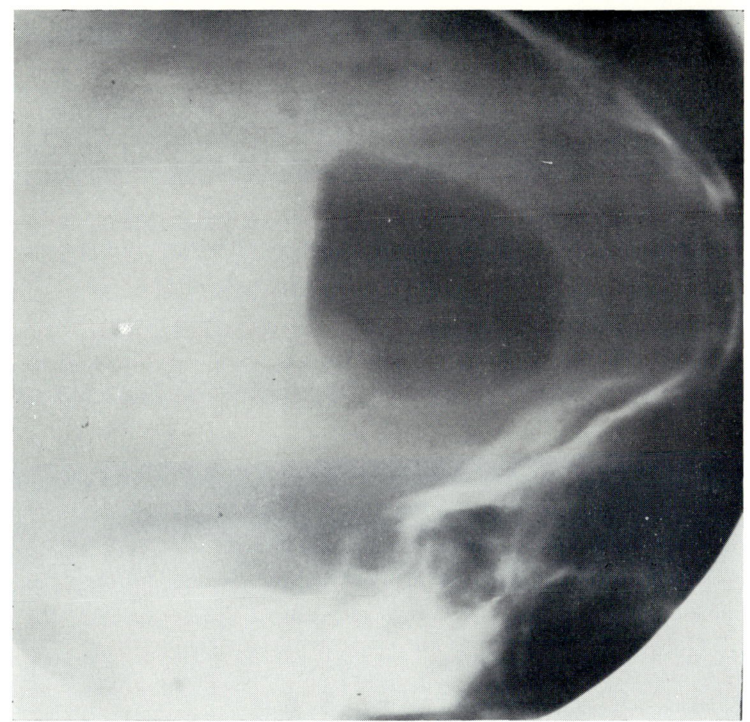

Figure 93 B.

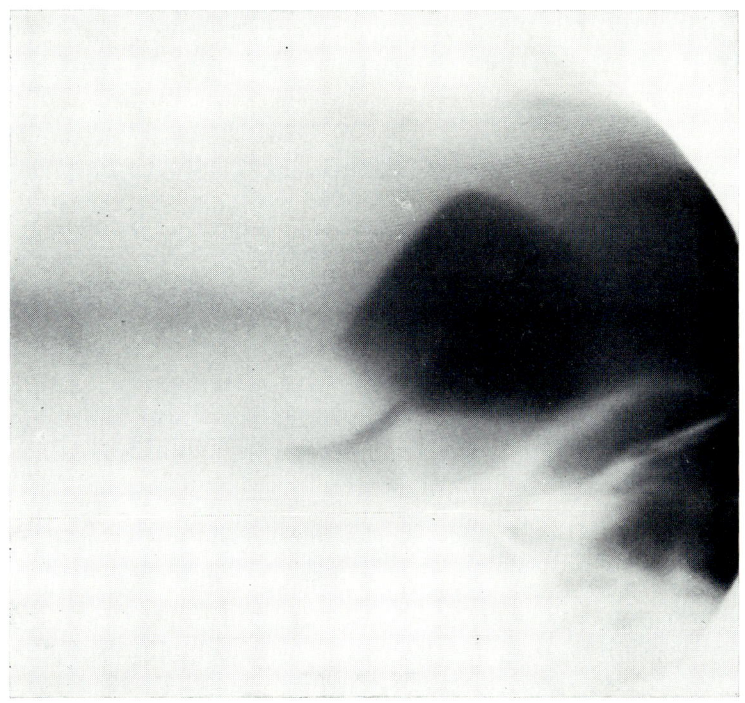

Figure 93 C.

tumor is common. The tumor is often quite smooth, but may be lobular. Visible calcification may be evident. The usual bony changes associated with dural meningiomas are absent. The tumor most often occurs in young women. There has been noted a certain predilection for the left ventricle. Ventricular obstruction and intracranial hypertension occur. Headaches may be ipsilateral, and contralateral homonymous hemianopia, hemiparesis and hemisensory deficits can be present. Variable speech deficits may accompany large dominant-sided tumors.

(d) Intracerebral tumors with lateral ventricular tumor extension.

Cerebral gliomas, either astrocytomas or ependymomas, occur in childhood and may result in ventricular block and hydrocephalus. Intracranial hypertension is common. While headache is often present, vomiting is not nearly as frequent as in the cerebellar-fourth ventricular tumors of childhood. Papilledema of low grade is usually present. Motor deficits and other focal cerebral signs are frequent. Focal or generalized seizures may occur. A large intraventricular extension suggests ependymoma. It is a grossly irregular tumor which involves both the cerebrum and lateral ventricle. There is usually no x-ray evidence of calcification. This tumor is even more common in the fourth ventricle in childhood, and may involve the third ventricle as well. The cerebral astrocytoma commonly involves the corpus callosum and may also invade the septum, thereby separating the lateral ventricles. The astrocytoma often distorts the ventricular system and does not ordinarily possess a prominent intraventricular component. Compression of the ipsilateral ventricle with enlargement of the opposite lateral ventricle is common. Obstruction of a portion of a lateral ventricle with sequestration and enlargement of a ventricular horn may be present. Calcification visible on plain x-ray is usually absent.

The oligodendroglioma may not involve the ventricular system, in which case it presents as a calcified cerebral tumor in an adult. Focal cerebral seizures are commonly associated. However, the oligodendroglioma may present as a bulky, irregular lateral ventricular mass with hydrocephalus. The oligodendroglioma may present as an asymmetrical septal mass as well. The oligodendroglioma may be a mixed astrocytoma. Cerebral astrocytomas of various grade are also common in adult life. The most common adult glioma is the glioblastoma multiforme. This tumor may extend into the lateral ventricle and present as an irregular ventricular mass. Compression of the ipsilateral ventricle and extension into the corpus callosum often occur. Calcification is not ordinarily visible.

(e) Intraventricular hematoma.

Intracerebral hemorrhage as a result of arterial hypertension, ruptured aneurysm or AVM, or head trauma can result in rupture of clot into the ventricular system. The multilobulated, irregular hematoma can sometimes be visualized within an air-filled ventricle. The ipsilateral ventricle is often compressed by the mass of intracerebral hematoma. The opposite lateral ventricle is shifted and may be compressed or dilated. The aqueduct may be obstructed by third ventricular clot or by extension of intracerebral hemorrhage into the midbrain.

B. Cerebral edema

Cerebral edema is clinically encountered in two basic forms: generalized and localized. In either instance, the patient may be stuporous or comatose. When edema is bilateral, diffuse and severe, depressed consciousness is the rule, while more limited forms of brain swelling may be compatible with the alert state. A clinical indicator of the presence of significant edema is the neurological response to steroids and diuretics. Reduction of cerebral edema may lead to improvement in the level of consciousness and to diminution of neurological deficit. However, such improvements are only possible under limited circumstances and may be quite transient. Cerebral edema is commonly seen in neurological surgery as a result of intracranial neoplasm, infection, hemorrhage and trauma.

1. Cerebral edema and brain tumor (Fig. 94).

Brain tumors produce intracranial hypertension as a result of one of several factors.

a. Tumor bulk alone.
b. Tumor bulk plus significant cerebral edema.
c. Tumor bulk plus hydrocephalus.
d. Tumor bulk plus brain herniation.

When edema is operative, the focal signs of the mass tend to be magnified. If a tumor occupies a "silent" brain region, local surrounding edema may reflect the involved cerebral lobe. As the edema becomes more extensive, falsely localizing signs may appear which

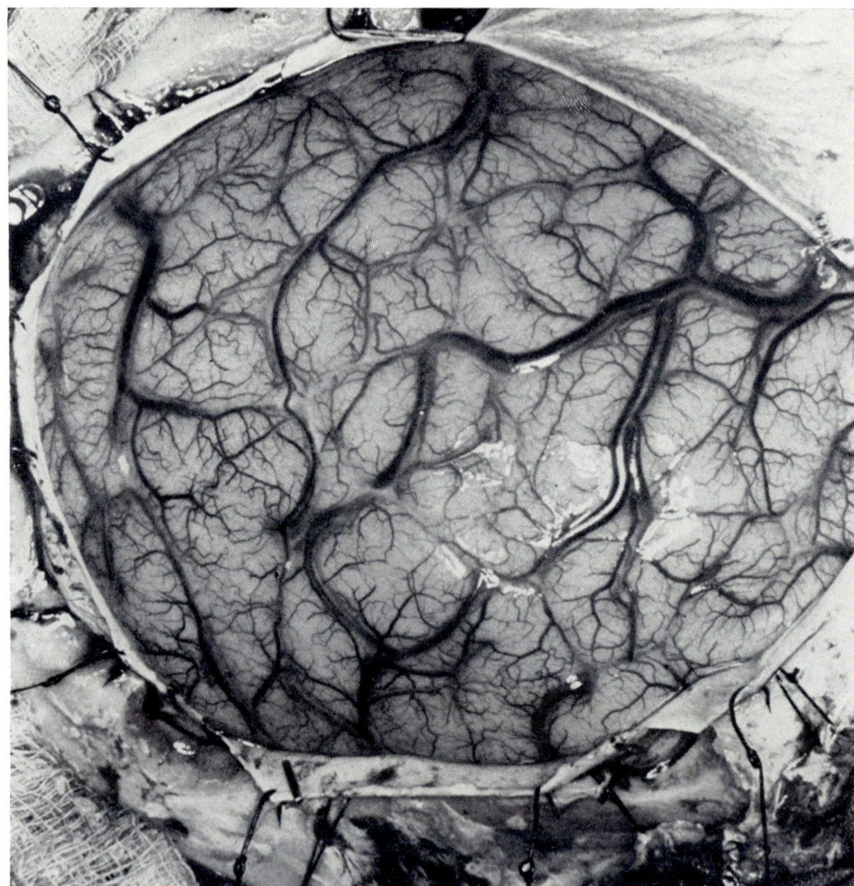

Figure 94. Cerebral edema. The brain is swollen, the gyri are widened and the sulci are narrowed. A deep cerebral glioma was present.

lead one away from the actual tumor site. Unilateral cerebral edema typically results in subfalcial shift across the midline. Bilateral cerebral edema may not produce midline shift even when intracranial tension is high. Either unilateral or bilateral brain swelling can result in transtentorial herniation. Unilateral edema of gradual development may produce marked subfalcial shift without much transtentorial shift. Unilateral edema of rapid development has a greater tendency to produce transtentorial herniation with or without marked subfalcial midline shift. Brain swelling may be minimal with slowly growing extracerebral meningiomas, and maximal in the rapidly growing glioblastomas. The "butterfly" glioblastoma of the corpus callosum extending into deep cerebral regions is often associated with bilateral edema. The low-grade astrocytoma of the cerebral hemisphere may occur with minimal edema. Cerebral edema is especially prominent in metastatic carcinoma, even when the deposit is relatively small. Multiple bilateral deposits accompanied by massive swelling of both hemispheres is typically reflected by initial drowsiness, an initially good response to steroids with diminishing hemiparesis, and eventually progressive intracranial hypertension. The initial drowsiness does not necessarily imply multiplicity or even bilaterality of deposits, although this is often the case. Any caudal cerebral tumor which translates its pressure to the vein of Galen is apt to produce marked cerebral edema. Tentorial meningioma is an example.

2. Cerebral edema and intracranial infection.

Marked edema is also evident in the acute brain abscess. In contrast, the edema may be relatively slight in chronic brain abscess with a thick abscess capsule. The edema may be limited to the frontal or temporal lobe if the abscess is secondary to frontal sinus or middle ear infection. Otitis or mastoiditis may be complicated by either temporal lobe or cerebellar abscess. Temporal lobe abscess with its surrounding cerebral edema can readily produce intracranial hypertension and transtentorial herniation. Cerebellar abscess with obstructive hydrocephalus can also result in intracranial hypertension with tonsillar herniation. Sixth nerve palsy occurring with otitis media or mastoiditis does not necessarily indicate intracranial hypertension. It occurs with petrositis and extension of infection to the inferior petrosal sinus. In Gradenigo's syndrome, it may be associated with trigeminal involvement. Rarely, a cerebellopontine abscess can occur with production of an angle syndrome with seventh and eighth cranial nerve palsies, with or without trigeminal, cerebellar and pressure signs. Infective thrombosis of the sigmoid and transverse sinuses associated with middle ear infection can lead to otitic hydrocephalus. Sagittal sinus thrombosis when acute, whether infective or noninfective, results in massive cerebral swelling typically with intracerebral hemorrhage. Gradual sinus occlusion may occur without significant edema. Bilaterally diffuse cerebral edema due to intracranial infection may indicate the multiple abscesses of hematogenous origin, diffuse cerebritis, or thrombophlebitis of a major venous sinus. Acute subdural empyema can lead to cerebral edema with marked unilateral predominance. Progressive deterioration in consciousness may also reflect brain abscess with transtentorial herniation, rupture of an abscess into the lateral ventricle with acute purulent ventriculitis, uncontrolled meningitis or septicemia, or an acute meningitic hydrocephalus. Hydrocephalus is usually a postmeningitic complication, but can occur acutely when the basal cisterns are filled with purulent material.

3. Cerebral edema and primary subarachnoid hemorrhage.

Intracranial hemorrhage is a common source of brain swelling of generalized type. Subarachnoid hemorrhage due to ruptured aneurysm or arteriovenous malformation is often associated with spasm of cerebral arteries (Fig. 95). When spasm as severe, diffuse bilateral brain swelling occurs and is manifested by stupor or coma (Fig. 96).

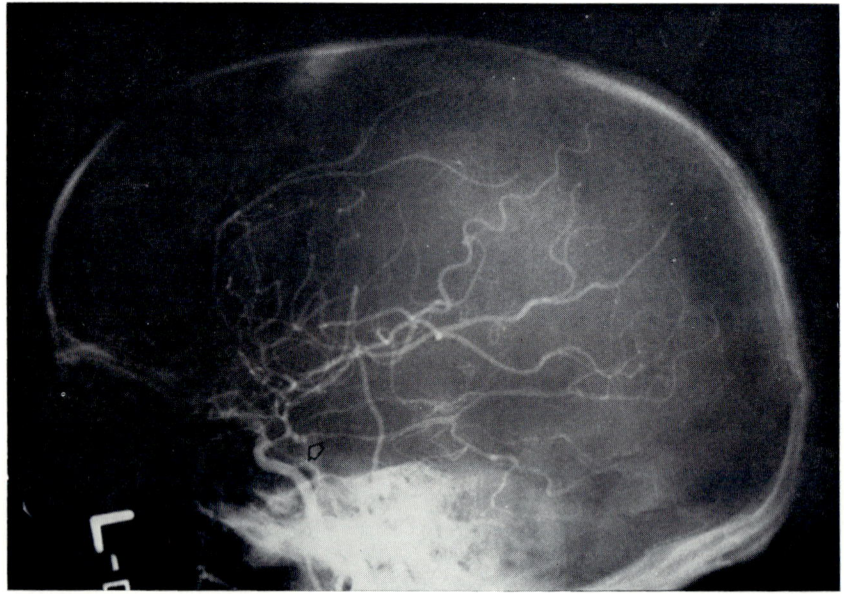

Figure 95. Subarachnoid hemorrhage with arterial spasm. The intracranial arteries are narrowed due to spasm. Arterial narrowing is particularly evident in the vicinity of the ruptured aneurysm (arrow).

Other sources for impairment of sensorium in such patients include intracerebral hematoma, intraventricular hemorrhage, and ischemia or hemorrhage within the upper brain stem. Arterial spasm can also be localized resulting in focal cerebral infarction or limited brain swelling unaccompanied by obtundation. Evidence of spasm and brain swelling may be entirely absent (Fig. 97), the patient remaining fully alert. Primary (i.e. nontraumatic) subarachnoid hemorrhage is much more commonly the result of ruptured aneurysm than bleeding arteriovenous malformation. Both result in signs of meningeal irritation with headache, photophobia and stiff neck. Headache may

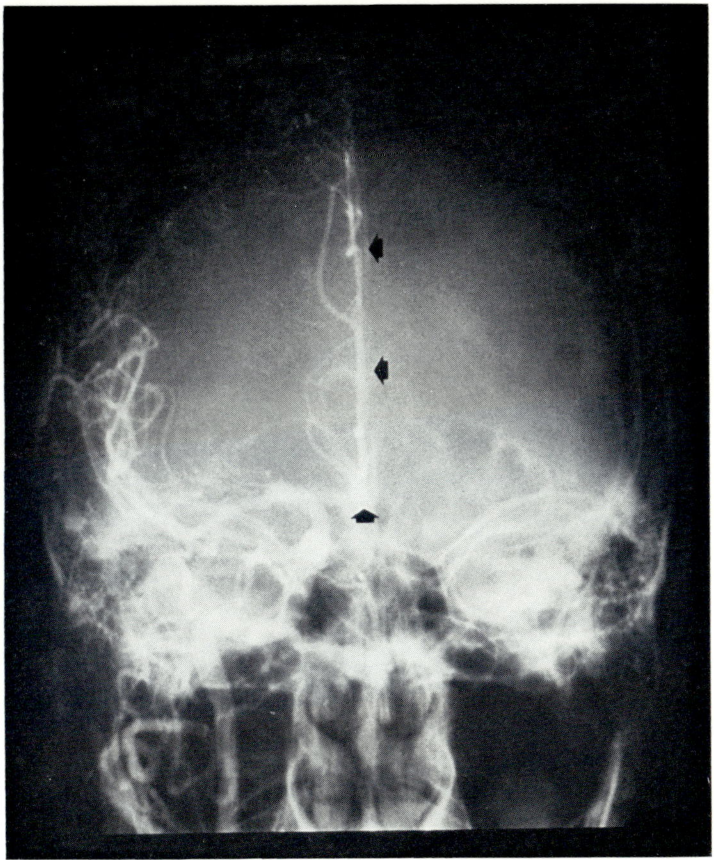

Figure 96. Intracranial hypertension. There is marked arterial straightening due to elevated intracranial pressure. The cardinal angiographic signs of intracranial hypertension are generalized arterial straightening, delayed circulation time and evidence of brain herniation. These signs are superimposed upon the angiographic features of the localized intracranial mass. Angiographic evidence of hydrocephalus may or may not be accompanied by intracranial hypertension.

be frontal, generalized or suboccipital. Occasionally, pain is limited to the posterior cervical area. The pain of intracranial hemorrhage is often severe, but is occasionally mild. Progressive obtundation is often associated with diminishing headache. Even nuchal rigidity may subside in the deeper comatose stages.

a. Hemorrhage due to arteriovenous malformation (AVM).

If the patient is an adolescent or a child, AVM should be suspected. This is especially true if there is a past history of epilepsy or past evidence of repeated subarachnoid hemorrhages. The latter may be manifested by previous sudden episodes of head-

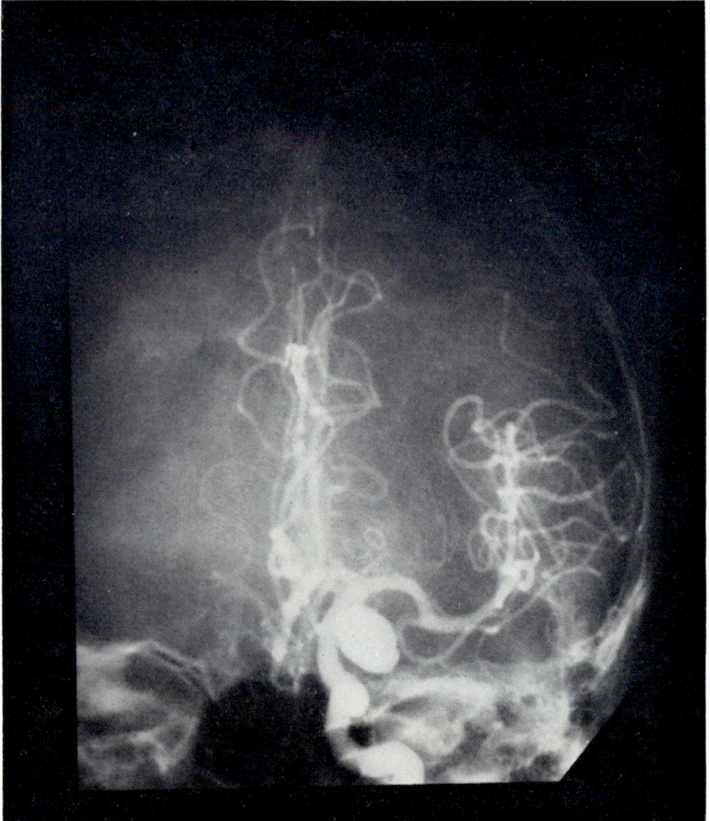

Figure 97. Carotid aneurysm. This aneurysm presented with subarachnoid hemorrhage. There is no angiographic evidence of spasm or brain swelling. The arteries are not narrowed and they take their usual undulating course.

ache or collapse. Previous bleeding episodes may have been misinterpreted as recurrent bouts of meningitis. Subarachnoid hemorrhage is twice as common a sign of AVM than is epilepsy. Hemorrhage or seizures may occur entirely without a history of the other. They also may occur in the same patient. Seizures may be focal or generalized. Since the usual AVM is in the middle cerebral distribution, focal clonic attacks beginning in the face or hand on the opposite side are not infrequent. Arteriovenous malformations may also clinically present later in life, in young or middle-aged adults when ruptured aneurysm is a many times more common event (Fig. 98 A-C).

b. Hemorrhage due to ruptured aneurysm.

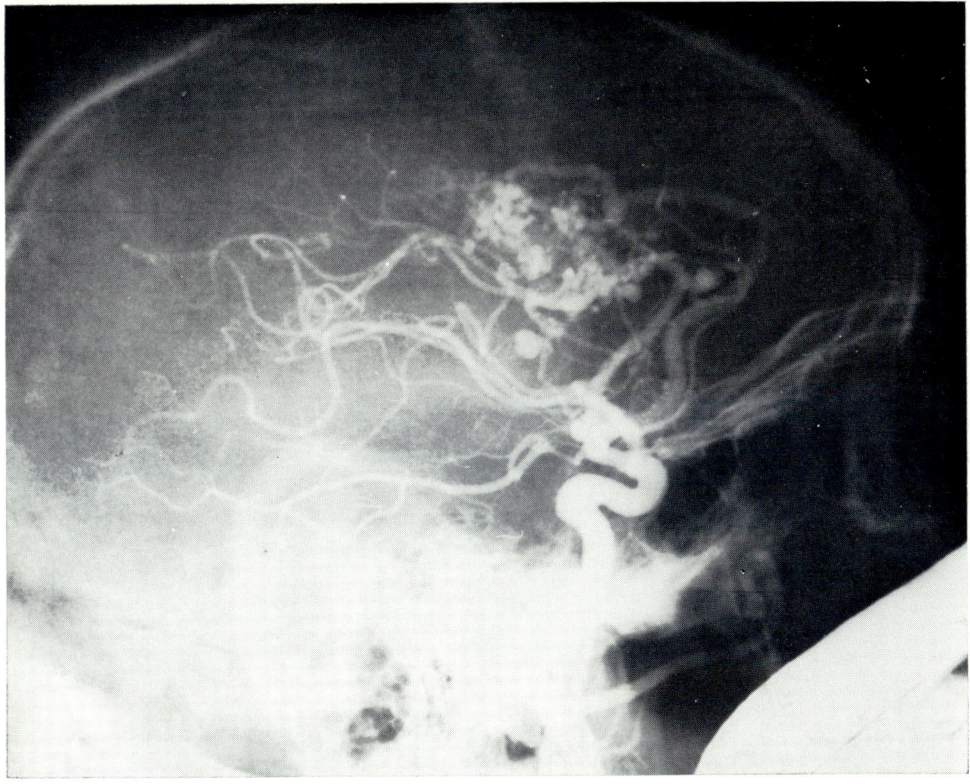

Figure 98. *(A)* Arteriovenous malformation with multiple aneurysms. This vascular abnormality presented with subarachnoid hemorrhage in a fifty-year-old man. Stupor and bilateral Babinski signs were present. The lateral arterial phase shows dilated anterior cerebral supply, the vascular anomaly and discrete aneurysms as well. *(B)* Later in the lateral sequence, dilated venous channels draining the anomaly are seen. *(C)* The AP view shows the midline location of the malformation.

Bleeding from a berry aneurysm is uncommon in childhood, the usual patient being a young or middle-aged adult. There is usually no previous history of hemorrhage at the time the patient presents. In some cases, a "premonitory headache" occurs within hours of the sudden onset of more severe headache. Such premonitory symptoms may reflect a "minor leak." There may be a previous history of nonspecific headaches, but previous collapse or severe cranionuchal pain in the past is relatively uncommon. A past history of epilepsy is unusual at the time of the initial aneurysmal rupture. The onset of symptoms may or may not coincide with an episode of exertion. A past history of chronic hypertension

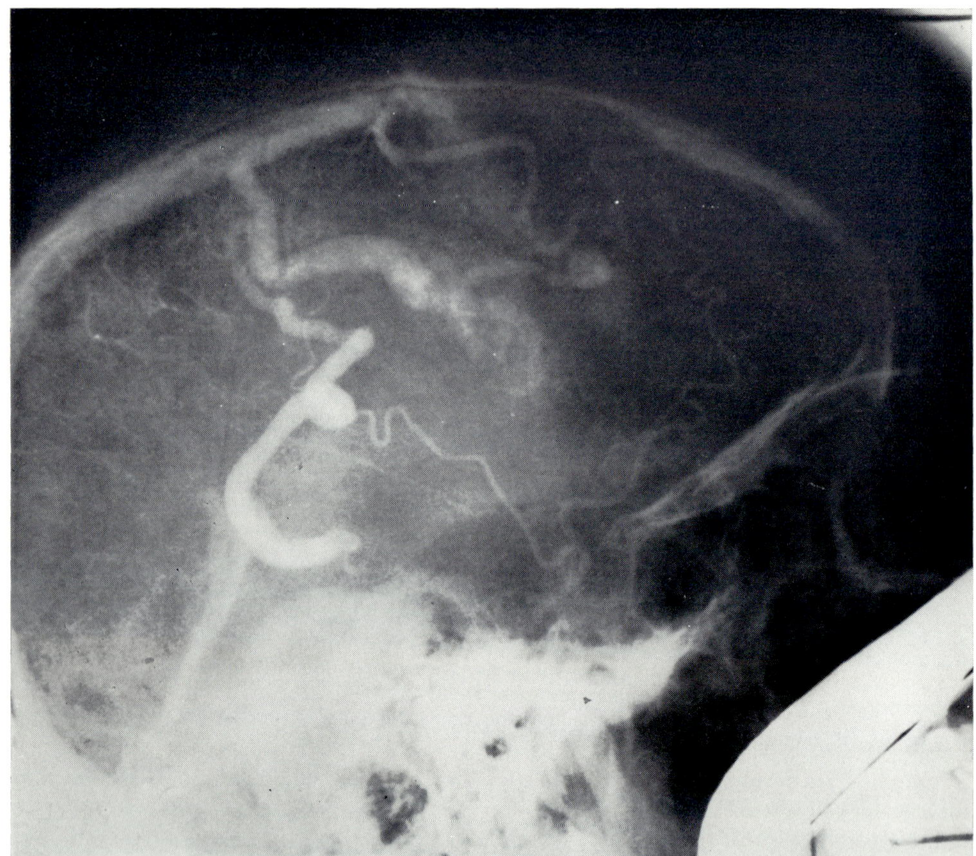

Figure 98 B.

is relatively uncommon, although acute arterial hypertension is frequently present following the hemorrhage. The patient with a ruptured aneurysm may be admitted at any level of consciousness from alert to deeply comatose (Fig. 99 A,B). Many aneurysms rupture with an apparently total lack of focal signs and are revealed only by angiography. However, certain localizing features suggest aneurysms at certain sites.

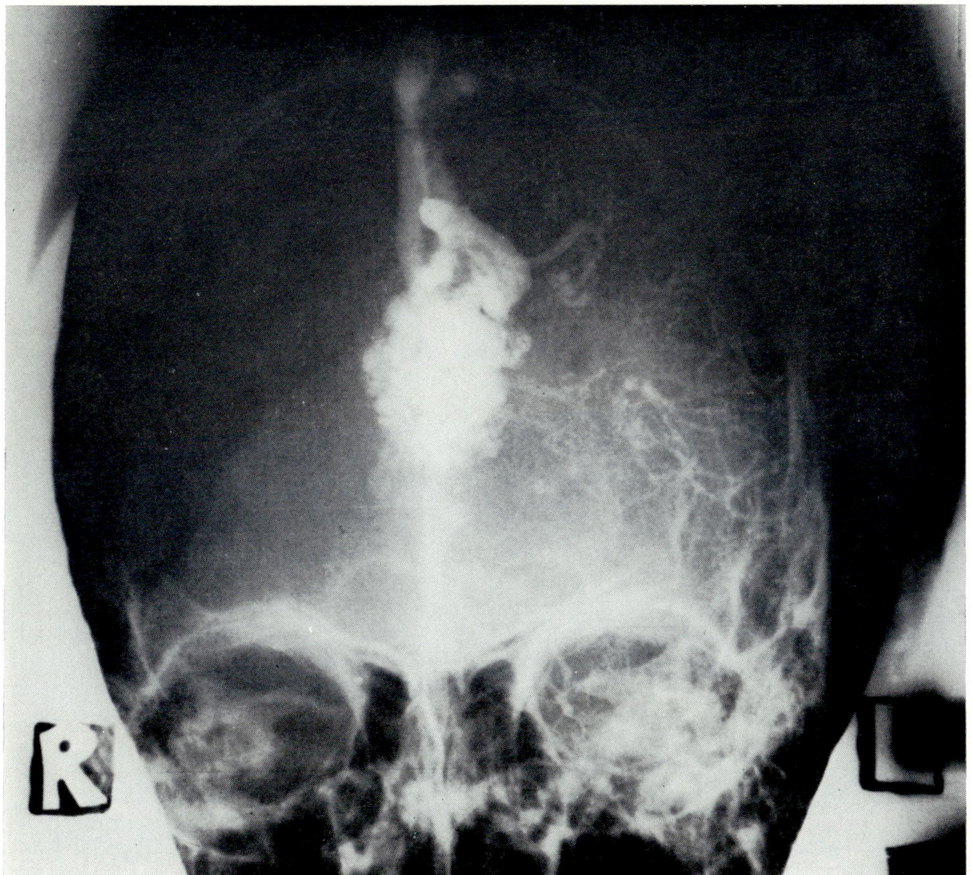

Figure 98 C

(1) Oculomotor palsy.

If the patient is alert, a dilated pupil suggests an internal carotid aneurysm at the posterior communicating level (Fig. 100). If the patient with subarachnoid hemorrhage is comatose, transtentorial herniation due to intracerebral hematoma should be ruled out first. Such a clot is more common following rupture of a middle cerebral aneurysm (Fig. 101). Rarely, a basilar bifurcation aneurysm may present with oculomotor palsy. When no subarachnoid hemorrhage has occurred, a dilated pupil may indicate a posterior communicating aneurysm or an intracavernous carotid aneurysm. Impairment of cranial nerves four, five and six favor the latter.

(2) Abducens palsy.

Lateral rectus weakness in cases of subarachnoid hemorrhage

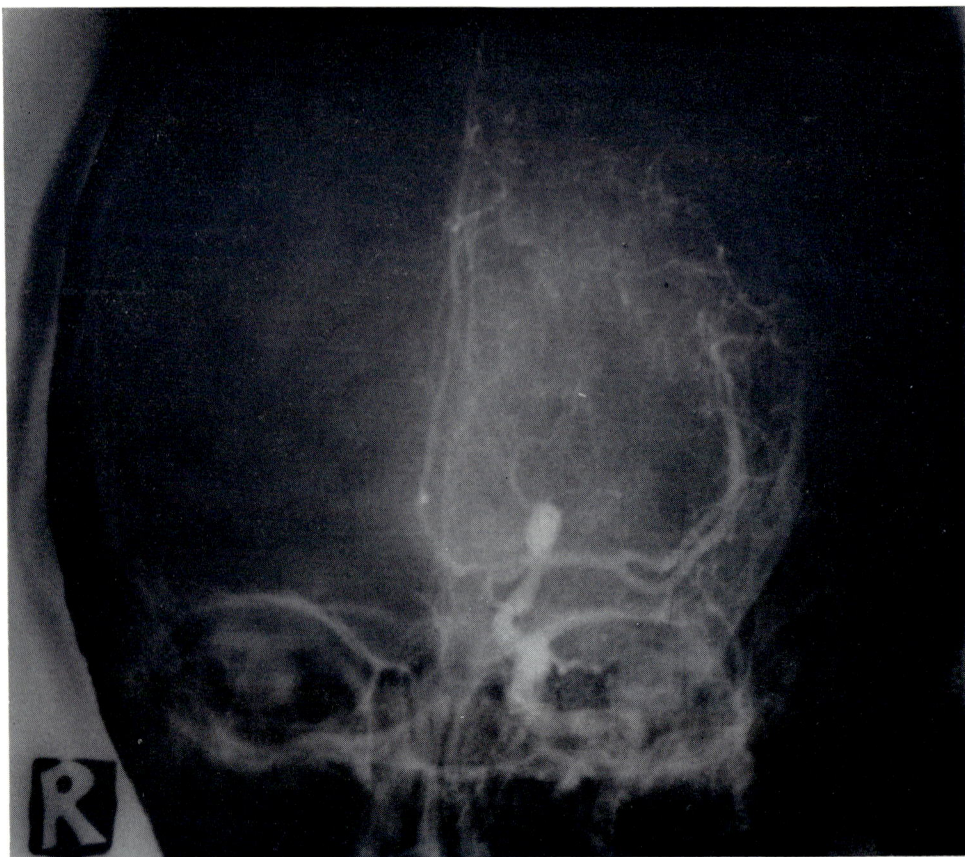

Figure 99. Bifurcation aneurysm. The patient presented in deep coma with hemiplegia following rupture of this aneurysm of the carotid bifurcation. The fundus of the aneurysm points upward in the direction of the basal ganglia (A), and there is widening of the distance between the anterior and middle cerebral arteries on the AP view. This aneurysm of the carotid apex (B) is less common than the typical carotid aneurysm at the posterior communicating level (see Fig. 100). The carotid bifurcation aneurysm should also be differentiated from the middle cerebral trifurcation aneurysm (see Fig. 101).

usually is a reflection of intracranial hypertension, rather than a localizing sign. However, when bilateral carotid angiograms are negative, abducens palsy may be the only indication of an infratentorial aneurysm.

(3) Visual symptoms, such as transient blindness.

This may occur with rupture of an anterior communicating aneurysm. Blurring or diplopia due to extraocular motor palsy must be differentiated from such visual loss. Transient blindness may occasionally occur with rupture of a basilar aneurysm

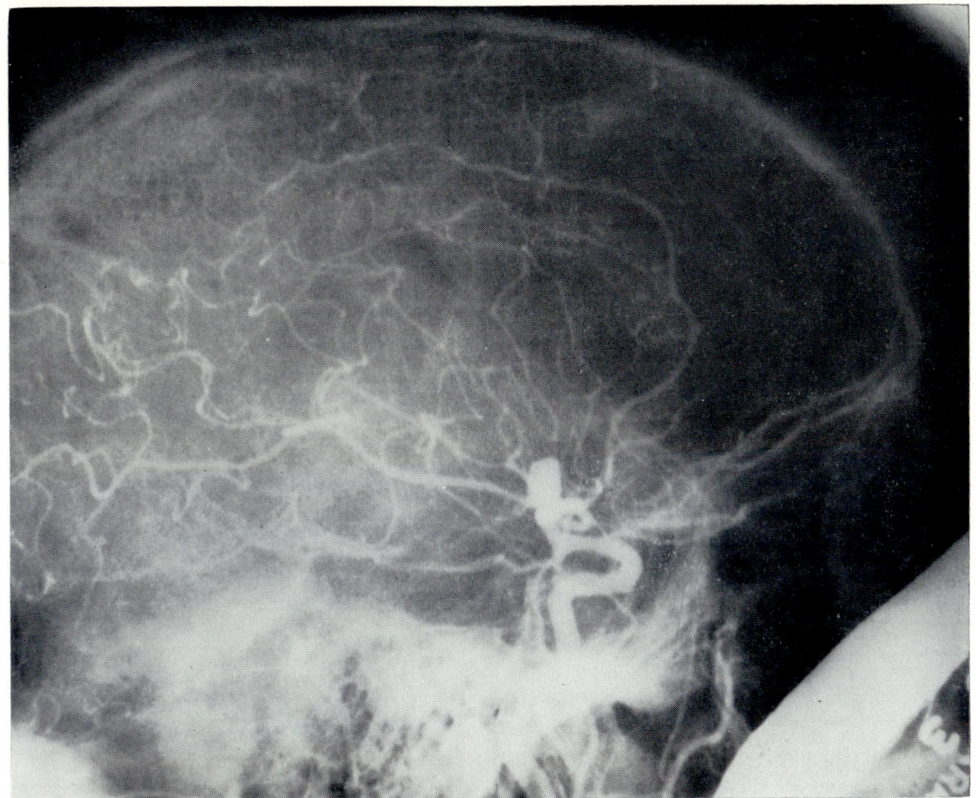

Figure 99 B.

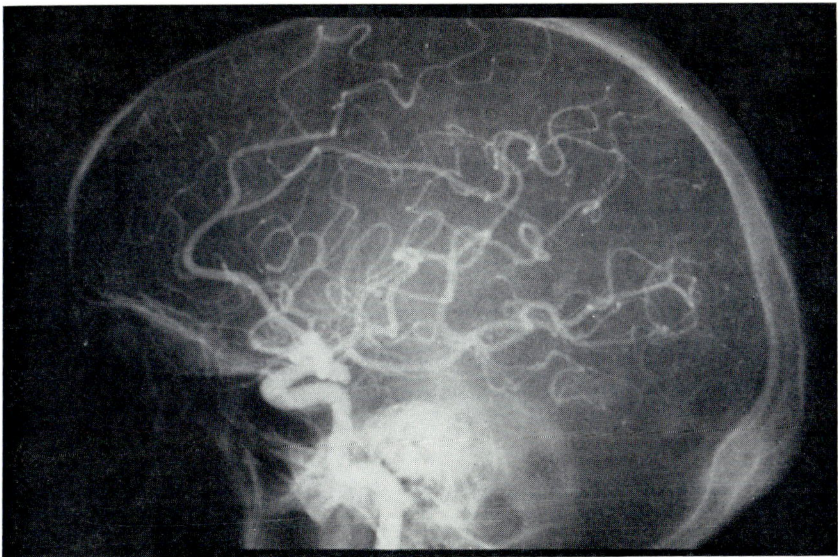

Figure 100. Posterior communicating aneurysm. This aneurysm presented with subaraachnoid hemorrhage and ipsilateral oculomotor palsy. There is no spasm (compare with Fig. 95).

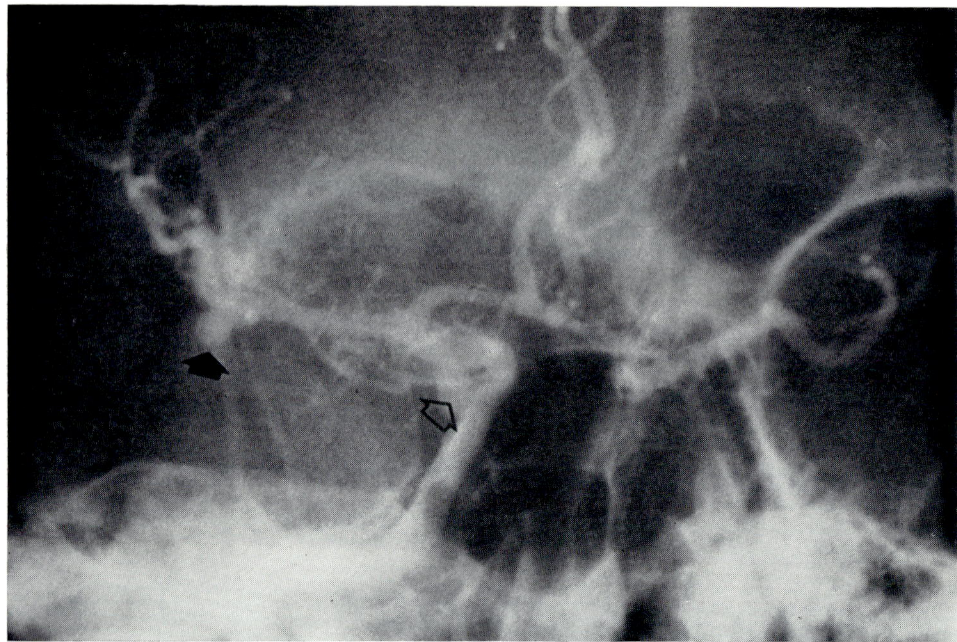

Figure 101. Multiple aneurysms. A middle cerebral aneurysm (black arrow) and a carotid aneurysm (white arrow) are shown. Multiple aneurysms occur in approximately one in every five or six patients presenting with spontaneous subarachnoid hemorrhage. Bilateral carotid angiograms are positive for a single aneurysm in the great majority of primary subarachnoid hemorrhages. Nonfilling of an aneurysm may result from focal spasm, thrombus in the fundus of the sac, or location of the responsible aneurysm on the vertebrobasilar tree. In the multiple aneurysm case, decision as to the site of rupture should rest on the size of the aneurysm, signs of focal spasm or surrounding hematoma, and localizing clinical signs if present.

associated with posterior cerebral arterial spasm. The anterior communicating aneurysm, like those of carotid or middle cerebral origin, is much more common than the aneurysm of the vertebrobasilar system.

(4) Transient loss of consciousness without any lateralizing or localizing signs.

This is a common hallmark of the ruptured anterior communicating aneurysm (Fig. 15). When bilateral carotid angiograms are negative, aneurysm of the basilar bifurcation should be suspected (Fig. 76). Both anterior communicating and basilar bifurcation aneurysms (i.e. at the rostral and caudal extremes of the circle of Willis) may of course produce an initial loss of consciousness which progresses to deep coma without lucidity.

(5) Motor paralysis.

Hemiparesis is most often due to a ruptured middle cerebral aneurysm, and hematoma should be ruled out. Worsening hemiparesis with deepening obtundation should be regarded as evidence of clot until proven otherwise. Transtentorial herniation should be suspected. Hemiparesis which is transient may reflect spasm of the middle cerebral or internal carotid arterial tree, and is most common with middle cerebral or supraclinoid carotid aneurysms. Dense, flaccid hemiplegia noted at the outset may reflect either intracerebral hematoma or spasm of lenticulostriate arteries with capsular infarction. Rarely, hemiparesis may be due to an acute subdural hematoma secondary to rupture of an aneurysm into the subdural space. Paresis of one or both legs at the time of subarachnoid hemorrhage suggests rupture of an anterior communicating aneurysm with anterior cerebral arterial spasm.

(6) Decerebration.

Extensor rigidity may result from transtentorial herniation with midbrain compression. Decerebrate posturing associated with coma can thus be the result of an intracerebral hematoma. It can also be seen with massive intraventricular hemorrhage or in primary hemorrhage or infarction of the upper brain stem.

(7) Acute seizures.

While a past history of epilepsy is relatively uncommon, acute focal cerebral seizures may herald a subarachnoid hemorrhage, usually from a middle cerebral aneurysm. Generalized attacks may also be associated with severe brain swelling due to extensive arterial spasm. Tonic seizures may accompany decerebration.

4. Cerebral edema and head trauma.

Another source of bilateral generalized brain edema is craniocerebral trauma. Cerebral contusion is often diffuse, although localized areas such as the frontal and temporal poles may be contused more severely. Significant trauma combines brain swelling with hemorrhage as a source of intracranial hypertension. The acute subdural hematoma syndrome is often associated with a relatively thin subdural hematoma and relatively major brain swelling and contusion. Acute focal and generalized seizures after head injury suggest cerebral contusion. They do not rule out the possibility of an associated intracranial hematoma. The general clinical course of most severe cerebral contusions, most acute subdurals and the majority of acute epidurals is one of progressive deterioration in consciousness with intracranial hypertension. Hemiparesis can be due to cerebral contusion with brain swelling as well as to intracerebral or extracerebral hematoma. The motor deficit associated with cerebral contusion is usually present immediately upon cranial trauma, so that a newly appearing or worsening hemiparesis should be interpreted as evidence for clot until proven otherwise. This applies as well to oculomotor palsy, development of systemic hypertension or other signs of deterioration. The presence or absence of subarachnoid blood does not materially aid in the differential between traumatic brain swelling and acute intracranial hematoma. Significant head injury is commonly associated with subarachnoid bleeding whether or not an intracranial clot is present. There is a great hazard in lumbar puncture in this acute phase after head injury because of the possibility of transtentorial herniation due to unrecognized hematoma.

Cerebral edema usually reaches a peak three to four days following craniocerebral trauma. During this period, initial deficits may worsen. This deterioration due to brain swelling may be simulated by a previously unrecognized hematoma. Such hematomas are often eccentrically located extracerebral clots which may have been missed without oblique views on initial carotid angiography. The late onset of deterioration after a number of days of stability following cerebral trauma may be due to late onset brain swelling. This is unusual and an unrecognized hematoma should be suspected. Meningitis due to basal fracture should be considered as a source of late deterioration. Communicating hydrocephalus of late onset may complicate the traumatic subarachnoid hemorrhage.

Cranial trauma to the vertex, with or without recognizable fracture, can produce thrombosis of the sagittal sinus on an acute basis. Bilateral cerebral edema with intracerebral hemorrhage, seizures and motor deficits are characteristic. A large depressed skull fracture can itself result in intracranial hypertension due to reduction in intracranial capacity. These are commonly associated with brain laceration, contusion and edema. Cerebral laceration, contusion and edema can also occur without significant depression. Depressed fracture increases the risk of dural laceration, CSF leak and meningitis. Cerebral laceration of nonsilent cortex, like contusion, leads to focal neurological deficit immediately upon cerebral trauma. Such laceration may result in subdural or intracerebral hematomas which magnify the initial deficit. Acute convulsions are commonly associated with laceration, contusion and traumatic cerebral edema whether these injuries are combined or in relative isolation.

C. Subdural hematomas

The usual age of clinical presentation of bilateral subdural hematomas is five or six months of life. The infant presents in one of four common ways.

1. Failure to thrive.
2. Convulsive disorder.
3. Pseudohydrocephalus.
4. Battered child.

There may be no history of cranial trauma. At times, a history of a breech delivery or prolonged labor is available. Symptoms may be quite nonspecific with a failure to gain weight, irritability, vomiting, dehydration and fever. Anemia may be noted. Seizures are common. They may be generalized or focal. They may be the first sign to focus attention on the nervous system. They may be mistaken for febrile convulsions. Seizures occur with or without fever when subdural hematomas are present. The seizures have little lateralizing value in infancy. The subdurals are bilateral in the large majority of infantile cases. This is quite the opposite of the adult subdural which is most often a unilateral mass. The bilateral subdurals may be asymmetrical in thickness. They usually extend over the entire cerebral convexity on each side. Seizures occur more frequently with subdural hematomas than in infantile hydrocephalus. This is an important point if cranial enlargement is noted, since cranial enlargement may be identical in both hydrocephalus and subdural hematomas. A bulging fontanelle and dilated scalp veins may occur in either case. Failure to thrive, vomiting and irritability are common to both the hydrocephalic and the infant with subdural hematomas. However, subdural hematomas usually do not become symptomatic until at least eight to ten weeks of life, and most cases are five to six months of age at the time of diagnosis. Therefore, abnormal cranial enlargement noted at birth or in the very early weeks of infancy is much more apt to be due to hydrocephalus. A history of a battered child with evidence of other injuries is sometimes obtained, and the possibility of subdural hematoma should be considered in these cases. A squint is commonly present, but is of little differential value. Papilledema is uncommon, but retinal and preretinal hemorrhages are common in infantile subdural hematomas, while unusual in infantile hydrocephalus. Optic atrophy can occur in either case and is a late sign. Spasticity is common in subdural hematomas and is more apt to be generalized. Spasticity also occurs in infantile hydrocephalus, in which it is usually more marked in the legs. The point is of little differential value, however. Paralysis may be quite marked postictally. Stupor is evidence of dangerously high intracranial pressure in these cases and may be misinterpreted as postictal depression. The diagnosis must be confirmed by subdural taps. Bilateral subdural hematomas constitute a very common cause of intracranial hypertension appearing in infancy. When cranial enlargement is not a prominent feature, the infant presenting simply a persistent failure to thrive, attention should be directed to the anterior fontanelle. Evident bulging and loss of normal pulsations, the infant being relaxed and held in the sitting position, may be the sole indicator of the presence of bilateral subdural hematomas.

The acute, subacute and chronic subdural hematomas of later childhood and adult life are most often unilateral lesions. In each case, the entire convexity of a hemisphere may be compressed by the hematoma. Alternatively, the bulk of the hematoma may occur over one of the cerebral poles. The acute subdural is at times a bilateral lesion. When bilateral, the associated acute cerebral contusion is often especially marked. Cortical laceration with cortical venous or arterial bleeding may be responsible for the acute subdural hematoma. Tearing of bridging veins is the most common source of subdural hematoma of any type. Tears extending into the sagittal sinus can occur with extensive bilateral subdural clots. Tears across the transverse sinus are also unusual, but can result in subdural collections both above and below the tentorium. Progressive coma with hemiparesis is the usual course in the acute subdural hematoma. Occasionally, a "lucid interval" similar to that more often seen in acute epidural hemorrhage can occur. The subacute and chronic subdural hematomas present a week or more following head injury. The great majority are unilateral. They commonly present a course of progressive intracranial hypertension with or without focal cerebral signs on the opposite side. Headaches and papilledema are common. Headaches may be ipsilateral. Focal cerebral seizures may occur and often have lateralizing value in contrast to those in infancy. Hemiparesis and other deficits, including stupor, may fluctuate. As in infancy, the history of trauma may be absent. This is especially true of the chronic subdural in the elderly, where minimal trauma may have been responsible months or even years before diagnosis (Fig. 102). The traumatic episode is commonly forgotten. The chronic subdural hematoma in this age group often mimics a "stroke." It also may present as a brain tumor syndrome with headaches and papilledema. It may occur as a dementia. The chronic subdural hematoma thus has a variable means of presentation at either extreme of life. Its one common feature

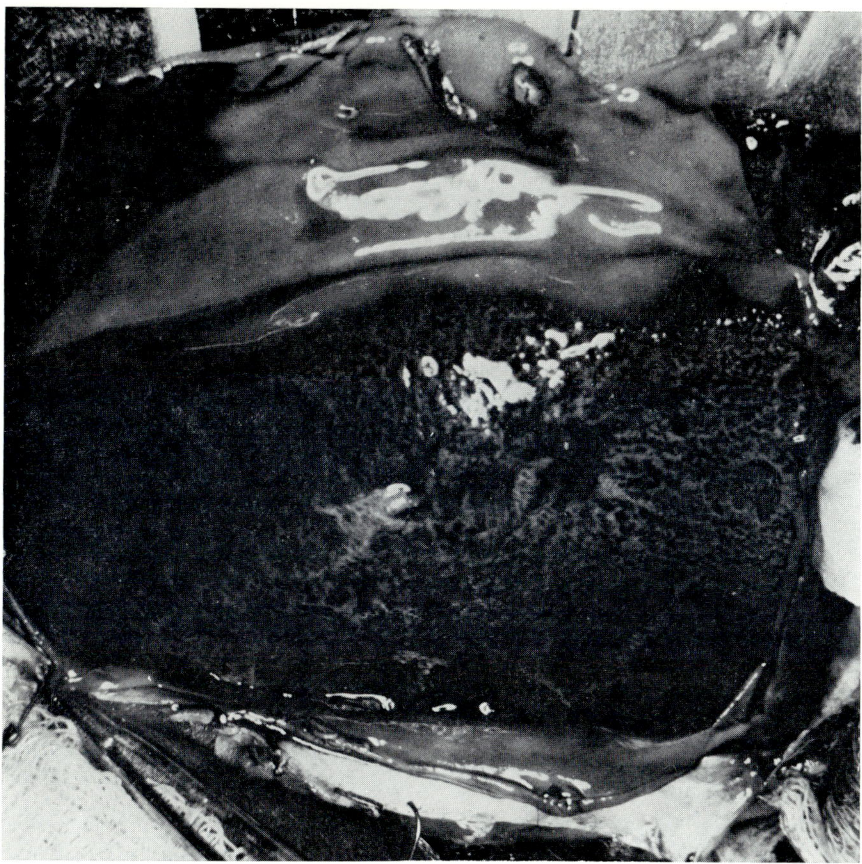

Figure 102. Chronic subdural hematoma. An old solid subdural hematoma with a thick outer membrane is evident. Liquid "machine-oil" fluid was also present. When a subdural hematoma is noted without any grossly visible membrane, the clot is usually less than two weeks old. By one month, the clot is usually liquified. The outer membrane approximates the dura in thickness at this time, and the inner membrane is about half as thick. By three months, the membranes are quite thick. Microscopic examination after this time reveals lysis of all red cells, unless secondary bleeding into the old hematoma has occurred. Hyalinization ensues, and ultimately, calcification may be present.

is its ultimate tendency in most instances to produce intracranial hypertension.

The subdural hygroma, with clear or xanthochromic fluid forming a subdural mass, may be unilateral or bilateral. The onset is usually of subacute or chronic type. Any age group may be affected. Cerebral compression with intracranial hypertension can occur. At times, a long history of focal cerebral or generalized seizures is obtained, and lobar or hemispheral atrophy without evidence of elevated intracranial pressure is noted.

In "hydranencephaly," large amounts of clear or straw-colored fluid can be obtained on bilateral subdural taps in early infancy. Cranial enlargement may be present at birth or begin in the first weeks of life, and is soon associated with markedly retarded development. The cerebral cortex is markedly thinned and may be largely absent. Bilateral congenital obstruction of the foramina of Monro may be responsible for huge ventricular size. Cranial transillumination reveals little if any opacity. Subdural taps are falsely positive in hydranencephaly because of the lack of significant cerebral mantle, the fluid being of ventricular origin.

Meningitis is common in infancy, and subdural effusion complicating nearly any form of bacterial meningitis is a frequent occurrence. Like the traumatic subdural hematoma of infancy, postmeningitic subdural effusion also is bilateral in most cases. Subdural taps in these effusions may reveal fluid which looks like subdural hematoma fluid with evidence of blood. The fluid may be clear as in a subdural hygroma. It may be obviously purulent as in subdural empyema. Cultures of subdural effusions may be positive or negative. Failure of a good clinical response to adequate antibiotic therapy, with evidence of persistent fever, convulsions or neurologic deficit should suggest this diagnosis.

D. Craniosynostosis

Generalized premature closure of cranial sutures in infancy characteristically leads to ultimate intracranial hypertension. Partial premature closure may or may not produce elevated intracranial pressure. A generalized mass effect is produced by a rapidly growing brain confined in a container too small for its projected growth. While prevention of the neurologically disastrous effects of prolonged intracranial hypertension (e.g. blindness, mental retardation) is the chief objective of early diagnosis and neurosurgical treatment, prevention of cranial deformity even in the absence of significant pressure is also important. Early diagnosis is the first prerequisite for successful treatment.

The normal pattern of craniocerebral growth exhibits the following milestones:

1. The normal rate of brain growth proceeds rapidly during the prenatal period and first two years of life. During this phase of rapid brain growth, the cranium grows at the edges of the bones of the vault. During the later phase of slow brain growth, the cranium grows by absorption of inner table bone and deposition of outer table bone. When brain growth stops, cranial growth stops. Cranial growth is thus normally a reflection of brain growth.

2. Prenatal period to birth—metopic suture closure usually occurs before birth. At birth, the cranial bones are normally separated since all other sutures remain open. Normal brain weight at birth is now approximately 400 grams. (*Note:* This has doubled by one year of age and tripled by six years. By twelve years, the adult brain weight of 1400 ± 300 grams is approached.)
3. Birth to three months—this is the period of the greatest brain and cranial growth rate. By three months, posterior fontanelle closure usually occurs; it may be closed at birth.
4. Six months—serrations visible on x-ray appear in the outer table, and a fibrous union of suture lines occurs.
5. Eight months—normal brain markings become visible on the inner table on x-ray examination.
6. Twelve months—cranial circumference has increased by more than 50 percent.
7. Sixteen to eighteen months—anterior fontanelle closure is usually complete on palpation of the skull.
8. Two years—the rate of brain growth now enters a distinctly slower phase. The anterior fontanelle is closed radiologically.
9. Seven years—ossification of the cranial base from ossification centers in cartilage is usually complete.
10. Fourteen to sixteen years—a functionally firm fusion of sutures of the cranial vault with effective cranial rigidity has usually occurred in most individuals by this period of adolescence.
11. Sixth to eighth decade—a solid bony union of all cranial sutures may be deferred until late adult life. As noted, cranial rigidity is effectively present by the middle of the second decade even without complete bony fusion.

Craniosynostosis is manifested clinically due to operation of the following factors:

1. Premature closure of cranial sutures usually occurs by the age of three months.
2. Premature closure of cranial sutures is often present at the time of birth.
3. Cranial deformity due to craniosynostosis becomes more accentuated during the first year of life.
4. Extreme cranial deformity only occurs when premature suture closure is present at birth.
5. The bone at the prematurely closed suture is abnormal and may form a palpable ridge.
6. Bone growth at right angles to the prematurely fused suture is reduced.

7. Bone growth in other directions is augmented.
8. Compensatory separation of nonfused cranial sutures occurs.
9. Most cases occur in males, and closure of the sagittal suture alone is most common.
10. Intracranial hypertension is most common when all cranial sutures are prematurely fused. The pressure syndrome can also occur when single sutures are prematurely fused, especially the coronal.

The clinical features of craniosynostosis include the following:

1. Cranial deformity.
2. Eye signs.
   a. Exophthalmos.
   b. Papilledema may or may not be present. When it occurs, it typically is not associated with retinal hemorrhages.
   c. Optic atrophy—a late sign.
   d. Squint—various forms of strabismus occur due to extraocular palsy and to orbital deformity.
3. Mental retardation.
4. Seizures—convulsions, like the eye signs and the development of mental retardation, are more common when intracranial hypertension exists. They are hence most common with generalized craniosynostosis and least frequent in closure of the sagittal suture alone.
5. Facial deformities—these are least common in isolated sagittal closure and most frequent in coronal or generalized craniosynostosis.

Definition of terms is important because of their continued descriptive usage.

1. Dolichocephaly (Fig. 103) or scaphocephaly—this is the long, narrow head due to craniosynostosis of the sagittal suture.
2. Brachycephaly (Fig. 104)—this is the wide, short head due to premature closure of the coronal or coronal and lambdoid sutures.
3. Acrocephaly—this is the broad, flat forehead occurring with brachycephaly.
4. Plagiocephaly—this is the cranial distortion due to an asymmetrical closure of one or more sutures; it includes the following:
   a. Unilateral coronal fusion.
   b. Unilateral coronal and squamosal closure.
   c. Unilateral lambdoid closure.

   Plagiocephaly produces a unilaterally flat forehead with facio-orbital asymmetry when due to coronal fusion. The posterior aspect of the head may be asymmetrically flat with either coronal or lambdoid closure.
5. Oxycephaly or turricephaly—this is a tower skull due to craniosynostosis of all sutures.

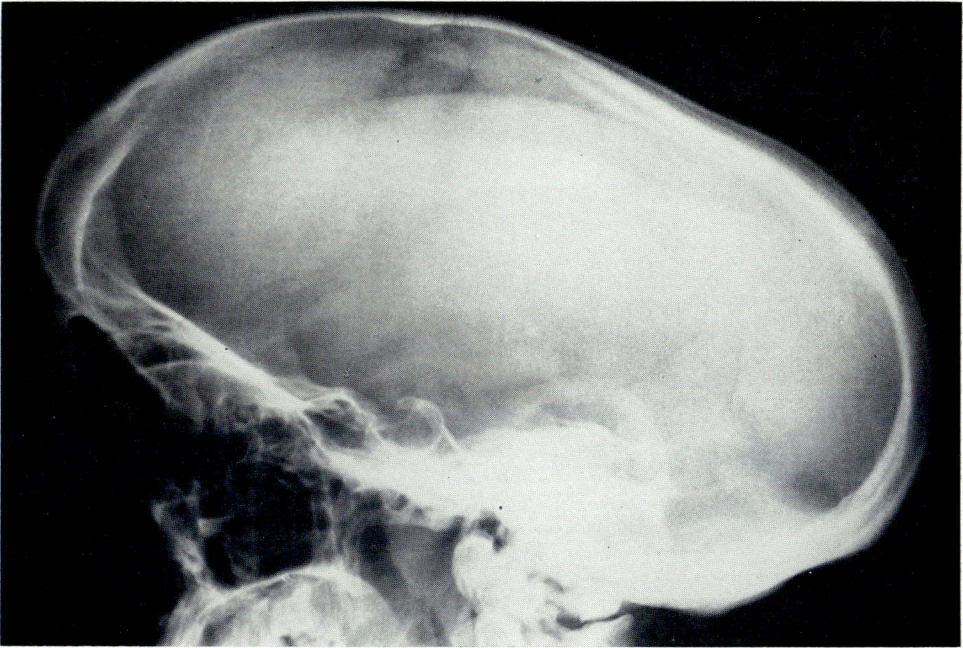

Figure 103. Dolichocephaly. Severe cranial elongation is present due to early premature fusion of the sagittal suture.

6. Trigonocephaly—this results from craniostenosis of the metopic suture with a vertical ridge in the midforehead. This is associated with hypotelorism or close-set orbits.
7. Late premature craniosynostosis—this occurs after the skull has reached nearly adult size and is not clinically important.
8. Craniosynostosis with other congenital anomalies—other anomalies are most commonly present in coronal craniosynostosis. They can occur in generalized closure and occasionally in sagittal fusion. The various types are as follow:
   a. Apert's syndrome or acrocephalosyndactylism—this is coronal closure with digital fusion.
   b. Crouzon's disease or craniofacial dysostosis—this is coronal closure with hypoplasia of the facial bones, frontal bossing, a hooked nosc, an upper lip shaped like an inverted "V," prognathism and kyphosis of the cranial base.
   c. Other congenital anomalies occurring with coronal closure include the following:
      (1) Cleft palate.
      (2) Choanal atresia with airway obstruction.

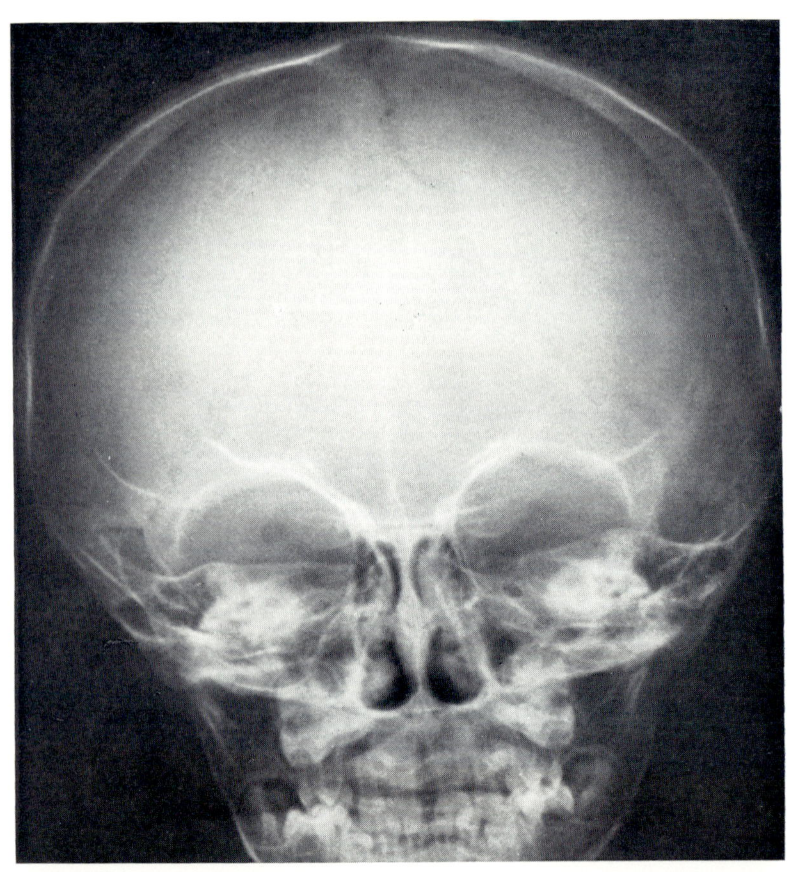

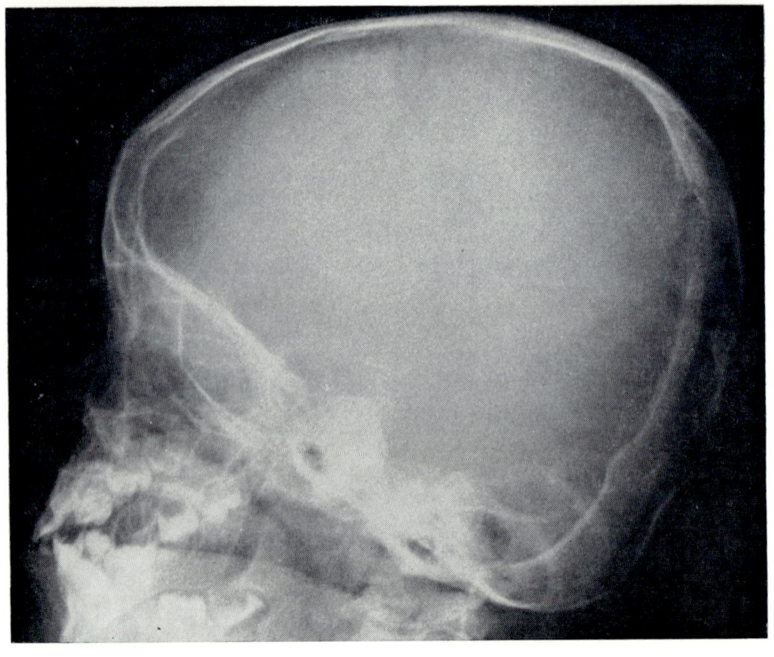

(3) A coronal syndrome with hypoplasia of the maxilla, proptosis and papilledema.
(4) Spina bifida or meningocele.
(5) Congenital heart disease, pyloric stenosis, imperforate anus, and so forth.

9. Hypophosphatasia and craniosynostosis—this is a familial disease presenting in infancy with multiple skeletal deformities and craniosynostosis. The clinical features include the following:
   a. Globular skull with premature fusion of cranial sutures.
   b. Prominent joints and costochondral junctions.
   c. Multiple fractures and skeletal softness.
   d. Failure to thrive.
   e. Vomiting.
   f. Convulsions.
   g. Generalized hypotonia.
   h. Cyanosis.
   i. Ultimate renal failure.
10. Pseudocraniosynostosis or microcephaly—microcephaly is defined by a completed brain weight of less than 900 grams and a secondarily small cranium. Fusion of cranial sutures may occur earlier than normally expected as a result of deficient brain growth. The head and brow are small and the scalp appears furrowed. The nose and ears may appear disproportionately large. Mental retardation and seizures reflect the primary brain damage and lack of cerebral development. Primary prenatal brain destruction with porencephaly may be responsible. Porencephaly indicates a brain cyst which communicates with the ventricle, the subarachnoid space, or both. If hydrocephalus does not develop, the head remains small and premature suture closure can occur. Familial forms of microcephaly are indicated by an elemental convolutional pattern of the small cerebrum. Jervis syndrome is a special form of microcephaly with diffuse cerebral calcifications visible on the skull x-ray.
11. Megacephaly—this term refers to an enlarged head of any etiology. The cranial enlargement usually reflects hydrocephalus occurring in infancy. It may result from any source of intracranial hypertension in infancy or early childhood. In unusual cases, megacephaly may reflect a megalencephalon with an unusually large brain, and without hydrocephalus.

Figure 104. Brachycephaly. Two views exhibit the cranial deformity due to premature fusion of the coronal suture.

12. Bathrocephaly—this refers to a normal variant in which there is overlap of the occipital bone in the region of the lambda. The overriding at the lambdoid suture is not clinically important. It should be distinguished from the prominent occiput with lambdoidal separation and elevation of the inion seen in the Dandy-Walker syndrome. It may also simulate a depressed fracture on x-ray examination.

Plain Skull X-rays in Intracranial Hypertension

1. Separation of the coronal suture—this is the most common sign of intracranial hypertension in childhood. Sellar changes are the commonest and earliest signs of increased intracranial pressure in the adult. Separation of the coronal suture due to elevated pressure may be seen as late as age sixteen and, rarely, even later. Separation of the sagittal suture and the lambdoid sutures may accompany coronal separation. After three years of life, suture separation of more than 2 mm is abnormal.
2. Cranial enlargement—indicates intracranial hypertension beginning in utero, in infancy or in early childhood. It can sometimes be seen in posterior fossa tumors of later childhood.
3. Exaggerated brain markings—normal convolutional markings can be seen as early as eight months. They may be absent until twelve to sixteen months. After two years, they are usually prominent throughout childhood and are often evident in the adult skull. Failure to develop normal brain markings suggests brain atrophy. Subdural hematomas of infancy can also prevent the appearance of brain markings, despite the presence of elevated pressure. Cerebral hemiatrophy is associated with absence of normal brain markings unilaterally with a smaller ipsilateral hemicalvarium. The bones of the vault on the side of the hemiatrophy are often thicker than those on the normal side. The "beaten silver" effect of exaggerated brain markings only indicates elevated intracranial pressure when other x-ray or clinical evidence of intracranial hypertension is present. It is a late sign of abnormal pressure. It may, however, be the only x-ray evidence of elevated pressure in craniosynostosis, when the prematurely fused sutures prevent sutural separation.
4. Thinning of cranial bones—diffuse thinning of the cranial vault commonly accompanies the cranial enlargement and sutural separation of infantile hydrocephalus. Craniolacunar skull with multiple areas of marked thinning and even absence of cranial bone suggests intracranial hypertension in utero. Hydrocephalus, meningomyelocele, encephalocele and other congenital anomalies are often associated.

Thinning of the bone of the cranial base in the region of the orbital plates, sphenoid and occiput is commonly seen in intracranial hypertension in infancy and childhood. Thinning of bone in the region of the sella is common in the adult with elevated pressure. A dilated third ventricle can produce similar sellar changes both in childhood and in adult life.

5. Sellar changes in intracranial hypertension—pressure atrophy of the sella is most prominently noted in the posterior sellar elements of the adult skull.
   a. Erosion of the rostral wall of the dorsum sella—the earliest sign.
   b. Erosion of the posterior clinoids.
   c. Progressive erosion of the entire dorsum and sellar floor with diffuse loss of cortical margins.
   d. Eventual sellar enlargement may occur.

   Sellar changes due to pituitary tumor differ. In most pituitary tumors, intracranial hypertension is absent. The pituitary tumor produces sellar ballooning early, with expansive erosion of both anterior and posterior sellar elements. The inferior surface of the anterior clinoid is thinned unilaterally or bilaterally early in pituitary tumor expansion, and the clinoids are sharpened and pointed upwards. Parasellar masses can also produce rostral changes in an anterior clinoid or tuberculum. The suprasellar mass with clinoidal erosion tends to point the clinoids downward. Third ventricular hydrocephalus can produce rostral sellar erosion. The cerebellar tumor of childhood with elevated intracranial pressure and obstructive hydrocephalus can in this way produce both sellar changes and suture separation. In the adult, early sellar changes posteriorly (i.e. dorsum, posterior clinoids, posterior sellar floor) are most often due to intracranial hypertension, commonly as a result of brain tumor. Chronic subdural hematoma or other source of increased pressure must be ruled out. These posterior sellar changes require at least a month and may take many months in slowly developing intracranial hypertension. In the adult, early sellar changes anteriorly (i.e. anterior clinoids, tuberculum, anterior or entire sellar floor) have greater localizing value. They are commonly due to pituitary and parasellar tumors and aneurysms usually without intracranial hypertension.

BIBLIOGRAPHY

Agee, O. F., Musella, R., and Tweed, C. G.: Aneurysm of the great vein of Galen. Report of two cases. *J. Neurosurg., 31:*346-351, 1969.

Ajmone-Marsan, C., and Ralston, B. L.: *The Epileptic Seizure.* Springfield, Thomas, 1957.

Allcock, J. M., and Drake, C. G.: Ruptured intracranial aneurysms—the role of arterial spasm. *J. Neurosurg., 22:*21-29, 1965.

Anderson, F. M., and Geiger, L.: Craniosynostosis: a survey of 204 cases. *J. Neurosurg., 22:*229-240, 1965.

Anderson, F. M., Gwinn, J. L., and Todt, J. C.: Trigonocephaly, identity and surgical treatment. *J. Neurosurg., 19:*723-730, 1962.

Bailey, P.: *Intracranial Tumors,* 2nd ed. Springfield, Thomas, 1948.

Bailey, P., Buchanan, D. N., and Bucy, P. C.: *Intracranial Tumors of Infancy and Childhood.* Chicago, U. of Chicago, 1939.

Bakay, L., and Bean, B. C.: Relative diagnostic value of air study and angiography in suprasellar masses. *J. Neurosurg., 20:*729-739, 1963.

Bakay, L., and Klein, D. M.: *Brain Tumor Scanning with Radioisotopes.* Springfield, Thomas, 1969.

Baker, A. B.: *Clinical Neurology.* New York, Hoeber-Harper, 1955.

Baldwin, M., Bailey, P., Ajmone-Marsan, C., Klatzo, L, and Tower, D.: *Temporal Lobe Epilepsy.* Springfield, Thomas, 1958.

Ballantine, H. T.: Brain abscess. In Gurdjian, E. S., (Ed.) : *Cranial and Intracranial Suppuration.* Springfield, Thomas, 1969.

Barnett, H. J. M.: Some clinical features of intracranial aneurysms. *Clin. Neurosurg., 16:*43-72, 1969.

Barone, B. M., and Elvidge, A. R.: Ependymomas. A clinical survey. *J. Neurosurg., 33:* 428-439, 1970.

Batzdorf, U., and Malamud, N.: The problem of multicentric gliomas. *J. Neurosurg., 20:*122-136, 1963.

Benson, D. F., LeMay, M., Patten, D. H., and Rubens, A. B.: Diagnosis of normal-pressure hydrocephalus. *N.Engl.J. Med., 283:*609-615, 1970.

Berger, E. C., and Elvidge, A. R.: Medulloblastomas and cerebellar sarcomas. A clinical survey. *J. Neurosurg., 20:*139-144, 1963.

Bergland, R. M., Ray, B. S., and Torack, R. M.: Anatomical variations in the pituitary gland and adjacent structures in 225 human autopsy cases. *J. Neurosurg., 28:* 93-99, 1968.

Bhandari, Y. S., and Sarkari, N. B. S.: Subdural empyema. A review of 37 cases. *J. Neurosurg., 32:*35-39, 1970.

Biemond, A.: *Brain Diseases.* Amsterdam, Elsevier, 1970.

Blom, S., and Ekbom, K. A.: Early clinical signs of meningiomas of the foramen magnum. A new syndrome. *J. Neurosurg., 19:*661-664, 1962.

Bogen, J. E., and Gazzaniga, M. S.: Cerebral commissurotomy in man. Minor hemisphere dominance for certain visuospatial functions. *J. Neurosurg., 23:*394-399, 1965.

Brain, W. R.: *Diseases of the Nervous System,* 6th ed. London, Oxford U. P., 1962.

Branch, C., Milner, B., and Rasmussen, T.: Intracarotid sodium amytal for the lateralization of cerebral speech dominance. Observations in 123 patients. *J. Neurosurg., 21:*399-405, 1964.

Bray, P. F., Carter, S., and Taveras, J. M.: Brainstem tumors in children. *Neurology, 8:*1-7, 1958.

Bray, P. F.: *Neurology in Pediatrics.* Chicago, Year Bk., 1969.

Bremer, F.: Cerveau isolé et physiologie du sommeil. *C. R. Soc. Biol.* (Paris), *118:* 1235-1242, 1935.

Brock, S., and Krieger, H. P.: *The Basis of Clinical Neurology,* 4th ed. Baltimore, Williams & Wilkins, 1963.

Brodal, A.: *The Cranial Nerves, Anatomy and Anatomico—Clinical Correlations.* Oxford, Blackwell, 1959.

Brodal, A.: *Neurological Anatomy in Relation to Clinical Medicine,* 2nd ed. London, Oxford U. P., 1969.

Brodal, A.: *The Reticular Formation of the Brain Stem, Anatomical Aspects and Functional Correlations.* Springfield, Thomas, 1957.

Brodal, A.: Spasticity—anatomical aspects. *Acta Neurol. Scand., 38:*9-40, 1962.

Brodin, H.: Extradural hematomas. A survey of cases covering a 20 year period with special reference to diagnosis. *Acta Chir. Scand., 102:*99, 1952.

Buchanan, A. R.: *Functional Neuroanatomy,* 3rd ed. Philadelphia, Lea & F., 1957.

Buchsbaum, H. W., and Colton, R. P.: Anterior third ventricular cysts in infancy. *J. Neurosurg., 26:*264-266, 1967.

Bucy, P. C.: *The Precentral Motor Cortex.* Urbana, Illinois, U. of Ill., 1949.

Bucy, P. C., Keplinger, J. E., and Siqueira, E. B.: Destruction of the "pyramidal tract" in man. *J. Neurosurg., 21:*385-398, 1964.

Busch, E. A. V.: Brain stem contusions; differential diagnosis, therapy and prognosis. *Clin. Neurosurg., 9:*18-33, 1963.

Camp, J. D.: The roentgenological aspects of lesions around the sella turcica. *Clin. Neurosurg., 4:*61-74, 1956.

Campbell, E., and Whitfield, R. D.: The incidence and significance of shock in head injury. *Ann. Surg., 138:*698-705, 1953.

Campbell, J. B., and Cohen, J.: Epidural hemorrhage and the skull of children. *Surg. Gynecol. Obstet., 92:*257, 1951.

Carton, C. A.: *Cerebral Angiography in the Management of Head Trauma.* Springfield, Thomas, 1959.

Castellano, F., and Ruggiero, G.: Meningiomas of the posterior fossa. Acta *Radiol.* (Stockh.), suppl. 104, *11,* 1953.

Caveness, W. F.: Onset and cessation of fits following craniocerebral trauma. *J. Neurosurg., 20:*570-583, 1963.

Chamlin, M., and Davidoff, L. M.: Ophthalmologic criteria in diagnosis and management of pituitary tumors. *J. Neurosurg., 19:*9-18, 1962.

Chou, S. N., Story, J. L., French, L. A., and Peterson, H. O.: Some angiographic features of brain abscess. *J. Neurosurg., 24:*693-696, 1966.

Chutorian, A. M., Schwartz, J. F., Evans, R. A., and Carter, S.: Optic gliomas in children. *Neurology, 14:*83-95, 1964.

Ciembroniewicz, J. E.: Subdural hematoma of the posterior fossa. Review of the literature with addition of three cases. *J. Neurosurg., 22:*465-473, 1965.

Cobb, W. A.: The EEG of specific lesions. In Hill, D., and Parr, G. (Eds.): *Electroencephalography, a Symposium on its Various Aspects.* London, MacDonald, 1963.

Cogan, D. G.: *Neurology of the Ocular Muscles,* 2nd ed. Springfield, Thomas, 1970.

Cogan, D. G.: *Neurology of the Visual System.* Springfield, Thomas, 1966.

Cohen, L., and MacRae, D.: Tumors in the region of the foramen magnum. *J. Neurosurg., 19:*462-469, 1962.

Collier, J., and Adie, W. J.: Intracranial tumors. In Price, F. W. (Ed): *A Textbook of the Practice of Medicine,* 2nd ed. London, Oxford U. P., 1926.

Collins, W. F.: Subdural hematomas of infancy. *Clin. Neurosurg., 15:*394-404, 1968.

Crawford, T.: Some observations on the pathogenesis and natural history of intracranial aneurysms. J. Neurol. Neurosurg. Psychiatry, *22:*259-266, 1959.

Crosby, E. C., Humphrey, T., and Lauer, E. W.: *Correlative Anatomy of the Nervous System.* New York, Macmillan, 1962.

Cuneo, H. M., and Rand, C. W.: *Brain Tumors of Childhood.* Springfield, Thomas, 1952.

Cushing, H.: *Intracranial Tumors.* Springfield, Thomas, 1932.

Cushing, H.: *Selected Papers on Neurosurgery.* New Haven, Yale, 1969.

Cushing, H.: Some experimental and clinical observations concerning states of increased intracranial tension. *Am. J. Med. Sci., 124:*375-400, 1902.

Cushing, H.: *The Pituitary Body and its Disorders.* Philadelphia, Lippincott, 1912.

Cushing, H.: *Tumors of the Nervus Acusticus and the Syndrome of the Cerebellopontile Angle.* Philadelphia, Saunders, 1917.

Cushing, H., and Bailey, P.: *Tumors Arising from the Blood-vessels of the Brain, Angiomatous Malformations and Hemangioblastomas.* Springfield, Thomas, 1928.

Cushing, H., and Eisenhardt, L.: *Meningiomas, Their Classification, Regional Behaviour, Life History, and Surgical End Results.* Springfield, Thomas, 1938.

Dandy, W. E.: *Benign Tumors in the Third Ventricle of the Brain; Diagnosis and Treatment.* Springfield, Thomas, 1933.

Dandy, W. E.: *The Brain.* Hagerstown, Maryland, Prior, 1966.

Dandy, W. E.: *Selected Writings.* Springfield, Thomas, 1957.

Daniel, P. M., Prichard, M. M. L., and Treip, C. S.: Traumatic infarction of the anterior lobe of the pituitary gland. *Lancet, 2:*927-931, 1959.

Davidoff, L. M., and Epstein, B. S.: *The Abnormal Pneumoencephalogram,* 2nd ed. Philadelphia, Lea & F., 1955.

Davidoff, L. M., Jacobson, H. G., and Zimmerman, H. M.: *Neuroradiology Workshop.* New York, Grune and Stratton, 1961, vol. 1,2,3.

Davis, L., and Davis, R. A.: *Principles of Neurological Surgery.* Philadelphia, Saunders, 1963.

DeJong, R. N.: *The Neurologic Examination,* 2nd ed. New York, Hoeber-Harper, 1958.

De La Torre, E., Alexander, E., Davis, C. H., and Crandell, D. L.: Tumors of the lateral ventricles of the brain. Report of 8 cases, with suggestions for clinical management. *J. Neurosurg., 20:*461-470, 1963.

Dempsey, E. W., and Morrison, R. S.: The production of rhythmically recurrent cortical potentials after localized thalamic stimulation. *Am. J. Physiol., 135:*293-308, 1942.

Denny-Brown, D.: Motor mechanisms—introduction: the general principles of motor integration. In Field, J. Magoun, H. W., and Hall, V. E. (Eds.): *Handbook of Physiology, sect. 1: Neurophysiology.* Washington, D. C., Am. Physiol. Soc., 1960.

Denny-Brown, D.: *The Basal Ganglia and Their Relation to Disorders of Movement.* London, Oxford U. P., 1962.

Dott, N. M.: Intracranial aneurysmal formations. *Clin. Neurosurg., 16:*1-16, 1969.

Dott, N. M.: Carotid-cavernous arteriovenous fistula. *Clin. Neurosurg., 16:*17-21, 1969.

Duvoisin, R. C., and Yahr, M. D.: Posterior fossa aneurysms. *Neurology, 15:*231-241, 1965.

Echlin, F. A.: *Head Injuries and Their Management.* Philadelphia, Lippincott, 1956.

Echlin, F. A., Sordillo, S. V., and Gaucy, T. Q.: Acute, subacute and chronic subdural hematoma. *J. A. M. A., 161:*1345-1350, 1956

Ecker, A.: Upward transtentorial herniation of the brain stem and cerebellum due to tumor of the posterior fossa. *J. Neurosurg., 5:*51-61, 1948.

Ecker, A., and Riemenschneider, P. A.: *Angiographic Localization of Intracranial Masses.* Springfield, Thomas, 1954.

Edwards, C. H., and Paterson, J. H.: A review of the symptoms and signs of acoustic neurofibromata. *Brain, 74:*144-190, 1951.

Elliott, F. A., and McKissock, W.: Acoustic neuroma, early diagnosis. *Lancet,* 1189-1191, 1954.

Elvidge, A. R.: Long term survival in the astrocytoma series. *J. Neurosurg., 28:*399-404, 1968.

Epstein, B. S.: *Pneumoencephalography and Cerebral Angiography.* Chicago, Year Bk., 1966.

Evans, J. P.: *Acute Head Injury,* 2nd ed. Springfield, Thomas, 1963.

Falconer, M. A., Bailey, I. C., and Duchen, L. W.: Surgical treatment of chordoma and chondroma of the skull base. *J. Neurosurg., 29:*261-275, 1968.

Falconer, M. A., Serfetinides, E. A., and Corsellis, J. A. N.: Etiology and pathogenesis of temporal lobe epilepsy. *Arch. Neurol., 10:*233-248, 1964.

Feindel, W., and Penfield, W.: Localization of discharge in temporal lobe automatism. *Arch. Neurol. Psychiatry, 72:*605-630, 1954.

Fields, W. S.: *Neurological Diagnostic Techniques.* Springfield, Thomas, 1966.

Finney, L. A., and Walker, A. E.: *Transtentorial Herniation.* Springfield, Thomas, 1962.

Fokes, E. C., and Earle, K. M.: Ependymomas: clinical and pathological aspects. *J. Neurosurg., 30:*585-594, 1969.

Foltz, E. L., and Shurtleff, D. B.: Five-year comparative study of hydrocephalus in children with and without operation (113 cases). *J. Neurosurg., 20:*1064-1079, 1963.

Frankel, S. A., and German, W. J.: Glioblastoma multiforme. Review of 219 cases with regard to natural history, pathology, diagnostic methods, and treatment. *J. Neurosurg., 15:*489-503, 1958.

Freeman, J. M., and Borkowf, S.: Craniostenosis, review of the literature and report of 34 cases. *Pediatrics, 30:*57-70, 1962.

French, J. D.: The reticular formation. In Field, J., Magoun, H. W., and Hall, V. E. (Eds.): *Handbook of Physiology, sect. 1: Neurophysiology.* Washington, D. C., Am. Psysiol. Soc., 1960.

French, L. A., and Chou, S. N.: Osteomyelitis of the skull and epidural abscess. In Gurdjian, E. S. (Ed.): *Cranial and Intracranial Suppuration.* Springfield, Thomas, 1969.

French, L. A., Chou, S. N., and Story, J. L.: Cerebrovascular malformations. *Clin. Neurosurg., 11:*171-182, 1964.

Fulton, J. F.: *Physiology of the Nervous System,* 2nd ed. London, Oxford U. P., 1943.

Furlow, L. T.: Metastatic tumors of the brain. *Clin. Neurosurg., 7*:63-78, 1961.

Gallagher, J. P., and Browder, E. J.: Extradural hematoma. Experiences with 167 patients. *J. Neurosurg., 29*:1-12, 1968.

Garcia-Bengochea, F., and Berk, M.: The so-called solid hemangioblastomas of the cerebellum and vertebral angiography. *J. Neurosurg., 22*:35-39, 1965.

German, W. J.: The gliomas: a follow-up study. *Clin. Neurosurg., 7*:1-20, 1961.

German, W. J., and Flanigan, S.: Examination and diagnosis in patients with head injury. *Clin. Neurosurg., 12*:38-55, 1964.

Gol, A.: Cerebral astrocytomas in childhood. A clinical study. *J. Neurosurg., 19*:577-582, 1962.

Gol, A., and McKissock, W.: The cerebellar astrocytomas. A report on 98 verified cases. *J. Neurosurg., 16*:287-296, 1959.

Gonzalez, D., and Elvidge, A. R.: On the occurrence of epilepsy caused by astrocytoma of the cerebral hemispheres. *J. Neurosurg., 19*:470-482, 1962.

Goodman, J. M., and Mealey, J.: Postmeningitic subdural effusions: the syndrome and its management. *J. Neurosurg., 30*:658-663, 1969.

Goody, P. D.: Extradural hemorrhage of the anterior and posterior fossae. *J. Neurosurg., 5*:294. 1948.

Gowers, W. R.: *Diagnosis of Diseases of the Brain and of the Spinal Cord.* New York, Wood, 1885.

Granholm, L., and Radberg, C.: Congenital communicating hydrocephalus. *J. Neurosurg., 20*:338-343, 1963.

Grant, F. C., and Jones, R. K.: A clinical study of 200 posterior fossa gliomas in children. *Clin. Neurosurg., 5*:1-24, 1957.

Grinker, R. R., and Sahs, A. L.: *Neurology,* 6th ed. Springfield, Thomas, 1966.

Grossman, C. C.: *The Use of Diagnostic Ultrasound in Brain Disorders.* Springfield, Thomas, 1966.

Hamby, W. B.: *Intracranial Aneurysms.* Springfield, Thomas, 1952.

Hamby, W. B., and Dohn, D. F.: Carotid-cavernous fistulas: report of 36 cases and discussion of their management. *Clin. Neurosurg., 11*:150-170, 1964.

Harrington, D. O.: *The Visual Fields, A Textbook and Atlas of Clinical Perimetry.* St. Louis, Mosby, 1956.

Hawkes, C. D.: Craniocerebral trauma in infancy and childhood. *Clin. Neurosurg., 11*:66-75, 1964.

Hawkes, C. D., and Ogle, W. S.: Atypical features of epidural hematoma in infants, children and adolescents. *J. Neurosurg., 19*:971-980, 1962.

Haymaker, W.: *Bing's Local Diagnosis in Neurological Diseases,* 15th ed. St. Louis, Mosby, 1969.

Haymaker, W., Anderson, E., and Nauta, W. J. H.: *The Hypothalamus.* Springfield, Thomas, 1969.

Hécaen, H.: Aphasic, apraxic and agnosic syndromes in right and left hemisphere lesions. In Vinken, P. J., and Bruyn, G. W. (Eds.) : *Disorders of Speech, Perception and Symbolic Behavior. Handbook of Clinical Neurology.* New York, Wiley, 1969, vol. 4.

Hécaen, H., and deAjuriaguerra, J.: *Left Handedness, Manual Superiority and Cerebral Dominance.* New York, Grune, 1964.

Henderson, W. R.: The anterior basal meningiomas. *Br. J. Surg., 26*:124-165, 1938.

Hendrick, E. B., Harwood-Hash, D. C. F., and Hudson, A. R.: Head injuries in children: a survey of 4465 consecutive cases at the hospital for sick children, Toronto. *Clin. Neurosurg., 11:*46-65, 1964.

Hess, W. R.: The Functional Organization of the Diencephalon. New York, Grune, 1957.

Higazi, I., and El-Banhawy, A.: The value of angiography in diagnosis of extradural hematoma of the anterior fossa. Report of two cases. *J. Neurosurg., 24:*765-771, 1966.

Holmes, G.: *Introduction to Clinical Neurology,* 2nd ed. Edinburgh, Livingstone, 1960.

Hook, O., and Norlen, G.: Aneurysms of the internal carotid artery. *Acta Neurol. Scand., 40:*200-218, 1964.

Hook, O., and Norlen, G.: Aneurysms of the anterior communicating artery. *Acta Neurol. Scand., 40:*219-240, 1964.

Howell, D. A.: Upper brain stem compression and foraminal impaction with intracranial space-occupying lesions and brain swelling. *Brain, 82:*525-550, 1959.

Huber, A.: *Eye Symptoms in Brain Tumors.* St. Louis, Mosby, 1961.

Hughes, R. R.: *An Introduction to Clinical Electro-encephalography.* Bristol, Wright, 1961.

Jackson, H.: Orbital tumors. *J. Neurosurg., 19:*551-567, 1962.

Jackson, I. J., and Thompson, R. K.: *Pediatric Neurosurgery.* Springfield, Thomas, 1959.

Jackson, J. H.: *Selected Writings, Vol. 1, On Epilepsy and Epileptiform Convulsions.* London, Hodder and Stoughton, 1931.

Jakubiak, P., Dunsmore, R. H., and Beckett, R. S.: Supratentorial brain cysts. *J. Neurosurg., 28:*129-136, 1968.

Jamieson, K. G.: Aneurysms of the vertebrobasilar system. Further experience with 9 cases. *J. Neurosurg., 28:*544-555, 1968.

Jamieson, K. G., and Yelland, J. D. N.: Extradural hematoma. Report of 167 cases. *J. Neurosurg., 29:*13-23, 1968.

Jansen, J., and Brodal, A.: *Aspects of Cerebellar Anatomy.* Oslo, Johan, Goundt, Tanum, Forlag, 1954.

Jasper, H. H.: Diffuse projection systems: the integrative activity of the thalamic reticular system. *Electroencephalogr. Clin. Neurophysiol., 1:*405-419, 1949.

Jasper, H. H., and Bertrand, G.: Thalamic units involved in somatic sensation and voluntary and involuntary movements in man. In Purpura, D. P., and Yahr, M. D. (Eds.) : *The Thalamus.* New York, Columbia, 1966, pp. 365-390.

Jefferson, G.: Discussion on the differential diagnosis of lesions of the posterior fossa. *Proc. R. Soc. Med., 46:*719-726, 1953.

Jefferson, G.: On the saccular aneurysms of the internal carotid artery in the cavernous sinus. *Br. J. Surg., 26:*267-302, 1938.

Jefferson, G.: *Selected Papers.* London, Pitman, 1960.

Jefferson, G.: The tentorial pressure cone. *Arch. Neurol. Psychiatry, 40:*857-876, 1938.

Jennett, W. B.: *Epilepsy after Blunt Head Injuries.* London, Heinemann, 1962.

Jennett, W. B., and Lewin, W.: Traumatic epilepsy after closed head injuries. *J. Neurol. Neurosurg. Psychiatry, 23:*295-301, 1960.

Jewesbury, E. C. O.: Parietal lobe syndromes. In Vinken, P. J., and Bruyn, G. W. (Eds.) : *Localization in Clinical Neurology. Handbook of Clinical Neurology.* New York, Wiley, 1969, vol. 2.

Johnson, E. W.: Auditory findings in 200 cases of acoustic neuromas. In House, W. F. (Ed.) : *Monograph II, Acoustic Neuroma. Arch. Otolaryngol., 88:6:*598-603, 1968.

Johnson, E. W., and Sheehy, J. L.: Audiological aspects of the diagnosis of acoustic neuromas. *J. Neurosurg., 24*:621-628, 1966.

Johnson, R. T., and Yates, P. O.: Clinico-pathological aspects of pressure changes at the tentorium. *Acta Radiol., 46*:242-249, 1956.

Jouvet, M.: Biogenic amines and the states of sleep. *Science, 163*:32-41, 1969.

Jung, R., and Hassler, R.: The extrapyramidal motor system. In Field, J., Magoun, H. W., and Hall, V. E. (Eds.) : *Handbook of Physiology, sect. 1: Neurophysiology.* Washington, D. C., Am. Physiol. Soc., 1960.

Kahn, E. A.: The clinical applications of brain scanning. *Clin. Neurosurg., 12*:23-37, 1964.

Kahn, E. A.: Tumors involving the third ventricle. *Clin. Neurosurg., 7*:79-99, 1959.

Kahn, E. A., Crosby, E. C., Schneider, R. C., and Taren, J. A.: *Correlative Neurosurgery,* 2nd ed., Springfield, Thomas, 1969.

Kamrin, R. P., Potanos, J. N., and Pool, J. L.: An evaluation of the diagnosis and treatment of chordoma. *J. Neurol. Neurosurg. Psychiatry, 27*:157-165, 1964.

Kelly, D. L., Alexander, E., Davis, C. H., and Maynard, D. C.: Intracranial arteriovenous malformations: clinical review and evaluation of brain scans. *J. Neurosurg., 31*:422-428, 1969.

Kernohan, J. W., and Sayre, G. P.: Tumors of the central nervous system. In *Atlas of Tumor Pathology.* Sect. X, Fasc. 35 and 37. Washington, D. C., A. F. I. P., 1952.

Kernohan, J. W., and Woltman, H. W.: Incisura of the crus due to contralateral brain tumor. *Arch. Neurol. Psychiatry, 21*:274, 1929.

Kestenbaum, A.: *Clinical Methods of Neuro-ophthalmologic Examination,* 2nd ed. New York, Grune, 1961.

Kiloh, L. G., and Osselton, J. W.: *Clinical Electroencephlography.* London, Butterworth, 1961.

Kinal, M. E.: Traumatic thrombosis of dural venous sinuses in closed head injuries. *J. Neurosurg., 27*:142-145, 1967.

Kindt, G. W.: The pattern of location of cerebral metastatic tumors. *J. Neurosurg., 21*:54-57, 1964.

King, A. B., and Chambers, J. W.: Delayed onset of symptoms due to extradural hematomas. *Surgery, 31*:839, 1952.

Kirshner, N.: The function of catecholamines in the brain. *J. Neurosurg., 24*:165-167, 1966.

Kiser, J. L., and Kendig, J. H.: Intracranial suppuration. A review of 139 consecutive cases with electronmicroscopic observations on three. *J. Neurosurg., 20*:494-511, 1963.

Krayenbühl, H. A.: Abscess of the brain. *Clin. Neurosurg., 14*:25-44, 1967.

Krayenbühl, H. A.: Unilateral exophthalmos. *Clin. Neurosurg., 14*:45-71, 1967.

Krayenbühl, H. A., and Yasargil, M. G.: *Cerebral Angiography,* 2nd ed. Philadelphia, Lippincott, 1968.

Kricheff, I. I., Becker, M., Schneck, S. A., and Taveras, J. M.: Intracranial ependymomas: factors influencing prognosis. *J. Neurosurg., 21*:7-14, 1964.

Krieg, W. J. S.: *Functional Neuroanatomy.* Philadelphia, Blakiston, 1942.

Kurze, T.: A neurosurgical conspectus of otology. *Clin. Neurosurg., 13*:238-251, 1966.

Langfitt, T. W.: Increased intracranial pressure. *Clin. Neurosurg., 16*:436-471, 1969.

Lanigan, J. P.: Middle meningeal hemorrhage in children. *Lancet, 2*:65, 1942.

Laurence, K. M.: The natural history of hydrocephalus. *Postgrad. Med. J., 36*:662-667, 1960.

Lawton Smith, J.: Some neuro-ophthalmological aspects of head injury. *Clin. Neurosurg., 12*:181-192, 1964.

Lee, W. M., and Adams, J. E.: The empty sella syndrome. *J. Neurosurg., 28*:351-356, 1968.

Leeds, N. E., and Taveras, J. M.: *Dynamic Factors in Diagnosis of Supratentorial Brain Tumors by Cerebral Angiography.* Philadelphia, Saunders, 1969.

Lloyd-Smith, D. L.: The electroencephalogram as a diagnostic aid in neurosurgery: a review. *Clin. Neurosurg., 16*:251-268, 1969.

Locksley, H. B., Sahs, A. L., and Knowler, L.: Report on the cooperative study of intracranial aneurysms and subarachnoid hemorrhage., Sect. II. General survey of cases in the central registry and characteristics of the sample population. *J. Neurosurg., 24*:922-932, 1966.

Locksley, H. B., Sahs, A. L., and Sandler, R.: Report on the cooperative study of intracranial aneurysms and subarachnoid hemorrhage., Sect. III. Subarachnoid hemorrhage unrelated to intracranial aneurysm and AV malformation. *J. Neurosurg., 24*:1034-1056, 1966.

Low, N. L., Correll, J. W., and Hammill, J. F.: Tumors of the cerebral hemispheres in children. *Arch. Neurol., 13*:547-554, 1965.

Lundrgen, A., and Olin, T.: Muco-pyocele of sphenoidal sinus or posterior ethmodial cells with special reference to the apex orbitae syndrome. *Acta Otolaryngol., 53*: 63-77, 1961.

Luria, A. R.: Frontal lobe syndromes. In Vinken, P. J., and Bruyn, G. W. (Eds.): *Localization in Clinical Neurology. Handbook of Clinical Neurology.* New York, Wiley, 1969, vol. 2.

Luria, A. R.: *Higher Cortical Functions in Man.* New York, Basic Books — Consultants Bureau, 1966.

MacCarty, C. S., Boyd, A. S., and Childs, D. S.: Tumors of the optic nerve and optic chiasm. *J. Neurosurg., 33*:439-444, 1970.

MacCarty, C. S., and Brown, D. N.: Orbital tumors in children. *Clin. Neurosurg., 11*: 76-93, 1963.

MacEwen, W.: *Pyogenic Infective Diseases of the Brain and Spinal Cord.* New York, MacMillan, 1893.

Magoun, H. W.: *Ascending Reticular System and Wakefulness.* Springfield, Thomas, 1954.

Magoun, H. W., and Rhines, R.: *Spasticity. The Stretch Reflex and Extrapyramidal Systems.* Springfield, Thomas, 1948.

Malamud, N.: The effect of trauma on the brain stem. *Clin. Neurosurg., 6*:177-197, 1958.

Marino, R., and Rasmussen, T.: Visual field changes after temporal lobectomy in man. *Neurology, 18*:825-835, 1968.

Martins, A. N., Hayes, G. J., and Kempe, L. G.: Invasive pituitary adenomas. *J. Neurosurg., 22*:268-276, 1965.

Martin, J. P.: *The Basal Ganglia and Posture.* London, Pitman, 1967.

Matson, D. D.: Hydrocephalus. *Clin. Neurosurg., 13*:324-343, 1966.

Matson, D. D.: *Neurosurgery of Infancy and Childhood,* 2nd ed. Springfield, Thomas, 1969.

Matson, D. D., and Crigler, J. F.: Management of cranopharyangioma in childhood. *J. Neurosurg., 30:*377-390, 1969.

Matson, D. D., and Salam, M.: Brain abscess in congenital heart disease. *Pediatrics, 27:*772-789, 1961.

McCormick, W. F., Hardman, J. M., and Boulter, T. R.: Vascular malformations ("angiomas") of the brain, with special reference to those occurring in the posterior fossa. *J. Neurosurg., 28:*241-251, 1968.

McCormick, W. F., and Nofzinger, J. D.: Saccular intracranial aneurysms. An autopsy study. *J. Neurosurg., 22:*155-159, 1965.

McDowell, F., and Wolff, H. G.: *Handbook of Neurological Diagnostic Methods.* Baltimore, Williams and Wilkins, 1960.

McKissock, W., Richardson, A., and Bloom, W. H.: Subdural hematoma, a review of 389 cases. *Lancet, 1:*1365-1369, 1960.

McKissock, W., Taylor, J. C., Bloom, W. H., and Till, K.: Extradural hematoma, observations on 125 cases. *Lancet, 2:*167-172, 1960.

McLaurin, R. L.: Subdural infection. In Gurdjian, E. S. (Ed.) : *Cranial and Intracranial Suppuration.* Springfield, Thomas, 1969.

McLaurin, R. L., and Ford, L. E.: Extradural hematoma. Statistical survey of 47 cases. *J. Neurosurg., 21:*364-371, 1964.

McLaurin, R. L., and Helmer, F.: The syndrome of temporal-lobe contusion. *J. Neurosurg., 23:*296-304, 1965.

McNaughton, F. L.: Diagnosis of headache. *Neurology, 13:*24-26, 1963.

McRae, D. L.: Focal epilepsy: correlation of the pathological and radiological findings. *Radiology, 50:*439-457, 1948.

McRae, D. L., and Elliott, A. W.: Radiological aspects of cerebellar astrocytomas and medulloblastomas. *Acta Radiol., 50:*52-66, 1958.

Mealey, J.: Acute extradural hematomas without demonstrable skull fractures. *J. Neurosurg., 17:*27, 1960.

Merritt, H.: *A Textbook of Neurology,* 3rd ed. Philadelphia, Lea & F., 1963.

Meyer, A.: Herniation of the brain. *Arch. Neurol. Psychiatry, 4:*387, 1920.

Miller, R. A., and Burack, E.: *Atlas of the Central Nervous System in Man.* Baltimore, Williams & Wilkins, 1968.

Milner, B., Branch, C., and Rasmussen, T.: Study of short-term memory after intracarotid injection of sodium amytal. *Trans. Am. Neurol. Assoc.,* 224-226, 1962.

Monrad-Krohn, G. H.: *The Clinical Examination of the Nervous System,* 10th ed. London, Lewis, 1954.

Moody, R. A., and Poppen, J. L.: Arteriovenous malformations. *J. Neurosurg., 32:*503-511, 1970.

Morley, T. P., and Barr, H. W. K.: Giant intracranial aneurysms: diagnosis, course and management. *Clin. Neurosurg., 16:*73-94, 1969.

Moruzzi, G., and Magoun, H. W.: Brain stem reticular formation and activation of the EEG. *Electroencephalogr. Clin. Neurophysiol., 1:*455-473, 1949.

Munro, D.: *Cranio-Cerebral Injuries, Their Diagnosis and Treatment.* London, Oxford U. P., 1938.

Murphy, J. P.: *Cerebrovascular Disease.* Chicago, Year Bk., 1954.

Murphy, J. T., Gloor, P., Yamamoto, Y. L., and Feindel, W.: A comparison of electroencephalography and brain scan in supratentorial tumors. *N. Engl. J. Med., 276:* 309-313, 1967.

Myles, S. T., Needham, C. W., and LeBlanc, F. E.: Alternating hemiparesis associated with hereditary hemorrhagic telangiectasia. *Can. Med. Assoc. J., 103*:509-511, 1970.

Nassar, S. I., and Mount, L. A.: Papillomas of the choroid plexus. *J. Neurosurg., 29*: 73-77, 1968.

Needham, C. W.: The reticular formation and generalized seizures. A thesis. McGill University, Montreal, Canada, 1968.

Needham, C. W., Bertrand, G., and Myles, S. T.: Multiple cranial nerve signs from supratentorial tumors. *J. Neurosurg., 33*:178-183, 1970.

Needham, C. W., and Dila, C. J.: Synchronizing and desynchronizing systems of the old brain. *Brain Research, 11*:285-293, 1968.

Nielsen, J. M.: Agnosia, apraxia, aphasia: Their value in cerebral localization. *L. A. Neurol. Soc., (Los Angeles)*, 1936.

Nielsen, J. M.: *A Textbook of Clinical Neurology,* 3rd ed. New York, Hoeber-Harper, 1951.

Northfield, D. W. C.: Rathke-pouch tumors. *Brain, 80*:293-312, 1957.

Nugent, G. R., Sprinkle, P., and Bloor, B. M.: Sphenoid sinus mucoceles. *J. Neurosurg., 32*:443-451, 1970.

Ojemann, R. G., Fisher, C. M., Adams, R. D., Sweet, W. H., and New, P. F. J.: Further experience with the syndrome of "normal" pressure hydrocephalus. *J. Neurosurg., 31*:279-294, 1969.

Olivecrona, H.: Acoustic tumors. *J. Neurosurg., 26*:6-13, 1967.

Ommaya, A. K.: Cerebrospinal fluid rhinorrhea. *Neurology, 14*:107-113, 1964.

Pagani, L. F.: The rapid appearance of papilledema. *J. Neurosurg., 30*:247-249, 1969.

Parkinson, D., Hunt, B., and Shields, C.: Double lucid interval in patients with extradural hematoma of the posterior fossa. *J. Neurosurg., 34*:534-536, 1971.

Paschkis, K. E., Rakoff, A. E., Cantarow, A., and Rupp, J. J.: *Clinical Endocrinology,* 3rd ed., New York, Hoeber-Harper, 1967.

Patton, H. D., and Amassian, V. E.: The pyramidal tract: its excitation and functions. In Field, J., Magoun, H. W., and Hall, V. E. (Eds.) : *Handbook of Physiology, sect. 1: Neurophysiology*. Washington, D. C., Am. Physiol. Soc., 1960.

Peach, B.: Arnold-Chiari malformation: anatomic features of 20 cases. *Arch. Neurol., 12*:613-621, 1965.

Peach, B.: The Arnold-Chiari malformation: morphogenesis. *Arch. Neurol., 12*:527-535, 1965.

Peet, M. M.: The cranial nerves. In Lewis, D. (Ed.) : *Practice of Surgery*. New York, Hoeber-Harper, 1968.

Penfield, W.: Engrams in the human brain. Mechanisms of memory. *Proc. R. Soc. Med., 61*:831-840, 1968.

Penfield, W. G.: Thoughts on the function of the temporal cortex. *Clin. Neurosurg., 4*:21-33, 1956.

Penfield, W., and Erickson, T. C.: *Epilepsy and Cerebral Localization.* Springfield, Thomas, 1941.

Penfield, W., and Jasper, H.: *Epilepsy and the Functional Anatomy of the Human Brain*. Boston, Little, 1954.

Penfield, W., and Kristiansen, K.: *Epileptic Seizure Patterns, A Study of the Localizing Value of Initial Phenomena in Focal Cortical Seizures.* Springfield, Thomas, 1951.

Penfield, W., and Milner, B.: Memory deficit produced by bilateral lesions in the hippocampal zone. *Arch. Neurol. Psychiatry, 79*:475-497, 1958.

Penfield, W., and Rasmussen, T.: *The Cerebral Cortex of Man, A Clinical Study of Localization of Function.* New York, MacMillan, 1950.

Penfield, W., and Rasmussen, T.: Vocalization and arrest of speech. *Arch. Neurol. Psychiatry, 61:*21-27, 1949.

Pitkethly, D. T., Hardman, J. M., Kempe, L. G., and Earle, K. M.: *Angioblastic* meningiomas, clinicopathologic study of 81 cases. *J. Neurosurg., 32:*539-544, 1970.

Plaut, H. F.: *Vertebral and Carotid Angiograms in Tentorial Herniations.* Springfield, Thomas, 1961.

Plum, F., and Posner, J. B.: *The Diagnosis of Stupor and Coma.* Philadelphia, Davis, 1966.

Pool, J. L.: Diagnosis and recent advance in treatment of subarachnoid hemorrhage. *J. A. M. A., 187:*404-409, 1964.

Pool, J. L., Potanos, J. N., and Krueger, E. G.: Osteomas and mucoceles of the frontal paranasal sinuses. *J. Neurosurg., 19:*130-135, 1962.

Pool, J. L., and Potts, D. G.: *Aneurysms and Arteriovenous Anomalies.* New York, Hoeber-Harper, 1965.

Poppen, J. L., and Marino, R.: Pinealomas and tumors of the posterior portion of the third ventricle. *J. Neurosurg., 28:*357-364, 1968.

Pribram, H. F. W.: Encephalography in diagnosis of posterior fossa tumors. *J. Neurosurg., 19:*269-276, 1962.

Raimondi, A. J., Samuelson, G., Yarzagaray, L., and Norton, T.: Atresia of the foramina of Luschka and Magendie: the Dandy-Walker cyst. *J. Neurosurg., 31:*202-216, 1969.

Ramon-Moliner, E., and Nauta, W. J. H.: The isodendritic core of the brain stem. *J. Comp. Neurol., 126:*311-326, 1966.

Rand, C. W.: *The Neurosurgical Patient, His Problems of Diagnosis and Care.* Springfield, Thomas, 1944.

Randall, R. V.: Endocrinologic aspects of nonfunctioning pituitary tumors. *J. Neurosurg., 19:*19-21, 1962.

Ranson, S. W.: *The Anatomy of the Nervous System,* 3rd ed. Philadelphia, Saunders, 1928.

Rasmussen, T., and Blundell, J.: Epilepsy and brain tumor. *Clin. Neurosurg., 7:*138-158, 1959.

Rasmussen, T., and Branch, C.: Temporal lobe epilepsy. Indications for and results of surgical therapy. *Postgrad. Med., 31:*9-14, 1962.

Ray, B. S., and Bergland, R. M.: Cerebrospinal fluid fistula: clinical aspects, techniques of localization and methods of closure. *J. Neurosurg., 30:*399-405, 1969.

Reeves, D. L.: Epidermoid (mixed) tumors of the central nervous system. *J. Neurosurg., 26:*21-24, 1967.

Reid, W. L., and Cone, W. V.: The mechanism of fixed dilatation of the pupil resulting from ipsilateral cerebral compression. *J. A. M. A., 112:*2030-2034, 1939.

Reigh, E. E., and Nelson, M.: Posterior-fossa subdural hematoma with secondary hydrocephalus. Report of a case and review of the literature. *J. Neurosurg,, 19:*346-348, 1962.

Reigh, E. E., and O'Connell, T. J.: Extradural hematoma of the posterior fossa with concomitant supratentorial subdural hematoma. Report of a case and review of the literature. *J. Neurosurg., 19:*359-364, 1962.

Reimenschneider, P. A., and Ecker, A.: Venographic clues to localization of intracranial masses. *Am. J. Roentgenol. Radium Ther. Nucl. Med., 72:*740-752, 1954.

Ring, B. A., and Waddington, M. M.: Angiographic identification of the motor strip. *J. Neurosurg., 26:*249-254, 1967.

Robb, P.: Epilepsy. A review of basic and clinical research. National Institute of Neurological Diseases and Blindness, Monograph No. 1, U. S. Public Health Service, 1965.

Roberts, M., and German, W. J.: A long term study of patients with oligodendrogliomas. Follow-up of 50 cases including Dr. Harvey Cushing's series. *J. Neurosurg., 24:*697-700, 1966.

Roberts, T. D. M.: *Neurophysiology of Postural Mechanisms.* London, Butterworth, 1967.

Robertson, E. G.: Cerebral lesions due to intracranial aneurysms. *Brain, 72:*150-185, 1949.

Roth, J. G., and Elvidge, A. R.: Glioblastoma multiforme: a clinical survey. *J. Neurosurg., 17:*736-750, 1960.

Rowbotham, G. F.: *Acute Injuries of the Head, Their Diagnosis, Treatment, Complications and Sequels,* 3rd ed. Edinburgh, Livingstone, 1949.

Rucker, C. W.: Ocular manifestations of pituitary tumor. *Clin. Neurosurg., 4:*34-60, 1956.

Russell, D. S., and Rubinstein, L. J.: *Pathology of Tumors of the Nervous System.* London, Arnold, 1959.

Sachs, E.: *Diagnosis and Treatment of Brain Tumors and Care of the Neurosurgical Patient,* 2nd ed. St. Louis, Mosby, 1949.

Sahs, A. L., Perret, G., Locksley, H. B., Nishioka, H., and Shutety, F. M.: Preliminary remarks on subarachnoid hemorrhage. Section I. *J. Neurosurg., 24:*782-816, 1966.

Schechter, M. M.: Angiography in head trauma. *Clin. Neurosurg., 12:*193-225, 1964.

Scheibel, M. D., and Scheibel, A. B.: Patterns of organization in specific and nonspecific thalamic fields. In Purpura, D. P., and Yahr, M. D. (Eds.) : *The Thalamus.* New York, Columbia, 1966, pp. 13-46.

Scheinberg, S. C., and Scheinberg, L. C.: Early description of chronic subdural hematoma. Etiology, symptomatology and treatment. *J. Neurosurg., 21:*445-446, 1964.

Schildkraut, J. J., and Kety, S. S.: Biogenio amines and emotion. *Science, 156:*21-30, 1967.

Schneider, R. C., Crosby, E. C., and Farhat, S. M.: Extratemporal lesions triggering the temporal-lobe syndrome. The role of association bundles. *J. Neurosurg., 22:*246-263, 1965.

Schurr, P. H.: Pituitary tumors in man. In Harris, G. W., and Donovan, B. T. (Eds.) : *The Pituitary Gland.* Los Angeles, U. of Calif., 1966, vol. 2.

Segarra, J. M.: Cerebral vascular disease and behavior, I. The syndrome of the mesencephalic artery (basilar artery bifurcation) . *Arch. Neurol., 22:*408-418, 1970.

Sherrington, C. S.: Decerebrate rigidity and reflex coordination of movements. *J. Physiol., 22:*319-332, 1898.

Sherrington, C. S.: *Selected Writings.* London, Hamilton, 1939.

Shulman, K., Martin, B. F., Popoff, N., and Ransohoff, J.: Recognition and treatment of hydrocephalus following spontaneous subarachnoid hemorrhage. *J. Neurosurg., 20:*1040-1049, 1963.

Smith, K. R., Weinburg, W. A., and McAlister, W. H.: Failure to thrive: the diencephalic syndrome of infancy and childhood. A case report. *J. Neurosurg., 23*:348-351, 1965.

Sprague, J. E., and Chambers, W. W.: Control of posture by reticular formation and cerebellum in the intact, anesthetized and unanesthetized and in the decerebrated cat. *Am. J. Physiol., 176*:52-64, 1954.

Spurling, R. G.: *Practical Neurological Diagnosis,* 6th ed. Springfield, Thomas, 1960.

Stein, B. M., Leeds, N. E., Taveras, J. M., and Pool, J. L.: Meningiomas of the foramen magnum. *J. Neurosurg., 20*:740-751, 1963.

Suzuki, J., Wada, T., and Kowada, M.: Clinical observations on tumors of the pineal region. *J. Neurosurg., 19*:441-445, 1962.

Symonds, C. P.: Concussion and its sequelae. *Lancet, 1*:1-5, 1962.

Symposium on head injury. *Clin. Neurosurg., 12*:38-394, 1966.

Tator, C. H., Fleming, J. F. R., Sheppard, R. H., and Turner, V. M.: A radioisotopic test for communicating hydrocephalus. *J. Neurosurg., 28*:327-340, 1968.

Taveras, J. M., and Wood, E. H.: *Diagnostic Neuroradiology.* Baltimore, Williams & Wilkins, 1964.

Taylor, L. B.: Localization of cerebral lesions by psychological testing. *Clin. Neurosurg., 16*:269-287, 1969.

Thompson, W. L., Swensson, N. L., and Buell, H.: *Radiologic Pathology Work Book, Central Nervous System.* Washington, D. C., Armed Forces Institute of Pathology, 1967.

Toglia, J. U., Netsky, M. G., and Alexander, E.: Epithelial (epidermoid) tumors of the cranium. Their common nature and pathogenesis. *J. Neurosurg., 23*:384-393, 1965.

Toole, J. F. and Patel, A. N.: *Cerebrovascular Disorders.* New York, Blakiston-McGraw-Hill, 1967.

Udvarhelyi, G. B., Khodadoust, A. A., and Walsh, F. B.: Gliomas of the optic nerve and chiasm in children: an unusual series of cases. *Clin. Neurosurg., 13*:204-237, 1966.

Ulrich, J.: Intracranial epidermoids. A study on their distribution and spread. *J. Neurosurg., 21*:1051-1058, 1964.

Van Buren, J. M., Poppen, J. L., and Horrax, G.: Unilateral exophthalmos. *Brain, 80*:139-175, 1957.

Vander Ark, G. D., and Kahn, E.: Spontaneous intracerebral hematoma. *J. Neurosurg., 28*:252-256, 1968.

Vieth, R. G., and Odom, G. L.: Intracranial metastases and their neurosurgical treatment. *J. Neurosurg., 23*:375-383, 1965.

Vincent, C., David, M., and Thiébaut, F.: Le cône de pression temporal dans les tumeurs des hemispheres cerebraux. *Rev. Neurol., 65*:536, 1936.

Vincent, C., Thiébaut, F., and Rappoport, F.: A propos du cône de pression temporal. *Rev. Neurol., 54*:116, 1930.

Vondra, J.: *Fractures of the Base of the Skull.* London, Iliffe, 1965.

Walker, A. E.: The art of selecting technical aids for neurological diagnosis of brain lesions. *Clin. Neurosurg., 13*:277-290, 1966.

Walker, A. E.: Brain herniations. In Vinken, P. J., and Bruyn, G. W. (Eds.) : *Disturbances of Nervous Function. Handbook of Clinical Neurology.* New York, Wiley, 1969, vol. 1.

Walsh, E. G.: *Physiology of the Nervous System.* London, Longmans Green, 1957.

Walsh, F. B.: Some ocular signs of cerebral tumors in children. *Clin. Neurosurg., 5*:166-176, 1957.

Walsh, F. B., and Hoyt, W. F.: The visual sensory system: anatomy, physiology and topographic diagnosis. In Vinken, P. J., and Bruyn, G. W. (Eds.) : *Localization in Clinical Neurology. Handbook of Clinical Neurology.* New York, Wiley, 1969, vol. 2.

Wartenberg, R.: *Diagnostic Tests in Neurology, A Selection for Office Use.* Chicago, Year B., 1953.

Wechsler, I. S.: *A Textbook of Clinical Neurology,* 7th ed. Philadelphia, Saunders, 1952.

Weir, B., and Elvidge, A. R.: Oligodendrogliomas. An analysis of 63 cases. *J. Neurosurg., 29:*500-505, 1968.

White, H. H.: Brain stem tumors occurring in adults. *Neurology, 13:*292-300, 1963.

White, J. C.: Aneurysms mistaken for hypophyseal tumors. *Clin. Neurosurg., 10:*224-250, 1962.

Whittaker, K.: Extradural hematoma of the anterior fossa. *J. Neurosurg., 17:*1089, 1960.

Williams, D.: Temporal lobe syndromes. In Vinken, P. J., and Bruyn, G. W. (Eds.) : *Localization in Clinical Neurology. Handbook of Clinical Neurology.* New York, Wiley, 1969, vol. 2.

Wilson, C. B.: Glioblastoma multiforme—present status. *Arch. Neurol., 11:*562-568, 1964.

Wilson, M.: *The Anatomical Foundation of Neuroradiology of the Brain.* Boston, Little, 1963.

Woodhall, B.: Osteomyelitis and epi-, extra-, and subdural abscess. *Clin. Neurosurg., 14:* 239-255, 1967.

Wright, R. L.: Traumatic hematomas of the posterior cranial fossa. *J. Neurosurg., 25:* 402-409, 1966.

Young, B. R.: *The Skull, Sinuses and Mastoids. A Handbook of Roentgen Diagnosis.* Chicago, Year B., 1948.

Zulch, K. J.: *Brain Tumors, Their Biology and Pathology.* New York, Springer, 1967.

INDEX

D

Q

R

S